Law, Ethics and Professional Issues for Nursing

This comprehensive new text book covers core ethical and legal content for pre-registration nursing students. It provides readers with a sound understanding of the interrelationships between the Nursing and Midwifery Council (NMC) code of conduct, standards and competencies, ethics and relevant sections of the English legal system.

The only truly integrated text in the field, it opens with overviews of law and nursing, and of ethical theories and nursing. It goes on to explore key areas of contention – such as negligence, confidentiality and consent – from legal and ethical perspectives, mapping the discussion onto the NMC code of conduct. The chapters include objectives, patient-focused case scenarios, key points, activities, questions, areas for reflection, further reading and a summary. Case law, statutes and ethical theories are presented where appropriate.

Written by an experienced nurse-lecturer with a law and ethics teaching background, *Law, Ethics and Professional Issues for Nursing* is essential reading for all pre-registration nursing students, as well as students of other healthcare professions.

Herman Wheeler is a Lecturer in Nursing and Health Sciences, University of Birmingham, UK. A trained mental health and adult nurse, he also holds a postgraduate diploma and MA in law and is a Chartered Psychologist. He currently teaches law and ethics to nursing and health students.

Law, Ethics and Professional Issues for Nursing

A reflective and portfolio-building approach

Herman Wheeler

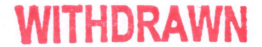

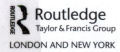 Routledge
Taylor & Francis Group

LONDON AND NEW YORK

First published 2012
by Routledge
2 Park Square, Milton Park, Abingdon, Oxon, OX14 4RN

Simultaneously published in the USA and Canada
by Routledge
711 Third Avenue, New York, NY 10017

Routledge is an imprint of the Taylor & Francis Group, an informa business

British Library Cataloguing in Publication Data
A catalogue record for this book is available from the British Library

Library of Congress Cataloging-in-Publication Data
Wheeler, Herman.
Law, ethics, and professional issues for nursing : a reflective and portfolio-building approach / Herman Wheeler.
p. ; cm.
Includes bibliographical references.
1. Nursing—Law and legislation—Great Britain. 2. Nursing ethics—Great Britain. 3. Nursing and Midwifery Council (Great Britain). Code. I. Title.
[DNLM: 1. Legislation, Nursing—Great Britain. 2. Clinical Competence—Great Britain. 3. Ethics, Nursing—Great Britain. 4. Nurse's Role—Great Britain. 5. Nursing Process—Great Britain. WY 33 FA1]
KD2968.N8W48 2012
344.4104'14—dc23
2011026480

ISBN13: 978–0–415–61888–5 (hbk)
ISBN13: 978–0–415–61889–2 (pbk)
ISBN13: 978–0–203–14474–9 (ebk)

Typeset in Times New Roman by Prepress Projects Ltd, Perth, UK

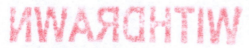

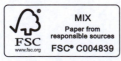

Printed and bound in Great Britain by the MPG Books Group

To my late mother and father, Olive and John Wheeler, both of whose genes have given me the drive I have to achieve what I set out to do. May God bless their souls!

Contents

15 Mental health law   290
    (WRITTEN BY HERMAN H. WHEELER AND CHRISTOPHER WAGGSTAFF)

Figures

Tables

Boxes

Acknowledgements

I thank my wife, Heather, who, as always, gave me much encouragement and inspiration to complete the manuscript for this book. I thank her also for using her knowledge and expertise as a Bachelor and Masters graduate and as a registered mental nurse, a registered general nurse, a registered midwife and a registered midwife tutor to provide me with helpful comments on some of the chapters and for researching and locating some of the theoretical sources that I drew on to write this book.

My thanks to Dr Duncan Randall (Lecturer in Paediatric Nursing and Coordinator of the Child Branch Programme within the Bachelor of Nursing (Hons) Degree in the School of Health and Population Sciences, College of Medical and Dental Sciences, University of Birmingham, UK) for reviewing and commenting on Chapter 14, 'Child protection: Legal, ethical and professional issues'. I take responsibility for any errors in the chapter.

My thanks to Christopher Wagstaff (Lecturer in Mental Health Nursing and Coordinator of the Mental Health Branch Programme within Bachelor of Nursing (Hons) Degree, School of Health and Population Sciences, College of Medical and Dental Sciences, University of Birmingham, UK) for agreeing at very short notice to contribute to the chapter on Mental Health Law.

Table of cases

Table of statutes and statutory instruments

1   Introduction
Value to nursing students

Objectives of this chapter

By the end of this chapter you should be able to:

- understand why I wrote this book and its importance to nursing students especially;
- understand relationships between law, ethics and the Nursing and Midwifery Council (NMC) code of conduct, nursing standards, behaviour and ethics;
- articulate how law influences the NMC's set-up and functioning;
- appreciate that there are other healthcare regulatory bodies apart from the NMC; the importance of healthcare regulatory bodies;
- appreciate that law, ethics and moral values have relationships with professional values, code of conduct and behaviour, and are central to your nursing role.

Why this book?

My undergraduate nursing students often tell me that there is a place in the market for a book that focuses on the needs of preregistration nursing students with respect to mapping *law*, *ethics*, *moral values* and *professional nursing standards and development issues* onto nurses' *professional code of conduct* (PCC). To this end I write from 'inside' nursing, as a nurse educator and a psychologist with appropriate legal qualifications and experience of teaching law and ethics to healthcare students, including nurses, physiotherapy and medical students. *Cost of the book* was a major consideration. The book addresses key knowledge components from law, linking it to key ethical principles, and with the NMC (2008a) Code, and with its standards and competence domains outlined in its publication *Standards for Pre-registration Nursing Education* (NMC, 2010a). Throughout the book I have tried to show the interactional and integral relationship between nursing and law, ethics, moral reasoning, nursing standards and code of conduct, all of which integrate to build up an epistemological and pragmatic knowledge framework that the student nurse needs to inform study and nursing practice. The subject matter will also help you as a registered nurse well beyond your student training. Although I wrote the book principally for pre-registration student nurses, irrespective of their chosen nursing branch, *children's*, *adult*, *mental health* or *learning disability nursing*, students of any of the health professions will find it useful, mainly because the legal, ethical, professional and health-related code of conduct principles it pursues are relevant and applicable to all the clinical disciplines: physiotherapy, medicine, radiography and so on.

I was determined to address the interaction between the disciplines of law, ethics, professional issues, standards and code of conduct guidance within one volume to make it relatively cheap for students to purchase in order to develop a good grasp of these elements from the same source, with direction to additional reading when and where required. Many existing legal texts aimed at nursing students, particularly, tend to cover *either* law *or* ethics in one volume, not usually both, which is more costly to students, some of whom are some-times strapped for cash. I believe it is important to show students that law does not stand alone; it informs nursing, just as it informs other aspects of their lives and other clinical pro-fessions such as physiotherapy, medicine, chiropody and radiography. For nursing students who have constantly asked me to write a book of this nature, the present text is my response. Many legal text books written for nursing and medical students are actually written by 'pure' lawyers whose understanding of these disciplines is, at best, second hand. This makes it that much more difficult to help healthcare students apply law, ethics and professional code of conduct principles to their clinical discipline through the framework of *reflective practice* and *professional portfolio* development as a *learning* and *clinical application tool*. This book addresses such a weakness by helping students develop their *law, ethics and professional issues portfolio* and their knowledge and working understanding of the notion of *reflective practice* by actually reflecting on clinical learning scenarios and applying them to patient care with a legal and ethical slant.

I chose to cover the mainly legal, professional and essential professional code of conduct and behaviour elements first, whilst making appropriate references to ethics, although a stronger focus on ethical theories linking to practice comes later in the book. I hardly make any apology for this arrangement, because to help students develop an appreciation of any of the key theoretical elements covered in the book it is important for subject elements to be covered in an orderly fashion, with the book helping the student to make appropriate links between the relevant elements of each of the subject disciplines. I recall one external examiner to the University of Birmingham, where I lecture, telling me that she felt that nurses needed a better understanding of relevant law and that, whereas there are several text books on law aimed at medical students and doctors, there were fewer available for nurses and other healthcare students such as those of physiotherapy and other clinical disciplines. The book addresses law, ethics and related professional code of conduct and behaviour issues, linking these to professional, legal and ethical standards of clinical practice. It relates the subject matter integrally to the NMC standards for the *competence domains* for pre-registration nursing students, setting all within the framework of professional portfolio building and reflective practice, the NMC standards of education and practice and its 2008 Code of Conduct.

Law, NMC standards for nursing and its Code of Conduct

Nurses are required to have an understanding of appropriate legal, professional and ethical framework for caring. In its *Standards for Pre-registration Nursing Education*, the NMC (2010a) states under *Domain 1: Professional Values* that nurses must practice according to *The Code: Standards of Conduct, Performance and Ethics* (NMC, 2008a), within 'recog-nised ethical and legal frameworks' recognising and addressing ethical challenges around patients' choices and decision-making. Moreover, nurses should act within the law when helping patients, their families and carers to find caring solutions to their needs. When you become a registered nurse you will need to undertake constant professional updating to maintain professional competence, being able to practice within safe, ethical, professional and legal frameworks. This book aims to help you to do so knowledgeably, competently and confidently.

Expansion of nursing role

The nurse's role continues to expand. With this comes 'expanded liability' (McHale, 2010, p. 317). Thus nurses need to be more aware than hitherto about legal, ethical and moral issues in caring. *Moral values* guide our *thinking* and *behaviour* and impact on our *ethical decision making* in relation to *caring*. Therefore the book has inclusively and relationally focused on how *moral values* are developed and how they can impact on our professional decision making. As a student nurse aspiring to become a mental health, children or adult nurse, you need a sound grasp of the NMC Code, which should remain a primary focus of your reading throughout your studies as a student and beyond. The book helps you to achieve this, making appropriate links between the Code principles, law, ethics and other professional concerns. Legislation applicable especially to mental health and children's nursing is covered mainly by focusing on the amendment of the 1983 Mental Health Act (MHA) by the 2007 MHA, and by looking at how the 2004 Children Act has amended in part the 1989 Children Act, particularly focusing on child abuse and child protection. These elements are covered in Chapters 14 and 15.

Drawing on what some of you may already know: your 'entry behaviour'

In some chapters, I have attempted to draw on some of what the student already knows, because none of you will have come to nurse training or other healthcare undergraduate programmes with an empty slate. You have all lived for at least 18 years, some of you for much longer, and therefore come to university with what psychologists call your 'entry behaviour': your knowledge, aptitude for learning, some skills perhaps, some moral values and beliefs and so on. In developing these attitudes, knowledge and behaviours, nursing would be insulting you if it did not assume you do have something to offer. Nursing and this book seek to build on your entry behaviour. From Chapter 2 onwards, therefore, I have occasionally asked you to undertake some *reflection*, identifying some of your already possessed knowledge, for example *what values you think you have brought with you into nursing*. I have then provided some answers, for example information on typical *caring values* that nurses are expected to develop and use in nursing care decision making; values which some of you may already have. In this sense, therefore, this text book is unique, since it has been my experience as an educator of healthcare students and a psychologist with a law and ethics teaching background that the vast majority of text books I have studied from or used to inform my teaching have tended to only 'dish out' large volumes of information, never assuming that students' interest can be heightened by stimulating their own thoughts; never finding out what students already come with (their *entry behaviour*) and then building on it with further knowledge. The chapter exercises are designed, therefore, to encourage your *reflection* and to encourage and will you on to *trust* yourself that you are not an empty slate, but a learner with a potential contribution to make. You already have some knowledge which you must build on, *taking responsibility for your learning*; one of the primary purposes of a good university education. As a student you must get into the habit of making use of your own pre-acquired knowledge (*entry behaviour*) and place your new learning in the context of prior knowledge and experience, using *reflection* to build up a more sophisticated knowledge base that you can use for many years to come to inform your clinical practice. Theory without application is incomplete. Theorising without meaningful reflection and clinical application of that theory is even more unfinished.

   In acknowledgement of this tested approach to meaningful learning and application of

that knowledge, most chapters contain student activities, including patient-focused scenarios, case studies, quizzes and questions which it is hoped you will use your *developing
academic and professional portfolio* to address.

Use of your portfolio

Use your *developing individual professional portfolio* to record your responses to the portfolio and reflective practice exercises posed. Portfolios are perhaps one of the most effective
learning tools that a student nurse can use to augment his/her learning. Your portfolio-based
personal reflection exercises will increase your aptitude and motivation for further learning and application of that learning to practice. You should also try out different reflective
practice models and select those that suit your purpose. There are many currently used in
nursing, for example Gibbs (1988), Schon (1983) and Kolb's (1984) experiential learning
model, to name a few.

Rising litigation costs to the National Health Service and implications for nurses

Increased litigation is currently very costly to the National Health Service (NHS) and can
be a source of anxiety for nurses and other healthcare professionals. The *Daily Telegraph* (9
June 2000) reported a doubling of cost of NHS negligence claims over 10 years. Moreover,
the *Daily Telegraph* (3 August 2010) reports that the cost of settling negligence claims in the
NHS increased to £15 billion, diverting much needed cash from patient care. In its annual
report the NHS Litigation Authority *Report and Accounts* (NHSLA, 2010) noted that in
2009/10 there were 6,652 claims, a 10 per cent increase over 2008/9, which in turn recorded
an 11 per cent increase over 2007/8. Nurses have a moral and professional responsibility
to give the highest standard of patient/client care, thus helping to reduce the number of
negligence claims against the NHS. High incidence of claims diverts money away from
patient care. Because of this, standards could fall. Healthcare practitioners must do their
best to prevent poor care due to negligent acts or omissions. We are into an increasingly
litigious public awareness culture in the UK, fast catching up with the culture in America.
An understanding of law can help the nurse navigate a safe legal course. Reading this book
will help you to become more knowledgeable about law, ethics and professional code of
conduct principles, including the *competence domains* you need to cover as a student.

Nursing and the place of law, ethics and Code of Conduct within it

As you embark on your journey to become a registered nurse it is important for you to
become aware of key aspects of the *nursing profession*, particularly how it is *regulated*,
its *primary functions* and what, in *legal, ethical* and *professional terms*, it requires of you.
By focusing initially on these points this book sets the scene to enable you to understand
the context and importance of *legal, ethical* and *professional code of conduct issues* and
principles relating to nursing care and your professional development to deliver nursing
care confidently and competently. A critical starting point is the realisation that nursing
must be practised within the law. Whichever country a nurse practises in, (s)he must operate
within the legal framework of that country. Some of you may work abroad after graduating.
You must learn about the law of that country and work within it. Some of you may even
undertake an overseas student elective. Legal accountability is also intrinsically tied in with
professional accountability, practice *competence, standards of conduct and behaviour* and
moral and ethical accountability if you are to give patients the best *holistic* care.

The very set-up and regulating of nursing by the Nursing and Midwifery Council is done by a legal order, the *Nursing and Midwifery Order 2001*, instituted by Parliament. As you will see throughout this book many elements of law – *statute* and *case* (otherwise called, *common*) law – relate to and control nursing practice in different ways.

Changing face of nursing demanding upkeep with law and professional standards

Demands on nursing are constantly changing and you need to keep up to date. Patients' and clients' needs are ever changing, particularly within the UK, which has a diverse mix of cultures within our patient population. Society is demanding more and more from its greater legal awareness. Publication of litigation cases and the availability of the internet have seen to this. This calls for up-to-date legal knowledge, as well as awareness of how ethical considerations influence nursing decision making. Some of the best evidence comes from *reflection* on experience, finding out what has worked best for us and our patient, drawing on *reflection* and the best *research evidence*. The law also changes frequently so you need to read to keep up. Even from the NMC, we see that the *standards of proficiency* that were in place for preregistration students have changed to new *standards for competence – generic and field*, which students coming into nurse training and education programmes in autumn 2011 need to achieve. An all-graduate nursing profession is indicated. So things change rapidly in both professional and legal circles and we all need to adopt and adjust positively, very quickly.

The *ethical* and *moral codes* we use to view situations, how we conduct our lives, how we relate to patients, clients, their relatives and the wider society are not static either. *Moral values* (our sense or values of *wrong* and *right* that we use to inform our decision making, our attitudes and behaviour in our daily lives) vary from one individual to the other, from one race to another, from one ethnic group to another, from one culture to another, even from country to country. Your individual *moral philosophy* is perhaps different from that of your patients/clients, tutors, lecturers and your peers with whom you study and work in the clinical settings. You must constantly assess whether your moral values are influencing you into adopting and carrying out best practice to the highest professional standards or those values are set to bring you into conflict with the law or your professional body.

Nursing, its regulation and implications for legal and ethical preparedness

If you want to talk about *ethical* and *legal* aspects and moral values within nursing, you need some understanding of what nursing is about – *definitions of nursing*. A former UK regulatory body for nursing (the United Kingdom Central Council for Nursing, Midwifery & Health Visiting) argued that 'a definition of nursing would be too restrictive for the profession' (UKCC, 1999, p. 18, para 2.19). If nurses were to take this view, literally, they would perhaps not be too certain of what was required of them professionally, legally, ethically, morally, emotionally or spiritually. Nursing has much to do with how it is defined. It has much to do with caring holistically for people. The above UKCC comment is vague and woolly, in fact hardly a definition; more of what I would call a 'cop out' of a useful definition. No nursing *standards* are spelt out in this vague statement. Vague approaches to defining nursing do not meet legal standards of what is *good* and *acceptable standard* of *nursing care*. This book explains what the law says about acceptable *standards of nursing care*. In regulating nursing the NMC lays down regulations, education and practice standards, including professional code of conduct, behaviour and ethics for nurses to work to. However we define nursing, nurses need to be clear of what is expected of them by their regulator and service users, principal focuses of this text book.

Place of law in setting standards of care for nurses

As a student or a qualified nurse you need to know some of the key benchmarks by which the law judges *acceptable* and *reasonable standard of patient care* by healthcare professionals, generally, not just nurses. The 'Bolam Test' defines key standards used by law to judge the *reasonableness* and *competency* of healthcare practice. We will return to this test under the chapter on negligence. However, briefly, the case of *Bolam v Friern Hospital Management Committee* [1957] 1 WLR 583 is an English *tort* (*civil wrong*) case that established appropriate standards of reasonable care by health professionals, including doctors, nurses, physiotherapists, radiographers and speech and language therapists. According to this test, if the health professional can show that the care given is based on a *reasonable*, *responsible* and *respectable* body of healthcare clinical discipline-specific opinion, then (s)he cannot be liable in negligence.

In the Bolam case Mr Bolam, a voluntary patient with mental health problems, agreed to have electro-convulsive therapy (ECT). He was not given muscle relaxant and his body was not restrained during treatment. His body jerked and flailed about violently and he sustained a fracture. He sued the hospital management for compensation, arguing that they were negligent in (a) not giving him muscle relaxants, (b) not restraining him and (c) not warning him of the risks involved. At the time of Bolam it was customary and very much the accepted practice for some doctors to give muscle relaxants prior to ECT, whereas others were opposed to doing so for fear of increasing the risk of fractures. The court ruled in favour of the hospital, with Judge McNeil saying that a health professional 'is not guilty of negligence if he has acted in accordance with a practice accepted as proper by a responsible body of medical men, skilled in that particular art'.

However, in a later case, *Bolitho v City & Hackney H.A.* [1999] 1 FLR 119 ECJ, the House of Lords (then the highest appellate court in England, now replaced in that role by the UK Supreme Court) stated that the expert opinion relied on in *Bolam* must be shown to follow *logically* and *reasonably* from specific circumstances, and that the issue of chosen treatment options must be weighed against *risks*. In other words nurses cannot just say: we are doing it this way because it has been done like this since Adam. Likewise nurses cannot just leave it at saying: we are doing it this way because it matches the acceptable body of professional nursing opinion. Nurses must now also ask themselves: does the care follow *logically given all the variables involved*? Have we taken into account the best *reflective practice* and *research* evidence and done everything possible to avoid (if possible) risks to patients? Have we followed all the guidelines of the National Institute for Health and Clinical Excellence (NICE)? Is the patient aware of the risks (s)he faces? If we can answer these questions in the affirmative, then we are heading in the right direction in providing care to a *reasonable* and *acceptable standard*; maybe even to the *highest standard* possible. At the time of the *Bolam* case it was not customary to warn patients of risks, particularly small ones. Today healthcare clinicians are required to inform patients of all possible risks, so long as they are known. Nursing needs to follow not only the best available *research evidence*, but also evidence arising from their *critical reflection* and analysis of their nursing practice. This includes evidence amassed from using portfolio to reflect on practice.

In delivering care to a satisfactory standard, nurses (and in fact all healthcare clinicians) must also follow guidelines from the NICE. Most of the guidance is based on research evidence. The Royal College of Nursing (RCN, 2003, p. 1) has pointed out that in the UK 'there is no legal definition of nursing', although most countries have a legal definition of the title 'nurse'. However, the Health & Social Care Act, 2001, defines 'registered nursing care' as distinguishable from 'social care' or 'personal care', although this is specifically for defining responsibility for provision and funding. Although this legal slant points to who could be held accountable for nursing provision and funding, it does not tell us much about nurses' *individual responsibility* and *accountability* in providing best nursing care, and therefore how the law, ethics and professional codes of conduct apply to the nurse.

Courts of law will be inclined to take into account professional responsibility, accountability, standards for competent practice, code of conduct and professional behaviour guidance, in judging nurses' practice standards and the way they have been applied to the patient. This means then that a judge could take these factors into account, as well as the *Bolam standards*, when deciding a case in which the nurse's practice was brought into question. So let us look at other *definitions of nursing* and see whether they suggest yardsticks that the law may deploy when judging nursing standards and performance.

Can we apply strict legal principles to Florence Nightingale's definition of nursing?

In her work *Notes on Nursing: What It Is and What It Is Not* Florence Nightingale (1859) stated: 'Nature alone cures . . . And what nursing has to do . . . is to put the patient in the best condition for nature to act upon him' (p. 74) This definition does not tell us about how we do so, the ethical, legal and professional skills and competencies we need to nurse, the parameters and scope of nursing or what the accountability factors within nursing are. Therefore, to apply strict legal or ethical frameworks to such a definition would not be all that helpful. This is because the law tends to apply defined rules and principles to what we do in our professional and even our private interactions. For example, the criminal law applies penance in the form of imprisonment if we are found guilty of intentionally killing someone. In the courts we would face a charge of murder, or less seriously manslaughter. We should respect people's privacy (see, for example, Human Rights Act, 1998, Article 8).

The law relating to *confidentiality* and *consent* demands that we respect confidentiality and protect data or information we hold on our patients (Data Protection Act, 1998); not discriminate unfavourably against people with disability (Disability Discrimination Act, 1995; Equality Act, 2010); seek people's consent before we treat them; and so on. However, looking back at Florence Nightingale's definition of nursing we could perhaps make the point that, although it does not supply us with parameters that we can apply strict legal principles to, it does nevertheless put an obligation on nurses to 'put the patient in the best position for nature to act upon him'; whatever that 'best position' is. A little vague for a legal test of certainty, but perhaps meaning do one's best to ensure that the patient's physical, social, psychological and spiritual needs are met, and leave the rest of his recovery to nature, fresh air, the right good foods, warmth and sunshine. Maybe even to God in a Christian world, to Allah in a Moslem world, and so on! The thing about these *nature* needs is that often patients need help from nurses to benefit from these natural healing sources and products, which the patient's illness may prevent him/her taking advantage of entirely by him-/herself.

Other definitions of nursing and indicators of good nursing

Other definitions of nursing are a little more precise, enabling legal, ethical and professional code of conduct principles to be more easily applied to aspects of practice. A formidable American nurse, *Virginia Henderson*, defined nursing as having a unique function:

The unique function of the nurse is to assist the individual, sick or well, in the performance of those activities contributing to health or its recovery (or to peaceful death) that he would perform unaided if he had the necessary strength, will or knowledge.

(Henderson, 1960, p. 15)

Although such a definition does not lay down any strict legal criteria by which nursing is defined, it nevertheless says something about the *role of the nurse*, what the nurse is supposed to do in the case of attending the person, *sick* or *well*. It implies that nurses have *obligations* towards their clients/patients in sickness, health and *even up to and at the point of the patient's death*. If the *law* and our *professional code of conduct* accept such a definition of nursing they may hold a nurse to such obligations. For example, if, having accepted the role of a nurse in relation to caring for patients/clients in *sickness and in health and up to the patient's death*, we demonstrate failure to care in an effective, compassionate and meaningful way, or fail to care to the professional and legal standards established and therefore expected, we could be held accountable *professionally*. This is because NMC policy standards use language such as that the nurse must 'deliver high quality essential care to all'; 'act with professionalism and integrity, and work within agreed professional, ethical and legal frameworks'; 'practise in a compassionate, respectful way, maintaining dignity' (NMC, 2010a). Later in her definition of nursing, Virginia Henderson goes on to say that nurses should *perform* this *unique function* in such a way as to help the patient gain 'independence' (p. 15). Moreover, the nurse must help the patient 'carry out the therapeutic plan as initiated by the physician' and in doing so must work 'as a member of a team' (p. 15), helping other health professionals to care, as they also help him/her to care for the patient/client. If we accept these views of nursing and our professional body embodies them and puts them into a *code of conduct*, then we are *obliged*, professionally, ethically and legally, to carry them out when nursing a patient. It is to be noted that one is not saying that Henderson's view of nursing constitutes a legal requirement. What is being said, though, is that, if a nurse's professional body establishes a code of conduct for nurses to work to, then the law of the land within which that nursing is being carried out could hold the nurse professionally and legally accountable. Similarly, the nurse's registration body (in the UK the NMC) could hold the nurse accountable for failure to carry out care to an acceptable standard. Let us see what this nursing regulatory body in the UK looks like, what its primary functions are and how it compares with other UK healthcare regulatory bodies.

The NMC compared with other UK regulatory bodies

One of the hallmarks of being a *professional* is to operate with *professionalism*, meaning to work to a *recognised professional code* of conduct, behaviour and ethics; to operate at a certain level and *standard* of *knowledge*, *skills* and *competence*, whilst *possessing* and *demonstrating* appropriate *attitudes*, *dress code* and *demeanour,* in *serving* the *clientele* that the professional was *educated* and *trained* to serve. Professionalism also implies the professional being dedicated, committed, diligent, hard-working, competent, *responsible* and *accountable* for his/her professional actions and omissions too, and for his/her behaviour on the job and in private life too. For *healthcare professionals* such as nurses, doctors, physiotherapists, dentists, clinical psychologists, radiographers, pathologists, dieticians, podiatrists, pharmacists and orthotics, to name a few, the *patients* and clients we treat are our *clientele*, better known as *healthcare consumers* and *service users*. Mental health and learning disability nurses often refer to their *service users* as *clients* whereas adult nurses tend to refer to theirs as *patients*. Each healthcare profession has its own *professional regulatory body*. In the UK the *Nursing and Midwifery Council* is the professional body with legal responsibility for the education, training and practice of nurses. Its remit was established under law, under a particular legal instrument called the *Nursing and Midwifery Order 2001*, although there are other pieces of legislation that govern how the NMC works and carries out its legal obligations. The Council's main responsibilities are to:

- Safeguard the health and wellbeing of the public; doing so by establishing and maintaining a register of all qualified nurses and midwives who practise in the UK. (Getting rid of bad nurses is implied!)
- Set and review standards for nursing and midwifery training, education, practice and conduct.
- Investigate allegations of impaired fitness to practise on grounds of professional misconduct, incompetence and ill-health. In this way the NMC calls on nurses and midwives to account for their practice and behaviour.

In October 2010 the NMC reported (http://www.nmc-uk.org/about) that there are presently 682,000 nurses, midwives and specialist community public health nurses on its register, making it the regulator for the largest group of healthcare professionals practising in England, Wales, Scotland and Northern Ireland. To reflect its strong, balanced and unbiased professional decision-making focus, the NMC is made of *registrant members* as well as *non-registrant members* of the *public*; the latter are known as 'lay members'. 'Registrants' are all qualified nurses and midwives who are registered with the NMC. A combination of professionals and lay people is a good mix to ensure standards because lay members may be likely to see things differently from professional nurses, and most certainly they will always have their own personal interests at heart, investing their time and energy to make sure nursing policies will deliver best care for them and their significant others and the public in general. Both views may build up strong professional guidance frameworks for nurses to work to. Purely self-regulation may not be healthy; a lay point of view may be needed.

Recommendation from your university for professional registration

When a student nurse qualifies in one of the *branches of nursing* (e.g. *adult, mental health, children's* or *learning disability nursing*) (s)he will need recommendation from the training institution to say (s)he is a fit person to gain professional registration. This implies that during your student nurse training you will be observed by your lecturers and clinical supervisors, who will in the end determine whether you are a suitable person to recommend to the NMC for professional registration – a point to bear in mind, constantly, during your education and clinical practice. You do not want to qualify and be unable to get registered. On your very last clinical placement, *sign off mentors* will work with your education and other placement staff to take responsibility to say you have achieved all the competences and are therefore suitable to be recommended for professional registration. These checks and balances all help to ensure that standards are maintained during your academic and professional development and, most importantly, that the public is protected and cared for by a competent professional work force.

Comparison of NMC with the Health Professions Council, and working within multidisciplinary teams

Some of you may be training alongside other health and social care students such as physiotherapists, speech and language therapists, clinical psychologists, art therapists, biomedical scientists, chiropodists, occupational therapists, radiographers and social work students.

These other professions, except for the last, social workers, are regulated by a different professional body named the Health Professions Council (HPC). Social workers and other social care providers are regulated by the General Social Care Council (GSCC). Doctors' training and practice are regulated by the General Medical Council. The HPC regulates the education, training and practice of about 15 health professions. As at January 2011, compared with the NMC's 682,000 registrants, the HPC regulated approximately 205,000 healthcare professionals. If you are not training alongside some of these other professional groups you will certainly meet them within the *multidisciplinary* healthcare team within the clinical practice areas. Like the NMC the HPC was set up by a legal order, known as the *Health Professions Order 2001*, as an independent health regulator. As a comparison, the HPC has similar roles and functions to the NMC, its primary duty being to protect the public. It is a crime to state that one is registered to any of these Councils if one is not so registered. As some of the students I teach are not just nurses, but physiotherapists, podiatrists and medical students, I have tried to make some of the patient-focused scenarios that I have written to help your learning actually inform incidents and situations that both nurses and other healthcare students, example physiotherapists, could become involved with and learn from.

Professional discipline and your regulatory body

Both the NMC and the HPC aim to maintain professional discipline, behaviour and competency in practice by ensuring proper standards of education, training and practice. In doing so every individual nurse is *responsible* and *accountable* for his/her behaviour *on* and *off* the job and for the standard of care given to his/her patients/clients. To assess the standards expected of you as a student nurse and a qualified practitioner you need to read the NMC's policy documents: *Standards for Pre-registration Nursing Education*, *Guidance on Professional Conduct for Nursing and Midwifery Students* and *The Code* (NMC, 2010a,b, 2008a), which are essentially aimed at guiding the practice, professional and ethical behaviour of nurses and midwives. You can locate these documents on the NMC website (http://www.nmc-uk.org).

Qualified nurses and midwives whose conduct and competency fall below acceptable professional standard could be removed from the professional register. The Councils' chief aim is to protect the public from poor practitioners, ensuring that the public receives the highest standard of healthcare. Like the NMC, the HPC can remove from its register any of its registrants found guilty of professional misconduct on or off the job. See http://www.hpc-uk.org/mediaandevents/pressrelease/index.asp?id=466 for examples of healthcare professionals who have been struck off by the HPC.

Disciplinary measures against poor standards

In its business of maintaining standards of education, training and practice and to protect the public from bad practitioners, each year the NMC receives approximately 1,500 complaints about its registrants' fitness to practice, conduct or health (http://www.nmc-uk.org/templates/pages/Search?q=cache:f8Wegjc5Y10J:www.nmc-u; visited November 2010). It treats these complaints very seriously. NMC panels of registrants and lay people consider allegations made about registrants deemed to be jeopardising public safety. These panels have a range of sanctions available to them, from issuing a *caution*, through *suspension from the register*, to *removing* registrants from the register. In 2004/5 the NMC struck off 106 registrants and cautioned 41.

The NMC reports a rising trend in the number of allegations against registrants brought to its attention each year. Registrants facing allegations against them have the right to a fair hearing and to satisfactory representation. In our country everyone has a right to fair professional hearing and to a fair legal trial in a court of law should this arise. Indeed the Human Rights Act 1998 states in Article 6 that everyone has a right to fair trial, to a fair hearing and the right not to be punished without fair hearing. Article 3 states that no one should be subject to inhuman and degrading treatment or punishment. Therefore for the NMC or HPC to punish one of their registrants without according them these rights would be to breach their registrants' fundamental human rights.

Students' obligation to give high-quality care within the framework of proper indemnity insurance cover

As a student nurse the patient is still entitled to expect a very high quality of care from you. You have a moral, professional, ethical and legal obligation to provide care to a high standard. A patient/client is entitled to expect high-quality care irrespective of who is delivering that care. As a patient in hospital you would expect the same. A patient who is injured by poor-quality care from a student nurse is unlikely to say, 'oh well, she was only a student, so I will put up with this' or 'he is only a student so I won't bother to sue the Trust'. It is for this reason that we ask student nurses and other healthcare students such as physiotherapists to join a professional organisation such as UNISON or the Royal College of Nursing, or, in the case of physiotherapy, the Chartered Society of Physiotherapists (CSP), for example, in order to secure protective indemnity insurance. This is done just in case you unwittingly injure a patient through careless or negligent practice. If you fail to join one of these professional organisations, you could leave yourself and your patient vulnerable in the event that your practice unwittingly harms a patient. Of course, patients are more likely to sue the health professional's employer under *vicarious liability* (see Chapter 7 on negligence) than to sue an individual healthcare professional, but you never know. So be indemnified by proper insurance protection before you care for patients.

Necessity to seek professional guidance

It is also for the reason above (i.e. aiming to give the best care and trying not to hurt patients) that as a student you are advised to make sure you know what you are doing for the patient before you do it. If as a student you are unsure of what care you should provide, you should consult with, and get directions from, your mentor, clinical educator or supervisor, or other appropriately qualified professional. As a student you owe it to your patients to be responsible and safe in meeting their needs. You have a duty to give patients safe and competent nursing care. You cannot say, 'oh well as a student I am not accountable for what I do'. Indeed you have professional, moral and legal duty of care to the people you care for. You are responsible for what you do from the first day you enter training. Equally, when you qualify and start to delegate to junior staff, you have a responsibility and an obligation to ensure that those to whom you delegate have the necessary ability to carry out the care safely and competently.

Indemnity insurance for registered practitioners

The NMC recommends that, as a registered nurse caring for patients/clients, you have professional indemnity insurance cover. This is in your best interest and that of your patients/clients, should a patient bring a professional negligence claim against you. This is even more important if as a nurse you are off duty and decide to help someone in your capacity as a nurse and in the process negligently harm them. When you are working for an employer such as an NHS Trust that trust will most certainly carry vicarious liability for any negligent act or omission on your part and that of other employees. However, it is important to note that vicarious liability does not normally extend to nursing activities undertaken outside your employment. In any case a patient can, if (s)he sees fit, bring a negligence claim against a health professional directly, although this is unlikely to happen as the health professional's employer has more financial muscle than the employee. If this happens you need to be sure you are covered by your personal indemnity policy. So from when you become a healthcare student till the day you retire from professional practice as a registered practitioner be sure you are always covered by a suitable indemnity insurance policy. When working outside your employer's authority you are personally accountable for your own indemnity insurance should you negligently hurt your 'patient'. The NMC (2008a) makes this particular point in its Code:

> If unable to secure professional indemnity insurance, a registrant will need to demonstrate that all their clients/patients are fully informed of this fact and the implications this might have in the event of a claim for professional negligence.

Qualified nurses as independent practitioners

Qualified nurses are independent practitioners in their own right. They carry personal accountability for their individual practice, even though nurses on the whole have to work within a multidisciplinary team and must therefore cooperate with other healthcare professionals for the good of their patients/clients. When you become a registered nurse you are accountable to your employer, client/patient and professional body to deliver the highest standard of care to your patients. You must ensure you can deliver care competently. Work within the limits of your competence and take *life-long learning* steps to develop added competences you do not have at a given point in time. Such behaviour will help to secure proper standards of nursing care that is unlikely to hurt patients and drive up the NHS legal liability bills due to health professionals' negligent practice. While you are a student the mentors who supervise your work have a professional responsibility to ensure that they do not delegate to you tasks and responsibilities that are beyond your capability. However, you the student also have a responsibility to make sure you are able to deliver the care you have been delegated to do in a careful, competent and safe way. If you are not sure, ask your mentor for guidance. Do not jump in blind.

Extended role duties

In recent years nurses have taken on many *extended role duties* that doctors traditionally carried out. A sound understanding of law, ethics and professional responsibilities will help to ensure that in delivering extended duties your practice is sound and not open to legal challenge. Nurses also need to be aware of the ethical complexities and dilemmas in their practice. Only nurses who are knowledgeable about healthcare law and ethics will be able to address important *legal, moral and ethical questions thrown up by clinical practice*. Understanding some law will also help students and qualified nurses in their personal private lives where knowledge of some aspects of law is required. Before I embark on Chapter 2, I must implore you to read and gain further understanding of the NMC (2008b) Code of Conduct, found at: http://www.nmc-uk.org/Nurses-and-midwives/The-code/The-code-in-full/. Furthermore please read *Guidance on Professional Conduct for Nursing and Midwifery Students* (NMC, 2010b), found at http://www.nmc-uk.org/. . ./Guidance/Guidance-on-professional-conduct-for- nursing-and-midwifery-students-September-2010.PDF.

Summary and conclusion

This chapter has provided an overview of the rationale for writing this book and outlined its potential value to all pre-registration nursing students. It has sought to establish key links between the NMC standards for pre-registration nursing education and practice and law, ethics and nurses' code of conduct. It has highlighted the rising cost of negligence claims on the NHS and how this could impact on nursing and nurses. The chapter makes the point that nursing and its practices are intrinsically tied into the law and ethics. Nurses must practise in accordance with the law of the country they work in. The increasingly changing face of nursing brings greater complexity to the nurse's widening and deepening role, exposing nurses more than ever before to the risk of liability in negligence, especially as the population nursing serves is becoming increasingly aware of legal issues that make people more litigious. As constant *change* in nursing is a reality, nurses must be aware of the growing need for them to keep up to date legally, ethically and in terms of professional competence. A few nursing definitions were examined; although useful in their indications of what nursing is about, they do not supply clear standards of practice, yet the law itself sets very clear standards of acceptable healthcare practice. A study of law will enable nurses to understand their legal professional obligations. Where definitions and standards of nursing practice are woolly and unclear, nurses could be put on a collision course with the law and could behave unethically.

As a nurse you must ensure you maintain high professional, ethical, moral and legal standards in nursing practice and personal behaviour even off the job. The NMC expects all nurses, students included, to follow its code of conduct, performance, ethics and behaviour. As a student you must learn the principles set out in the Code and be guided by them. You must also make sure you conduct your professional life with integrity and appropriate and acceptable moral values. The NMC is just one of the bodies responsible for regulating health and social care practice provisions. There are other professional bodies such as the HPC, the GSCC and the British Medical Council (BMC), all of which principally aim to protect the public by ensuring the highest standard of patient/client care. Regulating health and social care practices is an obligatory legal imperative, but also a personal professional and ethical obligation.

2 Applying professional codes, laws and moral principles

Objectives of this chapter

After reading this chapter you will have an understanding of:

- the concept of nurses' personal and professional responsibility and accountability;
- how the NMC's Code of Conduct guides professional standards, behaviour and practice within a safe legal, moral and ethical framework;
- the interaction of the NMC Code and standards of behaviour with law, ethics and moral values within the caring process, drawing on written patient-centred scenarios and common law cases;
- how to start building a law, ethics and professional standards and code of conduct portfolio;
- the concept of *duty of care* and the complexity and moral dilemma involved in making practical nursing decisions.

Introduction

We noted in the preceding chapter the importance of nurses understanding law, ethics and PCC and the fact that every nurse must abide by the law within which (s)he practises. We need to do this to provide safe care and also to prevent our employers and ourselves becoming *respondent*s in patients' negligence suits because of poor care that harms patients. We also noted that nurses need to be able to work within multiprofessional teams as different healthcare professionals have different roles to play. This is because patients have different needs and different healthcare professionals need different, as well as some overlapping, skills and competencies to help meet these needs. However, all healthcare professionals are required to work together, in partnership, and to their own professional code of conduct. This is one of the factors that entitle health and social care professionals to claim the label of *professionalism*. *Whatever competencies we claim to have as health professionals, we should be able to deliver them within a safe and acceptable legal and ethical framework.*

As stated earlier, in the UK the NMC determines the professional standards nurses and midwives must work to. The Council's most important responsibility is to protect the public as consumers of healthcare. It does so by ensuring its registrants are fit for purpose, being able to provide care competently. Your university and the NMC expect that as a student nurse you will behave professionally within your academic institution, in the clinical setting and in all aspects of your life, private and public. Behaving professionally includes behaving within the framework of the law. It means behaving professionally and legally whether you are shopping, partying, or caring for patients. The NMC stresses 'good health', 'good character', and 'fitness to practice' as preconditions to students gaining professional registration. In its policy document *Guidance on professional conduct, for nursing and midwifery students* the NMC (2010b) further states: 'When you have successfully completed your programme, your university will let us know that you have met the education and practice standards and are of good health and good character'. Moreover, 'It's important that you're aware that your behaviour and conduct, both during your programme and in your personal life, may have an impact: your fitness to practise . . .' (NMC, 2010b).

The NMC expects you to successfully undertake your programme's allotted theoretical and practical hours of training, of which roughly half is made up of clinical experience, and the other half theory.

The purpose of this chapter is first to examine the notions of *professional responsibility and accountability* and then to tease out some of the *professional standards* of *behaviour* expected of you as a student and a registered nurse. This chapter therefore provides you with knowledge, but at the same time it periodically calls on you to identify and reflect on situations and come up with some answers. This is designed to challenge you, to stimulate you to 'build' some knowledge yourself, as a means of stimulating and motivating your learning and readiness to build on prior acquired knowledge. In the process of learning, each successive level of knowing acts as a prerequisite to the next level of knowledge and understanding. You are encouraged, therefore, to become *engaged* with *each reflective student activity* presented before looking at answers provided by in the chapter. If you go to what the writer proposes as possible responses to each reflective question first, you will find it more difficult to think up answers for yourself in respect of these exercises and in your wider learning and clinical practice.

Nurses' accountability and responsibility

The interrelationship between law, ethics and PCC calls for an examination of the notions of *professional responsibility* and *accountability*. Nursing is about accepting and demonstrating *responsibility* – responsibility to self, your studies as a student nurse, your peers you study and work with, health professionals who supervise your learning and development of proper skills and competencies within clinical practice, and of course the patients and clients whom your entire education is preparing you to care for. We start by asking the question, what do we mean by *responsibility* and *accountability?*

To be *responsible* one has to have the prerequisite capabilities to produce responsible conduct and behaviour. One also has to be put in a situation requiring responsible behaviour. Studying to be a nurse and actually caring for clients and patients is one such position. Life experiences may teach responsibility, so that as a student entering training you may have already come possessing a caring, responsible attitude derived from personal life experiences, your personality make-up, your genetic predisposition, prior teaching, reading and the varied experiences of growing up that you come with. This sense of responsibility – personal moral, ethical, professional obligation to care for others – needs to be built upon by your nurse training. By the end of your course you will be a different person in the sense of having new knowledge, skills, competencies, attitudes and maybe even belief systems. What you believe in influences your behaviour and conduct towards others. Hold onto this point for a minute; we will return to it below.

Accountability

The fact that we are entrusted with responsibility and we accept responsibility necessarily means that we must at some point account for, or give a reckoning of, what we have done. Nursing requires you to be accountable for what you do. Accountability is our obligation to give explanation for our actions and omissions. You can see therefore that *responsibility* and *accountability* are integrally linked; *responsibility* leads to *accountability*.

Reflective activity

As a new first-year nursing student, please stop for a minute or two and consider some of the responsibilities you feel that becoming a student nurse has brought you. List these in Box 2.1, in no particular order. After you have done so go to Box 2.2, which has been completed for you to show some of the responsibilities I believe becoming a nurse student has placed upon you. Compare the areas of responsibilities and accountability with those you identified for yourself.

Student portfolio activity

To further your learning and development in relation to your understanding of the new student nurse's responsibilities and accountability please undertake the work in Box 2.3.

Categorising accountability

In looking closely at what I wrote in Box 2.2, I realised that I could categorise 'account-ability/responsibility' into a number of *domains*. For example, one area of a student's responsibility is to him/herself. For example you have responsibility for your own learning. You have responsibility to other people, agents, interest groups and so on, beyond 'self', for example to the university or placements.

Reflective question

Reflect on whether you feel the student nurse has responsibility to other sources/agents/persons apart from oneself. What are they? In response to the above exercises, you may have thought of the sorts of sub-groups/classifications/domains/areas or sub-divisions of *accountability/responsibility* that I have come up with under Figure 2.1.

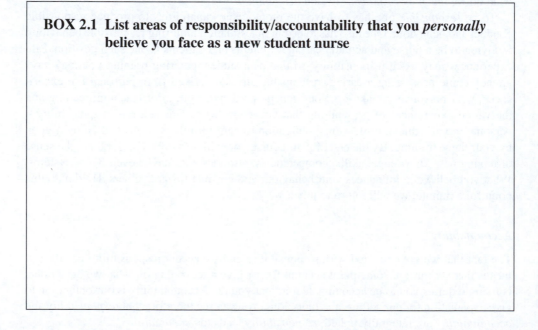

BOX 2.1 List areas of responsibility/accountability that you *personally* believe you face as a new student nurse

BOX 2.2 Some of the responsibility/accountability the writer believes the new student nurse takes on when (s)he enters student nurse training

- Responsibility to register/enrol on the nursing course (university registration).
- Responsibility for learning/organising learning – you will not be spoon fed!
- Responsible conduct in halls/privately rented accommodation, for example towards people and property; for instance avoid malicious damage to halls/landlord's property.
- Obtain, read, understand and follow study timetables, locating rooms and getting to lectures, demonstrations, seminars and the like on time.
- Budgeting responsibilities: balance your budget, for example buying meals and books, paying for accommodation and entertainment – achieving the famous 'making ends meet'!
- Balancing time between studying, working in clinical placements, eating, playing, resting and so on.
- Keeping in touch with others, for example personal tutor, welfare tutors, family, friends, peers you will be working with; building and preserving team spirit that is so intrinsically part of nursing.
- Responsibility to identify and obtain university/other resources, such as libraries (books, journals, newspapers, computer database search resources, e-journals, NMC reading materials e.g. the NMC Code and *Standards for Pre-registration Nursing Education*), computer clusters, shops, bank, booksellers, canteen and dining rooms, post office, games rooms/gymnasium, other useful places/entertainment/recreational facilities that all healthy students will need.
- Being present at all mandatory teaching-learning sessions, for example fire lectures, manual handling, health and safety talks, cardio-pulmonary resuscitation classes.
- Responsibility to buy some course books/other learning materials, not just rely solely on university resources.
- *Diligently* attend lectures and practical demonstrations, seminars and so on.
- *Make use of* university support clubs, university-wide/school student support/welfare services and so on.
- Ascertain location of clinical placements, means of transport and so on.
- Getting self to and from placements safely and in good time.
- Join the necessary trade union/professional organisation, such as RCN or UNISON, for the necessary insurance indemnity cover you need for your clinical placement.
- Conduct self professionally, legally, ethically at university/clinical placements/home/public places. Responsibility to study NMC guidelines on professional and personal behaviour.
- Develop appropriate and effective study habits, motivation to study and do well
- Cultivate sound ethical and caring values, appropriate professional attitudes, and gain the necessary competencies, skills and knowledge required of you as a student nurse.
- Achieve learning outcomes/objectives, competencies, in university/clinical placement modules.

- Follow appropriate professional guidance from mentors/supervisors/clinical educators.
- Work within the limits of one's competence, providing patients with the highest standard of nursing care, through proper mentor supervision and recognising personal limitations.
- Accountability: for example to self, university, clinical staff, tutors, parents/others; legal, professional, ethical accountability and so on.

BOX 2.3 Personal reflection and portfolio building

In reflecting on the areas of responsibilities/accountability of a new nursing student, as required to above, write up your reflection in the law/ethics and PCC section of your developing individual professional portfolio. Be sure to address the following:

- Set out clearly what you are trying to do: your aims and objectives.
- Select an appropriate reflection model or some other strategies and techniques for reflection; that can help you to achieve your reflection outcomes. There are many reflective models available to you, for example online ones, or those in your nursing text books, such as Gibbs (1988) or Schon (1983), or any other recognised reflective model. Briefly explain the model and say something about how it helped your reflection.
- Say whether you worked with others to achieve your reflection. If you did explain your and their contribution.
- Say whether you read materials/sources on the notion of nurses' responsibilities/accountability.
- Generate your ideas.
- What have you learned about (a) responsibility and accountability; (b) student nurses' responsibilities/accountability; (c) responsibilities and accountability of healthcare professionals in general; (d) how you see yourself taking responsibility for your learning at university, including in the practice setting; (e) yourself as a person, your knowledge, aptitude for learning, willingness and motivation to learn, learning style; (f) who you consider you are accountable to as a student nurse?
- How has the exercise contributed to your new knowledge/awareness and feeling?
- How has the learning helped with your personal academic and professional development?
- What additional things do you propose to do to further your learning about nursing responsibilities and accountability?
- What else did you learn in the process of this reflection?
- How do you now feel about the profession you have chosen to join?
- Do you feel you need to make any personal changes or adjustments to move forward in your academic and professional development? If yes, what?
- What does the NMC Code tell you about responsibility, accountability and professional and personal behaviour?

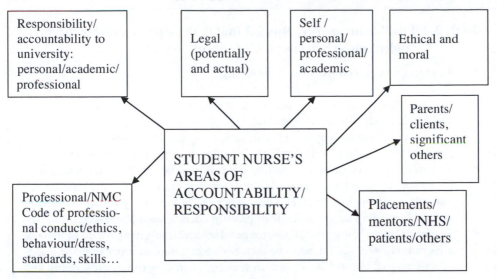

Figure 2.1 Domains of the student nurse's areas of *responsibility* and *accountability*.

Reflect a little further and see which items from Box 2.2 you could logically fit under the domain: *responsibility/accountability to the university*. An outline answer is provided for you in Box 2.4. Some are worded slightly differently from the wording used in Box 2.2 but their sense remains intact. I have also done this to encourage your thinking.

Failure to demonstrate responsibility may be linked to such things as non-attendance at lectures, practical demonstration sessions and/or clinical placements. Non-achievement may also be linked to failure to achieve specified learning outcomes and objectives related to clinical and academic course work that the university has set you. Failure to maintain a sense of responsibility may be the reason why a student may be referred to the *University's Fitness to Practice Committee*. When you qualify and register as a nurse you will need to continue to grow professionally, being able to maintain the competencies and standards of practice required of a registered nurse by an increasingly demanding and knowledgeable public. Failure to do so may be the reason why a registered nurse may be referred to a *NMC's Fitness to Practice Panel*. You will need to continue to involve yourself in continuing professional development (CPD) and *life-long learning* to ensure your competency to practice at the requisite level and to the requisite standard is maintained.

Justification for the 'accountability/responsibility' categories

The intention here is not to provide, at this point, a detailed justification for each item placed under specified *sub-groupings*/categories, for e.g. *University Accountability*, but to provide you (the reader) with *some* ideas of how justification could be made. So as an example, in relation to the item 'To register/enrol on my course at university', you may have thought of justification ideas such as:

*   I have a personal responsibility for my own learning, including enrolling at university.
*   The university has to account to other interested parties, such as NHS commissioning agents and the NMC, for all the nursing students it takes onto its nursing courses.

BOX 2.4 Possible items from Box 2.2 that may be placed under the student nurse's accountability to university

- To register/enrol on my course at university.
- To be a responsible house/dormitory mate, for example in halls of residence. For example, do not damage halls of residence/my private landlord's property.
- To keep in touch with my personal tutor.
- To balance my work/study and play, in such a way that neither my studies nor my personal physical and recreational needs suffer; in fact ensure both benefit.
- To ensure I have or can obtain or locate the appropriate study resources such as books (library-held books, as well as my own that I have personally purchased), journals, newspapers, computer database search resources, e-journals, the necessary NMC reading materials, code of practice documentation and so on.
- To ensure I attend diligently all teaching and information-giving sessions, and not miss out on essentials I need to be aware of/engaged in, in order to make a success of my studies, such as fire lectures, manual handling procedures, health and safety talks, cardio-pulmonary resuscitation courses, university welfare and student support services, my lectures and so on. All these are critical to my success.
- [Ascertain] Where/when my first clinical placements will be, and how I will get to and from them?
- To make sure I join/enrol with the necessary trade union or professional organisation, pay the required fees to secure the necessary insurance indemnity cover, in case I am cited for negligent practice with personal, university or NHS Trust liability for an injury to a patient I was involved in caring for.
- To conduct myself in a professional manner at all times, in the university, in clinical placements, public places, at home and so forth.
- To develop appropriate and effective study habits, caring attitudes, competencies for sound professional practice, the right ethical and caring values and ethics.
- To make sure that when I go to placement I achieve the learning objectives and competencies outlined for me by the university, learn as best I can, and follow appropriate professional guidance, respect the limits of my competence and provide my patients with the highest standard of care.

- It has to provide agents such as the NHS Students Grants Unit with information that may enable students to satisfactorily obtain their training bursaries, loans and the like, where these apply.
- The university can be called upon by NMC reviewers to provide information about students' performance, progress and attrition in relation to the course.
- It must provide agents such as Strategic Health Authorities/other commissioners with information about student numbers, attrition rates, success or failure on their programme.
- At the end of the programme, the university must provide the NMC with the necessary information to enable the NMC to decide if those applying for professional registration are worthy of this.
- Other quality assessment agencies, for instance the Higher Education Funding Council, responsible for monitoring standards of education and research in universities may seek such information from the university

- The university is obliged to provide a valid programme of pre-registration nursing education to all its pre-registration nursing students. After all it collects tuition fees from the Department of Health for teaching the nursing students. It has a responsibility and obligation to deliver high–quality education programmes.

Across the university, there are parallels to the last point made above. For example, non-nursing students across the university are equally entitled to education (and, in some cases, training) at the appropriate level and to the required standard. It does not matter that in the case of most nursing and, say, physiotherapy students their fees may be paid by the Department of Health. The important principle is that the university does not provide free education. It must therefore account for the standard of education it provides at a cost, irrespective of the professional and/or academic discipline the student comes from. So, indeed, you are not alone in being obliged to maintain standards, being responsible and accountable for your work.

This sense of responsibility and accountability goes on in the clinical practice settings too, where for example you will be responsible to your mentors and to the patients and their families for whom you care. The university and the placements have to work together to provide my nursing education and training and I am responsible to play my part in this.

To meet its own obligations then, the university has the right to call students to account for their academic and practical performance. This includes being successful in the necessary assessments prescribed for a module and/or your entire programme of study. As a student nurse, you have a responsibility to make sure you register/enrol at the university. In any case if you are not officially enrolled you are not a legitimate student and certainly will not have your loans or tuition fees paid. Neither will you be entitled to any tuition or facilities offered to bona fide students. You will not even get a council tax exemption letter from your university to pass to your landlord or your local council to exempt you from paying council tax.

As a student you have the right to expect your academic institution to provide you with a very high standard of education and clinical practice experience, although the universities organise these through various agencies such as NHS Trusts that provide patient care.

Other domains of responsibility/accountability and the overlapping nature of these

With respect to, for example, 'appropriate behaviour and conduct in halls of residence', the university can hold you accountable if you damage its property. So can your landlord if you live in private accommodation and demonstrate careless behaviour and conduct. Areas of your responsibility and accountability may fall within other category *domains* within Figure 2.1, apart from *university*. For example, your accountability may be *legal, professional, ethical and personal*. Here, one may point out the obvious, that there are interrelationships between the boxes of accountability in Figure 2.1. For example, as can be seen, the university does have links with the NMC and can therefore report adverse happenings related to a nursing student's conduct whilst on the course. As a student therefore you must take all steps to make sure your conduct and behaviour are of a good standard or you could find yourself being thrown off your programme of study.

Students have been known to be thrown off their degree and diploma programmes for such things as academic cheating (plagiarism; passing off other people's work as one's own). You must always acknowledge other people's work in your course work and examinations. University students may be expelled for other forms of unprofessional behaviour such as:

- violence and aggression;
- drinking and getting drunk;
- cheating and lying;
- engaging in fraudulent practices;
- failing their academic and clinical courses;
- damaging university property;
- shoplifting;
- public disorder.

As a student you must make sure your behaviour and conduct is beyond reproach. Conduct yourself professionally and enjoy your time at university to the fullest. Every good way you conduct your life in a private or public context outside nursing is an actual precursor to being able to conduct your professional behaviour within nursing to an acceptable, honourable and professional standard. Once you enter a profession such as nursing your total life is under scrutiny and this must be so because your professional body, the NMC, exists to make sure the public is protected. To do so it must ensure those who are registered as nurses are able to practise nursing with skill, competence, honour and integrity. Throughout your training and beyond please ensure you attain and maintain this level of behaviour and conduct. Patients are indeed vulnerable and cannot be left at the mercy of individuals who are unscrupulous, untrustworthy, volatile and professionally incompetent. When you see these characteristics in colleagues who call themselves nurses you have an obligation to blow the whistle on them. The profession, the patients, clients and their relatives expect no less from caring nurses.

Professional/NMC accountability/responsibility

Under 'Professional/NMC accountability' within Figure 2.1, you must remember that the NMC lays down *standards* to guide your professional and personal conduct and behaviour. Make sure you read the NMC (2010b) guide for students of nursing and midwifery, which can be found on its website. The NMC itself has legal responsibility and obligations, being charged under the Nursing and Midwifery Order 2001 [Article 5(2) (a)] to establish and maintain proper standards for nursing education and practice in England, Scotland and Wales. To meet its own obligations it robustly establishes and monitors standards of nurse education and practice. The NMC is accountable to Parliament and the public for the quality of nurse education and practice, being committed to maintain public safety and confidence in the nursing profession. You have an obligation to play your part in the larger picture. In the case of pre-registration nursing students, 50 per cent of their programme is theory and the other 50 per cent is practice. The education and training institution must satisfy the NMC that when nursing students complete their programme they have satisfied the 50 per cent theory/practice requirement and have fulfilled the *standards required for competent practice*. Until you achieve these you are not eligible to seek NMC registration. Clearly, this puts responsibility on students to complete the theory/practice requirements to the satisfaction of both the university and the NMC.

Student activity

Undertake the tasks in Box 2.5.

BOX 2.5 Student activity on responsibility

1   In an appropriate section of your portfolio, reflect on:
   - the role of the university regarding your training;
   - your responsibility regarding your training;
   - the responsibility of the NMC regarding your training;
   - responsibility of placements regarding your training;
   - the implications of students and registered nurses failing to meet the standards of profession training and practice;
   - the guidance provided the student by the NMC Code;
   - implications of student nurses failing to study and abide by the NMC Code.
2   download a copy of NMC Code, study it, assimilate it and put it in the professional development section of your portfolio.

NMC guidance on professional conduct

In the policy document *Guidance on Professional Conduct for Nursing and Midwifery Students* the NMC (2010b) states that the Code has four main principles:

1. Make the care of people your first concern, treating them as individuals and respecting their dignity.
2. Work with others to protect and promote the health and wellbeing of those in your care, their families, carers and the wider community.
3. Provide a high standard of practice and care at all times.
4. Be open and honest, act with integrity and uphold the reputation of your profession.

Now let us focus on the first principle statement above:

Make the care of people your first concern, treating them as individuals and respecting their dignity.

Hopefully, in the requisite section of your portfolio, you have come up with, and written down key points such as, when working with people:

- Treat them humanely, as individuals who are sensitive and deserving of respect.
- Treat as you would like to be treated. In other words be empathetic towards patients.
- Make the identification of the patient's needs and problems, the setting of realistic care plans to meet their needs, and the implementation and evaluation of those plans be your central priority.
- Make the care of your patient/client your central concern and demonstrate that they are important and you intend to do all you can to help them achieve their treatment objectives, be these health promotion objectives, rehabilitative goals such as relief of pain and suffering, learning to walk again, sit up, eat, drink and other activities of daily living, or overcoming stress and anxiety or other forms of mental and psychological illnesses.

- Treating people as individuals with holistic, bio-psychosocial needs, with interdependences with others, such as family members, carers and the wider community.
- Accept that patients have an important part to play in their care and that their views are important in decision making related to their care. In other words they are *autonomous* beings and because of this we should always first gain their consent before we treat them.
- The patient's or client's own views are central to the caring decision making.
- Maintain patients' and clients' privacy and dignity. For example, when attending to a patient or client, avoid undue invasion of personal space; for instance, if the patient is being cared for in an individual room, knock on the door before entering.
- If a patient is being private behind a curtain, avoid pulling back the curtain without first indicating your intension to enter the patient's private space.
- If appropriate, nurse patients in individual rooms, not on traditional Nightingale ward where it is difficult to maintain their privacy (DoH, 2005a).
- Address patients by their preferred names and titles.
- Avoid talking over patients or talking about them as though they do not exist.
- When speaking to your patients maintain eye contact with them and show that you are interested in their well-being, as this is likely to make them feel respected and valued.
- Appreciate that patients may be embarrassed about your attention to their bodily needs, for example washing them, drying them, feeding them, emptying their bed pans and urinals and perhaps attending to other facets of their personal hygiene.
- Demonstrate sensitivity in maintaining patients' privacy and dignity.

Even a patient who may be unable to speak, or who may be semi-conscious or fully unconscious, needs to be cared for in a sensitive and respectful way. There can be nothing more disrespectful than to take a fellow human being for granted, forgetting that, irrespective of whether one is ill or well each person is entitled to respect. If you ask a patient a question be sure to demonstrate that you are interested in an answer. Do not walk away as though you had just asked a rhetorical question, not deserving of a reply.

I recall being treated in a hospital for a chest infection. On the ward sister's round one morning, having arrived at my bed, she asked what sort of night I had. Before I could answer, she briskly proceeded to look at my charts at the end of the bed. There was no eye contact with me. Realising that sister's question was a rhetorical one, I decided not to answer to see if she would notice. She did not. That was an example of disrespect and an indication of sister 'going through the motion', but having no real interest in what I as the patient had to say. There was no real and sincere contact with me as a patient. My charts were more important than me or any reply I could give the sister!

If you ask a patient a question it should be because you want an answer, which could tell you something about how the patient felt, the sort of night (s)he thought (s)he had. Such response from the patient may form part of your report about the patient to the next shift of nurses. In that report the patient's direct words could be quoted to show his/her real perception of the night and the progress made. How patient-centred would such a report be? Maintaining eye contact and listening to your patient's reply can also help to establish effective interpersonal communication and sound therapeutic rapport and relationships.

It is important to remember that patients in hospitals are there because they are ill. Their morale may be low, their energies drained and altogether they may not just feel physically ill but be psychologically experiencing anxiety, depression and loneliness, as well as worrying about their significant others and whether they will recover from their illness. These things can reduce patients' capacity to cope, heal and recover. We should always remember to accord respect, privacy and dignity to our patients.

In reflecting on the NMC's caring principle, *make the care of people your first concern, treating them as individuals and respecting their dignity*, hopefully you have come up with, and written into your law, ethics and professional values portfolio, some of the points mentioned above. Now, let us consider how law, healthcare policy issues, staff attitudes, ethics, moral values and professional code of conduct principles apply to, or can support, the picture we have painted.

First the *Human Rights Act 1998, Article 8*, demands that we respect people's right to privacy and personal family life, part of the process of maintaining dignity. The law relating to privacy, dignity and confidentiality demands that we do not disclose patients' confidential information without their consent, although there are exceptions to this rule as we shall see later. The Equality Act 2010 calls on us to respect diversity and avoid unfair discrimination against people. Irrespective of our gender, race, ethnicity, social class, age or other category, we are all entitled to privacy and dignity.

Case law (*common law*) also protects patients' privacy. In a New Zealand case, *Furniss v Fitchett* [1958] NZLR 396, a doctor was successfully sued by a woman (who was one of his patients) for disclosing confidential information about her to her husband, who used the information to his advantage, which the woman claimed damaged her. Such behaviour denied the professional value to keep patients' information confidential. As a nurse you are not legally permitted to disclose a patient's confidential information to a third party without that patient's consent, even if the person to whom the information is disclosed is a relative of the patient. As you read further you will, however, find that there may be the extreme rare occasion when you may safely reveal certain information without the patient necessarily sanctioning it or giving you permission to do so. For example if you are confident that a patient in your care intends to harm or harm a known third party, you may be obliged to inform that party (*Tarasoff v Regents of the University of California*, 1976); yes, an American case that could have persuasive credibility in a British court. However, clearly while you are a student if you have concerns that one of your patients is seriously threatening to harm a known third party you must report your concerns to your mentor or some other senior member of staff.

The issue of confidentiality is a very important one however, and you would need to have very, very strong grounds on which to breach it without getting into trouble. In an English case, *X v Y* [1988], a court prevented a newspaper from identifying two doctors who had AIDS. The court held that confidentiality principle involved in protecting the doctors' identity and therefore patients' confidential hospital records was more important than protecting the public against 'theoretical' risks of AIDS and a newspaper's freedom to publish such information.

In terms of policy issues, in its publication *Elimination of Mixed-Sex Accommodation in Hospital*, the Department of Health (DoH, 2005b) gave a clear public commitment to eliminate mixed-sex wards in hospitals, and to organisational arrangements to secure patients' privacy and dignity, for example provision of segregated washing and toileting facilities for male and female patients. Safety would be a major consideration in providing such facilities in mental health settings. However, maintaining patients' privacy and dignity is not just about segregation. Staff attitudes and behaviour are critical influencing variables in according respect to patients, and in valuing their right to autonomy, consent and confidentiality. We should demonstrate sensitive caring attitudes by doing everything possible to ensure patients enjoy self-worth and self-esteem. Maintaining privacy and dignity is also about attending to individual needs, respecting people's cultural value systems, including their individual and cultural differences. The NMC Code states that we must treat people with dignity and respect, and take special care when dealing with vulnerable people, such as the elderly, the very young, disabled people and those suffering from learning disability and who may have lost their mental competence and be unable to consciously engage in self- or nurse-led care.

The *ethic* of *autonomy* (right to self-determination) (Beauchamp and Childress, 2008) demands that nurses respect right of the adult mentally competent to accept or reject treatments offered. An individual has an autonomous right to reject or agree to be touched by a healthcare professional. The *autonomy* principle also gives patients the right to be active participants in their care decision making; a right that also accords patients their right to self-respect, dignity and confidentiality.

Please complete the exercise in Box 2.6 and then go to the bullet points below:

- Attending to your patient's individual needs competently must be your top priority.
- Attend to the patient's individual needs with a sense of priority, dealing with more urgent needs first, for example, attend to a patient's breathing and bleeding problem over lower priorities such as washing, feeding and dressing.
- Respect the patient's cultural values, beliefs and religious needs; as far as is professionally and humanly possible do everything in your power to enable the patient to meet these needs.
- Value diversity and respect cultural differences and values in respect to your patients/ clients and their significant others.
- Accept that patients' cultural and religious values may differ from our own, and there may be even potential for clash of cultural values that could undermine effectiveness of nursing care.
- Avoid using one patient to judge another; they are two entirely different people with individual needs, and who may have entirely different values and beliefs.
- Remember that each patient has legal rights, including the right to life, the right to freedom from discrimination, torture and degrading treatment, and the right to privacy and personal family life.
- In your reflection be sure to address the proper ways of demonstrating politeness, courtesy, kindness and compassion to patients; then reflect on improper ways of doing these

---

BOX 2.6 Further student portfolio reflection exercise 2.1

In your further thoughts about the NMC's principle of 'making the care of people your first concern, treating them as individuals and respecting their dignity', the views expressed above tend to focus mainly on privacy and dignity. Now, apply further thinking to 'making the care of people your first concern', and write down in your portfolio the further ideas you have come up with. In doing this bear in mind notions such as:

- professional considerations;
- cultural concerns, thoughts and issues;
- social concerns, thoughts and issues;
- communication issues and concerns;
- legal considerations;
- ethical concerns.

After the above go to what I have written below and see if you came up with ideas similar to those I have bullet pointed below.

things. Practise the proper approaches in the clinical areas. You may want to practice in class on your friends and tutors, even before going to the clinical areas.

- Revise the relevant sections of the NMC (2008a) Code.
- Be polite to people and treat them as you would like to be treated, with politeness, courtesy, kindness and compassion.
- Appreciate patients' need for confidentiality, including gaining patients' consent to write about them in your portfolio or patient care studies, protecting their identity at all times. To this end use anonymity to protect patients.
- Do not disclose information that patients give you to unauthorised sources. Only persons involved with the patient's care and who have a need to know because they need to participate in the patient's care need to be told, and of course with the patient's consent.
- Protect patients' data and do not allow unauthorised persons to gain access to a patient's data without his/her consent. Patients' data are protected under the Data Protection Act, 1998. I recall as a student, a patient informing me that a visitor had been reading her notes placed at the bottom end of her bed!
- Follow established guidelines and procedures from your university, practice settings, professional code of conduct and mentors, as well as principles of law related to privacy and confidentiality.
- Only acceptable legal permitted confidential disclosure is permitted, for example through an order of the court.

Respecting patients' right to autonomy and autonomous decision making also means the unquestionable acceptance that patients have a right to confidentiality, privacy and dignity. The consent of the competent patient to investigation and treatment must be obtained at all times. So important are these principles that the NMC has issued advice on confidentiality. You can read the appropriate advice sheet online at http://www.nmc-uk.org/Nurses-and-midwives/Advice-by-topic/A/Advice/Confidentiality/. Moreover the NMC has also issued advice on consent. This can be read online at http://www.nmc-uk.org/Nurses-and-midwives/Advice-by-topic/A/Advice/Consent/.

Follow-up reflection

Have you seen evidence of improper conduct by nurses when they are dealing with patients? Reflect on the experiences and how you will endeavour to avoid such behaviour and conduct. Did you point out the improper or impolite behaviour to the nurses concerned? If not, why not? Even though you are a student, you too can make a difference. Even people who are senior to you can learn from you. Do not feel that you are so junior that you have nothing positive to give. Indeed you have, so do not feel hopeless or useless in these situations. In any case from the start of your training you are personally responsible for your conduct and behaviour. Such conduct and behaviour must always seek to put patients at the centre of care.

To further put patient at the centre of your professional activity, be sure to *cooperate with other healthcare professionals involved in the patient's care* to ensure the best patient care outcomes. To this end the NMC requires you to:

- be a good listener, responding appropriately to your patient's concerns and preferences;
- support people to achieve independence where possible, respecting the contribution they are able to make in the care decision making;
- give people clear information and advice in an intelligible way, to enable them to make choices and decisions about their care;

- collaborate with patients, their significant others such as family members and carers;
- value the fact that each *mentally competent* patient/client is an *autonomous* being with the right to make personal decisions relating to him-/herself, for example the patient/client can give, withhold or even withdraw consent relative to his/her treatment;
- gain the patient's consent to treatment before you attempt to provide it, to accord the patient his/her autonomous right to decide;
- not disclose patients' confidential information without their consent.

The last point may seem a little contentious. This is because you may be thinking, if I cannot tell my mentor what the patient told me, how am I going to ensure that continuity of the patient's care is achieved when I leave the patient care setting? This is a fair thought to engage in. To avoid any problems in this respect it is important that patients be informed initially that, because their care is provided by a team of healthcare professionals, including for example doctors, nurses, physiotherapists, pharmacists, maybe social workers, podiatrists and others, in order to provide them with the best multiprofessional care, information may sometimes have to be shared with other professional colleagues involved in the care. Be sure the patient is happy with this and that you have his/her consent to do so.

Relevant information needs to be passed to those *who have a need to know*, meaning other professionals who need the information in order to continue to work towards the best patient outcomes. Clearly people within the care situation who do not need to know the information should not have it. Such a decision has to be made through the best professional judgement and on the basis that the professional can justify that decision. As a student, if you are in doubt ask your mentor for guidance. It is always best to be cautious, careful and safe than to be otherwise.

You may be thinking also, what about patients who were once conscious and mentally competent to consent, withhold consent or even withdraw consent and were able to provide me with the information I needed to provide best care, but because of their unconsciousness or mental incompetence are now not able to communicate with me? What do I do here? In reality when patients are unable to communicate with you because they are unconscious or have lost mental competence to communicate, the healthcare professional must take decisions *in the patient's best interest*.

Additionally the NMC makes the point that you should:

- Make sure the patient knows you are a student. Respect the fact that patients have a right to request that their care be given by a registered health professional.
- Maintain and respect clear professional boundaries, for example:
  - be sure to end the professional relationship when you are no longer required to care for that person;
  - do not start a sexual relationship with your patient;
  - refuse gifts, favours and hospitality that may be interpreted by the patient as a means of securing preferential treatment;
  - do not accept the loan of money from patients or anyone related to them;
  - follow your professional guidelines in respect to maintaining clear professional boundaries with your patients. Visit http://www.nmc-uk.org for confirmation and further information on these points.

As so far we have been focusing on professional, ethical, legal issues and dimensions in care, you may want to continue to use such a framework to 'frame your thoughts' in identifying the issues and in deciding, with justification, how they ought to be handled, by you and/or others as you see fit.

In relation to the 18-year-old female patient in Box 2.7, it is quite normal to be thinking about questions and issues such as those set out below:

- Is this patient mentally competent? Examine section 2 of the Mental Competency Act 2005 and see how a patient's mental competency is determined. The NMC has also produced an advice sheet on the Mental Competency Act 2005; view this online at http://www.nmc-uk.org/Nurses-and-midwives/Advice-by-topic/A/Advice-Capacity-Act-2005/.
- This patient could bleed to death if I do not do something about her vaginal bleeding.
- She looks rather pale and her bleeding could be more serious than she thinks.
- She says there are blood clots present; sounds serious. What do I do? She wants me to tell no one! But what is my professional obligation and responsibility towards her? And myself for that matter?
- She is being treated for an acute chest infection and is perhaps coughing, which may be making her vaginal bleeding worse, as increased chest pressures during a fit of coughing can lead to increased abdominal and pelvic pressures.
- But isn't this awful for her? Feeling that she cannot talk to her mom or a senior member of the nursing staff about her situation.
- She may even be about to miscarry and I would not want to feel responsible for this. I would feel really guilty if I do nothing and the worst happens. Yet feel I ought to maintain her confidence and not tell any other member of staff. Such a moral dilemma! Such a professional, legal and ethical challenge for me!
- As an adult she has a right to miscarry if she chooses; she might not even want this child; on the other hand this poor unborn child has a right to live. But here again, her 'temple'/her body is her own and she has the (ethical) *autonomous* right to do as she pleases with it. But feel I owe her a professional, moral and legal duty to care for her to the best of my ability!
- However, I am aware that the law gives an expectant woman a right over those of her unborn child (*Paton v Trustees of British Advisory Service* [1978] 2 All ER 987). Mr William Paton of Liverpool had failed in his attempt to stop his wife from having an

---

BOX 2.7 Student portfolio reflection exercise 2.2

A patient scenario

You are located as a student on a medical ward. A female patient, 18 years old, being treated for an acute chest infection, reports to you that she is pregnant, but does not want her mother (who visits her daily) or the rest of the staff in the ward to know. She says she is bleeding per vaginam (PV) but that it is 'not serious'; she 'got through a similar problem two years ago'. Her current blood loss 'contains a few clots, but nothing to worry about. I just thought I would share this information with you as you seem such a friendly student nurse'. She further remarks, 'you can't say much to some of these other staff about your personal issues, because only yesterday I heard the staff nurse discussing with the sister the fact that a fellow patient, Mr Jarrett, has HIV and shouldn't be touched if it can be helped'. Your final thought as the patient finishes speaking to you is how pale she looks.

In an appropriate section of your portfolio, write down your thoughts on the issues of importance here, stating and justifying how you feel the situations in the scenario should be dealt with.

abortion. Under English law an unborn child is not a legal entity and has no right over its mother's decision to abort it. Once born alive, however, it can apply retrospective rights for criminal or civil wrong.

- Under the *Offences against the Person Act* 1861, s. 58, every pregnant woman who, with intent to procure her own miscarriage, unlawfully administers to herself any poison or other noxious thing, or unlawfully uses any instrument or other means, and whoever with intent to procure a miscarriage of any woman whether she be or not be with child shall unlawfully administer to her any poison or other noxious thing, or unlawfully use any instrument or other means, shall be guilty of a felony. However, this is not the case here. So what do I do?

- So do I let her lie here and abort if she wishes? But what of her health? I cannot allow her to just lie here and die. Can I persuade her to have herself examined by a doctor or senior nurse? [It is quite normal to be agonising with these rather ethical dilemmas.]

- She is 18 years old, an adult woman, in law a 'major' with the *mental competence* and autonomy to decide how she wants her situation to be handled, whom she wants to know about it, what she wants to do about her pregnancy and impending miscarriage, and so on.

- To reiterate, she seems mentally competent, not confused or having any learning disablement, so who gives me or anyone else any right to decide for her on the basis of taking a decision in 'her best interest'?

- She reported getting through 'a similar problem two years ago'; so perhaps she knows what she is dealing with. I wonder, however, what she meant when she said she 'got through a similar problem two years ago'? Aborted without complications? Aborted without anyone knowing? What did she mean by this?

- I feel good that this young lady feels she can share such an intimate problem with me; I must appear to her a person to be entrusted with her most confidential information.

- I must do nothing to sever this valuable nurse–patient relationship.

- The law, professional and ethical issues of *autonomy*, *justice*, *patients' right to informed consent* and *confidentiality* are stacked against me telling anyone else about this patient's condition without her consent. But morally and psychologically I am experiencing such *cognitive dissonance*, I really ought to tell someone else, perhaps a senior member of staff, what this young lady just told me.

- But here again I have learned that the ethics of *beneficence* states that patients should benefit from what I do. Not being hurt by my actions or omissions.

- The ethics of *non-maleficence* states that I ought to do nothing to hurt my patients. Here again if I do nothing this could hurt the patient more as she may miscarry or experience even more complications, perhaps even bleeding to death in that bed!

- If I tell the patient's mother what she told me without her consent, am I going to hurt this patient's feelings? Most probably! Most importantly I would have broken confidentiality and subjugated the patient's right to consent or refuse to consent by my divulging information about her, thereby fracturing our professional relationship. She could possibly even sue me for breaching her confidentiality, damaging her relationship with her mother and so on.

- If I disclose her confidential information this could damage the excellent professional relationship I have with her. She might tell me nothing else of significance in future.

- But surely this patient would/should have been told on admission that, although the staff will always respect and uphold her right to confidentiality, there is a need for staff caring for her to pass on information to other staff also caring for her so that the best care can be continued throughout her hospital stay.

- Perhaps her mother has a right to know; after all if she did not love her daughter and have her best interest at heart she would not come to visit her each day. But this would be against the law in relation to consent and confidentiality and would be unethical too, and against the NMC rule on confidentiality and consent.
- But the NMC Code states that I must put the patient at the centre of care, do nothing to hurt the patient, and provide her with the best care including respecting confidentiality, autonomy and her right to give and withdraw consent as she sees fit.
- The NMC Code also states that I should work with others to protect and promote the health and well-being of patients and their families and carers. So I have a real dilemma here, because if I 'tell on' the patient to her mother, I may think I am respecting the well-being of her mother as a family member, perhaps even enabling her to speak to her daughter about her problem and to help her, but disrespecting the patient's right to confidentiality and privacy, and may hurt my patient. I could also face the converse, upsetting her mother. Such a moral and ethical dilemma! What do I do?
- According to the patient, a named ward sister and a staff nurse behaved unprofessionally the day before, carelessly disclosing Mr Jarrett's confidential information. This must have upset this patient, making her particularly suspicious of the senior staff. This perhaps led to her telling me she wants me to hold the information of her pregnancy and vaginal bleeding strictly confidentially. On this point, perhaps I ought not to tell the sister and staff nurse about this 18-year-old young lady's bleeding problem.

Normal reactions to the above scenario issues

The above are just some of the normal reactions and feelings you may have to the issues in the scenario outlined above. I aim not to provide you with a line-by-line pointer to right or wrong actions, but to point out to you certain criticalities which a sensible professional in this situation would observe and even act on.

To start with, your first loyalty, professional responsibility and duty of care are to that 18-year-old patient. You owe your patient *a duty of care* in *law*, *ethics* and *moral values*, and *professionally*, to care for her to the best of your ability. You owe it to her to follow appropriate legal, ethical and moral guidelines, the NMC code of conduct, NMC guidance to student nurses, and health and safety guidelines, aiming always to achieve sound professional standards of care. It is important therefore to examine each question or issue set out above and decide for yourself, with appropriate justification, what you would/should actually do in relation to each question/issue. Use your portfolio to record your thoughts, possible actions and justifications.

Legal duty of care to this 18-year-old patient

When you have read the chapter on the English legal system, you will have a fuller picture of the legal elements in the scenario above. As a student nurse you own this patient *a legal duty of care*. All healthcare professionals owe their patients/clients a *legal duty of care* whilst those patients remain the responsibility of those professionals. This legal position comes from the case of *Donohue v Stevenson* [1932] AC 562. In this landmark *House of Lords* case, which examined whether ginger beer manufacturers owed a duty of care to the ultimate consumer of that beer, Lord Atkin stated that:

> You must take reasonable care to avoid acts or omissions which you can reasonably foresee would be likely to injure your neighbour. Who then in law is my neighbour?

The answer . . . persons who are so closely and directly affected by my act that I ought reasonably to have them in contemplation as being so affected when I am directing my mind to the acts or omissions which are called in question.

Applying Lord Atkin's reasoning above to your 18-year-old patient, that patient is your 'legal' neighbour; not the person who lives next to you, but a patient who is relying on your professional judgement and care, on the caring relationship of nurse to patient. You have a professional and legal relationship to that 18-year-old patient. Your duty of care to her exists because you can see that your actions or omissions are reasonably likely to cause her harm. You are probably now thinking, if I do nothing I could be liable for any harm that comes to her. On the other hand, if I betray the trust she places in me I am harming her and perhaps making myself liable for a possible breach of confidence. Such a moral dilemma! What do I do?

Under tort law, revealing confidential information could amount to negligence, but the patient has to prove that the revelation injured or damaged her. If you were a staff nurse who had signed a contract of employment and you breached it by disclosing the patient's confidential information you could be sued for breaching your contract of employment. Most NHS contracts of employment have confidentiality clauses built into them, with further conditions that staff who breach such clauses could be disciplined (DoH, 2003a). Note, however, NHS patients have no contract with the nurse, doctor or other health professional working within the NHS, and so cannot sue for breaching any contract with them. In English law, in the case of *Wainwright v Home Office* [2003] 3 WLR 1337, there is no tort (civil wrong) of infringing privacy. However, in the statute called the Human Rights Act 1998, a patient could sue for a breach of privacy under Article 8 of that Act.

It must be becoming clear to you now that in English law confidentiality is a complex area. Indeed confidentiality is not absolute and can be broken under certain circumstances. In the situation you are faced with in respect to your 18-year-old patient, you need to remember that, although you must do your level best to respect patients' confidence, there may be instances when you decide to breach them to protect others or the patient him-/herself. Does this apply here, do you think?

Professional duty of care

Hopefully, the staff would have done their job when admitting the patient, by telling her, and getting her agreement on the fact, that salient information relating to her problems, needs and care has to be shared with other healthcare professionals involved in her treatment. As a nurse you have a legal duty to inform your patient of her rights and what you are about to do for her, with her, on her. This does not suggest that you simply run off and inform the next nurse you see of what this patient has just told you. You do owe it to the patient, on a responsible professional level, to talk to the patient about what she has just disclosed to you, and what the implications could be for her if you did not pass the information up the chain of command to a more senior member of staff who may be able to help her. You have a professional, moral, ethical and legal obligation to talk to the patient and persuade her to let you relay her PV bleeding problem to your mentor or one of the doctors, who will be happy to talk with her and see what can best be done for her. You may feel that, given the patient's expressed lack of confidence in a named ward sister and staff nurse, because they breached another patient's confidentiality regarding his HIV status, it may not be appropriate to report the matter direct to the two staff named, for fear of further destroying the relationship you had built up with this patient. However, your primary concern must be to act in this patient's best interest, which must first be to persuade her to let you have her consent to pass such a critical piece of information on to the person(s) who can best help her. You should be able to persuade the patient that you are passing her confidential information up the chain of command not for the purpose of gossip, but to get her the best care in the circumstances she explained to you.

Other professional duty of care facets within this scenario include the following. The NMC does state in the 2008 Code that as a nurse you must make the patient 'your first concern', working with others to protect and promote 'the health and wellbeing of those in your care'; in doing so, 'act with integrity and uphold the reputation of your profession', and 'respect people's right to confidentiality', whilst at the same time informing people 'about how and why information is shared by those who will be providing their care'. Most importantly the NMC states that as a nurse 'you must disclose information if you believe someone may be at risk of harm, in line with the law'. The fact that this lady tells you she is bleeding clots, furthermore she looks pale, and she is already being treated for another serious condition, a chest infection, should ring important bells about the criticality of persuading this patient to accept professional help. You should of course not breach her confidence by disclosing her situation to her mother.

However, in the situation you are faced with, there is every likelihood if you told the patient that in her best interest (and yours too) you needed to report her serious problem to your mentor or the doctor, and actually proceeded to do so, and she were to take a legal action against you for breach of confidence, that action would be likely to fail. Why? You had taken all necessary steps to persuade her to let you get her medical help. You had determined that she was bleeding clots PV and looked very pale. You had assessed and decided that doing nothing including failing to persuade her to seek medical help was not an option. Moreover, omission on your part could be viewed as your failure to take the necessary steps to prevent more serious harm to her. The best course of action, however, must be to have the patient's consent to reveal her dilemma to your mentor and therefore to the medical staff who can help her. If you are in doubt how to behave professionally, in certain circumstances, such as in the scenario you are faced with here, always consult with your mentor, or even speak to your tutor. But be seen to act in the best interest of your patient. Avoid serious and obvious omissions in care. Risks that are reasonably foreseeable must be avoided. Moreover, always listen to your patients and respond to their concerns in a sensitive and caring manner.

Ethical and moral duty to this 18-year-old

Hopefully you would have weighed up your ethical duty to act in such a way as benefits the patient (ethics of beneficence, as per Beauchamp and Childress, 2008). Also, on a moral ground, hopefully you have considered that if you were in the position of this patient you would want some help from the nurses. Consider the place of the Mental Capacity Act (MCA) 2005, which requires health professionals to decide whether patients' decisions are competently arrived at, or made through irrationality, incompetence and mental confusion. Revisit the NMC advice sheet on the MCA 2005 online at http://www.nmc-uk.org/Nurses-and-midwives/Advice-by-topic/A/Advice-Capacity-Act-2005/.

It is not impossible for a patient who has lost a lot of blood to be confused and so their decision may not be competently arrived at. In such circumstances the healthcare professional has a legal, professional and ethical duty to act in the patient's best interest. You should do nothing to hurt your patient (ethics of non-maleficence), whilst at the same time respecting patients' right to autonomy, justice, fairness, equity and confidentiality. It would of course be out of line, illegal and unethical to tell the patient's mother what she told you, without the patient's consent. You may, however, want to persuade the patient to reconsider whether she wishes to share her problem with her mum, but that will be her decision.

Hopefully, from dealing with the issues above in relation to the scenario, you can see that taking the correct ethical, professional and even legal decisions in caring is not a simple task. It can be difficult and contentious, even proving a moral, legal and professional dilemma at times. Two critical points I believe you need to remember are your obligation to give the patient the best care possible, yet at the same time respecting her right to confidentiality, although there are times when confidentiality may not be seen as absolute. You are advised to read Chapter 6 in this book on confidentiality. Be sure to read the NMC guidelines on confidentiality at http://www.nmc-uk.org. In the case of *R v Department of Health ex p Source Information Ltd* [2000] 1 All ER 786, the Court of Appeal suggested that there is breach of confidence only if the breach affects the conscience of the person making the disclosure. Passing on essential client information to the team who have a need to know, in order to act in the patient's best interest, is not breaking confidence, because it is reasonable to expect that you have the patient's approval to pass on information affecting his/her care to the team. However, such approval must not be assumed; the patient must be told this right from the start, at the point of admission.

Writer's personal reflection

I recall when I was a third-year general (adult) nursing student an 18-year-old female patient informed me she had something to tell me. She proceeded to ask me to promise her that if she told me a 'secret' I would not tell anyone else. I was at that stage of my training alert and informed not to make any such promise, and told her so. That move on my part turned out to be particularly prudent, as the situation she told me was precisely the one in the scenario above, except the fact that the Mr Jarrett situation was not part of the real story. (I added the Mr Jarrett incident to extend the real-life case. Box 2.8 asks you to reflect on its implications.) I recall informing the patient that I could not make her a promise not to pass important information affecting her care to the senior staff, especially if I considered that failure on my part to pass the information to the team was likely to put her or any third party at risk.

How did I handle the real situation?

In that real event, I recall being very pleasant, very calm and caring, in telling the patient that she should think carefully about what she was about to tell me, as I might not be in a position to keep it secret if, for example, it would have any implications for her care, or that of other patients. I had further explained that I was professionally obliged to make sure she received the best care possible and that if what she was about to tell me seemed likely to pose a risk to her or a third party I would be obliged to pass the information to a senior member of staff in the hope that help could be found and impending risks averted. Because I had made no promise to keep secret what the patient was about to tell me, I was able to

---

BOX 2.8 Student portfolio reflection exercise 2.3

Regarding sister and staff nurse's careless revelation about Mr Jarrett's HIV diagnosis and advice to the staff not to touch him, use your portfolio to reflect on the issues involved and how you would handle them. In doing so, assess the extent to which this aspect of the scenario could have jeopardised nursing actions in relation to the first part of the scenario. Be sure to make your legal awareness, ethical principles, moral values, professional standards and knowledge of HIV causation and mode of transmission guide your reflections.

inform the ward sister what the patient had told me, although I had done so only after I had informed the patient of the need to let me share the information with a senior member of the nursing team and she had agreed. I was glad I passed the information to the sister, who acted immediately by getting a doctor to see the patient. The doctor examined the patient, with sister present, and concluded that the patient had lost a considerable amount of blood, was in a state of shock and had also started to develop septicaemia (severe blood poisoning). She was taken to the operating theatre as an emergency and operated on for a ruptured left fallopian tube. She had such a severe infection that she was administered intravenous antibiotics and fluids for nearly one week after her surgery. Thank God, her life was spared, even though she had lost one of her fallopian tubes. The patient did thank me for the action I had taken. On reflection, I was able to achieve a number of critical objectives. (1) I had maintained the patient's confidence in me and the integrity of our professional relationship, by actually persuading her to let me get her the help she needed, thereby not breaching her confidence. (2) I was able to get the patient the care she needed, thus averting the real risk of her dying from the haemorrhage or the septicaemia. (3) I had averted any possible risk of my being disciplined for failing to act professionally – competently, sensitively and caringly. (4) I had used my knowledge of professional standards, crucial ethical principles, moral values and safe legal principles relating to caring to guide my decision making.

Summary and conclusion

This chapter has helped you to understand the notions of *professional responsibility* and *accountability,* linked to code of conduct standards of behaviour and practice set out by the NMC. Links have been made between notions of professional, ethical, legal responsibility and accountability in relation to the role and responsibility of the new student nurse. Hopefully you are now starting to realise that the moral values and beliefs you brought to nursing are critical and can impact on nursing practice. The chapter also attempted to get you to think about critical legal, code of conduct and ethical principles within given scenarios and case law, using analysis of these issues and principles to start guiding your nursing decision making and in building your ethics, law and professional standards portfolio. In taking this approach you have been introduced to a number of legal and ethical concepts and principles, which the next few chapters will help you to develop. Chapter 4 in particular, on the English legal system, will help you put your legal learning into context.

3   Nurses and the law

Objectives of this chapter

After reading this chapter you should be able to:

*   link learning from this chapter to the NMC standard for pre-registration nursing education competency that requires nurses to 'Act with professionalism and integrity and work within agreed professional, ethical and legal frameworks and processes to maintain and improve standards';
*   define the concept 'law' and the principle of legal 'precedent';
*   relate law to the NMC Code and standards of nursing practice;
*   appreciate some of the things that may go wrong when nurses practise in disregard of proper legal and professional standards;
*   describe the benefits of legal awareness to student and qualified nurses.

Introduction

In its 2010 *Standards for Pre-registration Nursing Education* the NMC states (at page 5) that the public must be confident that all nurses will 'Act with professionalism and integrity and work within agreed professional, ethical and legal frameworks and processes to maintain and improve standards' (NMC, 2010a: p. 5). Furthermore, on page 11 we note, 'The nurse practises within a statutory framework and code of ethics delivering nursing practice . . . based on research evidence and critical thinking.' The necessity for nurse to practise within the framework of law is a recurring theme in this standards document, whether the NMC is talking about adult, mental health, children's or learning disability nursing practice.

This chapter poses and answers the question: what is law? It contrasts ancient religious 'laws' such as the Biblical Ten Commandments with current-day binding legal rules, principles and precedents, and considers the place of moral values and law. It then asks you to identify types of law you have heard about. It examines briefly the positive instructional feature of law, and explains the principle of *precedent* in English law. It then examines how the NMC *standards for competence – professional values*, *communication and interpersonal skills*, *nursing practice and decision making* and *leadership, management and team working* – relate to the law. The chapter cites examples of how nurses and other health professionals, globally, have infringed the law and disregarded their professional responsibility, obligation and accountability, in the process hurting, even killing patients. Hopefully, by learning about some historical illegal and cruel behaviour from health professionals such as nurses and doctors, you will ensure your professional conduct is above board and in accord, rather than discord, with the law. You are then asked to reflect on a patient-focused scenario using your knowledge and understanding of law, ethics and moral values. The chapter has used an American law case to show that as a nurse you may find you owe a duty of care not only to your patient but to a third party as well. The chapter looks at how a nurse following proper legal and professional standards and competences can keep out of trouble. It then demonstrates that not only is the very existence and foundation of the NMC grounded in law but so are its competencies for nursing and midwifery practice. Finally, the chapter identifies NMC Competency Domains, in particular *Domain 1: Professional values*, within all its branches of nursing – *general (adult) nursing, learning disability, mental health* and *children's nursing* – to see how they may offer guidance to areas of law that pre-registration nursing students need to focus on. This is considered a pragmatic prelude to Chapter 4, which focuses on the English legal system, primarily in terms of types and sources of law and the court system.

What is law (Box 3.1)?

I recall as a child playing in my school playfield and being told by my friends to stick to the 'law' of the game. As my friends' terms for playing the game were *not legally binding* on me, as a law would be, I would rather call the 'orders' that directed our games *non-binding* 'rules' rather than laws. Law may therefore be viewed as *imposed rules* that are *binding* on a population or community. That community has to follow those rules or suffer the *consequences* or *sanctions* linked to failure to follow the rules. In this sense law is an *authority* concept; a system of rules *enforced by legal principles* and *agencies* such as courts of law.

The Ten Commandments: are they laws?

Those of you who read the Bible will know that in the time of Moses a set of rules called the Ten Commandments were religious 'laws' for a particular community of people: *thou shalt not kill, commit adultery, envy thy neighbour* and so on. Today these norms are seen as sound social relationship values and rules, but, saving the act of 'killing', which is a common law offence for which we may go to jail, the law does not bind us to the values of not committing adultery or envying our neighbour. In other words it is not against the law to envy our neighbour; there are no legal sanctions for committing adultery. However, if, as the ex-nurses Beverley Allitt, Colin Norris and Benjamin Green or Dr Harold Shipman did, we kill our patients, we have committed a serious crime under *English common law*. We may even be immoral and sleep with our neighbours' or our friends' spouses or partners, but the law of England will not necessarily punish us for doing so. We may feel bad about engaging in these immoral acts because we have a conscience, but we have not broken the law.

I often ask first-year nursing students what values they come to university with that they use in their daily interactions. Often one gets responses such as to be kind, and considerate, caring, truthful to patients, honest, not judgemental, and so on. These are sound caring values or philosophical statements that are quite important in the nurse–patient relationship. We also use them to guide our social private life. However, you are, strictly, not *legally* bound by these caring values. You may be *morally* and *ethically* bound by them, but not legally. Law then is *rules with legal force*; law is a system of rules, enforced through certain institutions (police, courts, judges etc.), shaping society, politics and social order generally.

BOX 3.1 Student portfolio reflection exercise 3.1

In the law, ethics and professional issues section of your portfolio write down what you understand about the term 'law'. After doing this read what follows and see how near your answer is to my exposition.

Law prevents society from deteriorating into anarchy. The law decides rights, responsibilities and obligations and deals with complex issues such as equality and fairness. Law resolves conflicts between individuals, sometimes even prevents conflicts.

Types of law you may have heard about, even mentioned in your portfolio reflection

At a very simplistic level, *constitutional* law creates the framework for the creation of new law. *Contract* law regulates relationships between parties, binding parties to formal agreements that parties are bound by. *International law* regulates relationships between states. *Property law* regulates the transfer of property (*chattel*) between parties, for instance when you buy a house in return for which you hand over your money. *Administrative law* controls decisions of government agencies. But perhaps the two most important forms of law to the nurse and patient are the *criminal law* and the *civil law of tort*, which I will say more about below.

Instructional and positive legal rules

The law is usually more instructive and positive, telling you what to do, and what not to do. Examples of positive rules fitting the definition of law are:

*   Protect your patients' confidential data (data protection laws).
*   Do not discriminate on racial grounds or disability grounds (Race Relations Act; disability, equality legislation).
*   Girls under 16 (who are *'Gillick'* or *'Fraser' competent*) can have contraception advice without parental consent (*Gillick v West Norfolk and Wisbech AHA*), and may therefore also be able to agree to other forms of treatment without parental sanction.
*   Ensure that the standard of care given satisfies those founded on the *Bolam standards of care test* (as in the case of *Bolam v Friern HMC*).
*   You have a duty not to injure your patient by action or omission (*Donohue v Stevenson*).
*   Do not steal from your patient (a positive rule, breaking which is against the Theft Act of 1968).
*   Do not obtain consent for treatment and investigation from your patients without first providing them with the necessary information for informed decision (consent). If you did it would be a fraud; the consent you claimed to obtain legitimately would be ill-informed. Moreover, if you treat the patient without first gaining consent this constitutes trespass on the patient's person.
*   Do not abuse children or conceal abuse (Children Act 1989).
*   Do not touch a patient without first securing his/her consent (this is trespass in tort law, or criminal under the statute *Offences against the Person Act 1861*, e.g. actual bodily harm, offence under section 47, or wounding, sections 18 and 20).

Both the NMC Code and law are built upon normative or ethical rules, but those rules in themselves are not laws. Many of our ethical values pervade the law but the law does have agreed legal principles that we work to and must abide by.

Legal precedent

In the common (court- or judge-made) law of England we speak of the important principle of law called *precedent*: an *authority* derived from a legal case that has established a particular principle that binds future courts in making legal decisions where the material evidence (facts) of the later case are similar to those of the previous case.

In England, up to October 2009, the House of Lords was the UK's highest (domestic) appellate court, making decisions (precedents) binding the lower UK courts, such as the Court of Appeal, the High Court and subordinate courts below the High Court. However, since October 2009, the House of Lords acting as an appellate court has been reformed and replaced by the United Kingdom Supreme Court (rather like the American Supreme Court). Thus today the UK Supreme Court is the most senior domestic appellate judicial body in the UK. The judges who sit on this body are known as Justices of the Supreme Court. In your reading of landmark cases affecting nursing and healthcare standards generally, please look for landmark rulings either from the House of Lords before October 2009, or from the UK Supreme Court after October 2009.

In fact you will note that to date most seminal landmark cases having implications for standards in nursing and medical practice (e.g. *Bolam v Friern HMC*, *Gillick v Norfolk and Wisbech AHA* and *Donohue v Stevenson*) are rulings from the former House of Lords acting as the UK's highest appellate court. The House of Lords still functions today as a legislative body, working with the House of Commons to make new statute laws. However, its appellate function is now undertaken by the UK Supreme Court. However, it should be remembered that since Britain joined the European Economic Community (now the EU) in 1972 even the House of Lords (now the Supreme Court) is itself bound by rulings (precedents) of the European courts. For example, *Donohue v Stevenson* set out the principles underlying the bases on which a negligence case may be decided. For example, the patients must be able to show that:

- the nurse owes them a duty of care;
- the nurse breached that duty;
- the breach caused harm to the patient;
- the patient has evidence of that harm, for example it is obvious that the wrongful application of the splint caused the patient's pressure sore;
- the patient is therefore entitled to compensation.

Accountability in law and linking accountability to standards for competence

It is in every nurse's interest not just to understand what is meant by law but, in practice, to demonstrate real legal accountability in the context of caring. You must understand how the law can impact on and guide your nursing practice. Without legal understanding your practice as a student nurse and as a qualified nurse will fall short of legal expectations and standards. *Ensure you work within the framework of the law, as no one is above the law.* Those health professionals who operate as though they are above the law will soon feel the weight of the law. A criminal offence will be punished by the criminal law. A tort (a civil wrong) may find the offender being required to compensate his/her victim. UK nursing and medical history provides us with examples of health professionals who fell short of legal standards in healthcare practice; for example the infamous ex-nurse Beverley Allitt, who (in 1993) was convicted of killing four young children in her care and attempting to kill another three in Grantham, Lincolnshire, England. Nursing is not the only health profession with law breakers. Dr Harold Shipman, a GP, is perhaps the best-known serial killer in England. On 31 January 2000 he was found guilty of murdering 15 of his patients, jailed for life on the recommendation he never be released. He committed suicide in jail. Having pointing out these two negative examples, it is important for student and qualified nurses to know that the law is there to protect them as well as their patients. If you follow legal guidelines your practice should be sound and your career long. Break the law and you could be removed from the nursing register and probably jailed; maybe in the reverse order!

NMC code, standards and legal position

Nursing practice is informed by various philosophical and moral values such as honesty, kindness to your fellow humans, compassion and caring; in particular, UK professional regulation of nursing by the NMC is informed by the Council's *Code: Standards of Conduct, Performance and Ethics for Nurses and Midwives* (NMC, 2008a), and specified *standards for competent nursing practice*. These principles are themselves informed by sound philosophical values. The NMC's very foundation and existence is founded on law, in the sense that it was set up by a legal Order, the *Nursing and Midwifery Order, 2001*, so that its code of conduct and standards for practice have *legal force* behind them. The NMC is legally accountable to Parliament for standards of nurse training and practice. It has an obligatory (legal) duty to protect the public. It makes sense therefore to remind you, the student nurse (and indeed all registered autonomous practitioners), of some of the key standards for competence laid down by the NMC, as a prerequisite to helping you understand law relating to these standards.

In the UK professional standards in nursing education and practice must respect and operate within the UK legal framework. Similarly when you qualify, if you decide to work abroad, you must abide by the law of the country you are practising in. In its *Standards for Pre-registration Nursing Education* policy document, the NMC (2010a) sets out a number of *standards for competence*:

*   professional values;
*   communication and interpersonal skills;
*   nursing practice and decision making;
*   leadership, management and team working.

Of the above standards, it might be immediately apparent that the first, third and fourth offers direct scope for application of law, as there are clear instances where law influences *professional values*, *standards of nursing decision making and practice*, *management*, *leadership* and *team working*. For instance, the NMC (2008a) Code says 'make the care of people your first concern, treating them as individuals', a fundamental professional value. Additionally, patients have rights to *confidentiality*, *privacy*, *dignity*, *not to be discriminated against*, *not to have staff cross their sexual boundaries*, to *safe care and limited exposure to risks*, and *not to be treated with partiality and disrespect*.

Correspondingly, *human rights law* tells us that as individuals we have individual rights, such as to *life*, *privacy*, *freedom from discrimination*, *not to be enslaved or treated inhumanely or degradingly*, to *freedom of thought* and *free speech*, *to be a partner in contributing to nursing decision making regarding individual care*, *to have property brought with us to hospital protected, put into safe keeping or sent home in line with hospital policy*, as the case might be, *not to be punished by nursing staff*, and *not to be detained against our will unless under a legal order*, such as the Mental Health Act. Most of the above rights are enshrined in the Human Rights Act 1998. Moreover, patients have a right not to have their valuables stolen by nurses or others. If as a student you steal a patient's property you have committed a crime: theft, an offence against the Theft Act 1968.

How departing from nursing standards has hurt or killed patients: implications

As stated above, patients have a right not to be hurt or murdered by anyone, least of all by nurses and doctors who have a legal, professional and ethical duty of care not to harm their patients. It is a pity that the infamous (Dr) Harold Shipman and (ex-nurse) Beverley Allitt and other health professionals who have in the past murdered patients did not work to the obligation of their professional body to deliver care to the highest standard. It is equally a pity these individuals infringed the law to their own cost and above all their patients'.

Some details about professionals mentioned earlier who have killed patients

Dr Shipman, a GP, is probably the most prolific English serial killer, having 218 murders positively attributed to him, although it is thought that he probably killed many more. In January 2000 a UK court found Shipman guilty of murdering 15 of his patients. He was committed to prison for life, but killed himself by hanging in January 2004 (BBC News, 13 January 2004). In its sixth report the Shipman Inquiry (2002) concluded that 'Shipman killed about 250 patients between 1971 and 1998'. Of these 218 were 'positively' ascribed to him (*The Shipman Inquiry*: http://www.the-shipman-inquiry.org.uk/6r_page.asp?ID=3401). About 80 per cent of his victims were women. From various accounts the conclusion may be drawn that Dr Shipman was a callous, evil and calculating murderer. A coroner, John Pollard, described him as one who 'simply enjoyed viewing the process of dying and enjoyed the feeling of control over life and death, literally over life and death' (BBC News, 13 January 2004). It seems Dr Shipman killed most of his patients by injecting them with the drug diamorphine, a powerful opiate.

Beverley Allitt was a state-enrolled nurse, born 4 October 1968. Working as a nurse on a paediatric ward at Grantham and Kesteven Hospital, between February 1991 and April 1991 she murdered four children and injured nine others. She murdered her victims by injecting them with potassium chloride, which caused their hearts to stop. In some cases she killed by injecting her victims with insulin. In 1993 she was sentenced to life imprisonment at Nottingham Crown Court.

Whatever the motive of Allitt and Shipman, there can be no doubt that they demonstrated utter disregard for the sanctity of human life. They departed from proper moral standards and from the ethics of beneficence and justice; most of all from a proper humanitarian code of behaviour, totally disregarding their professional code of conduct to preserve life, not take it. They engaged in evil practices against the very helpless and vulnerable patients they were supposed to protect and care for. As a student you are obliged to report to proper authority if you suspect any health professional is abusing and harming patients in any way.

Nurses as a heterogeneous group

Nurses are not a homogeneous group of people. We come from all walks of life, each with our own idiosyncratic view of life, each with our own moral values, some good, some bad, some acceptable, some unacceptable to the nursing profession. However, one of the objectives of professional training is to ensure that all those who enter nurse training are properly trained and have developed caring, moral views and attitudes and have developed the necessary professional competencies to meet the needs of patients in a very caring and human way. Sadly, some rotten apples get through the admission gate or the training has failed to make the raw product into a caring professional nurse. Alternatively, somewhere along the line some caring people have become deranged and evil for any number of reasons. For these reasons, therefore, we as professional nurses must be on the alert for people who are ready to subjugate proper professional standards, replacing them with evil, cruel intentions and practices that harm patients.

Hurting your patient *deliberately* is a *crime* that will attract the appropriate punishment under the criminal law. If you feel you have a pathological tendency to hurt people, then nursing is not for you; get out and seek professional help. I have used the word 'deliberately' since a patient could be hurt or could even die at the hands of a careless (negligent) health professional, without that professional deliberately setting out to hurt or kill the patient. If our careless (negligent) practice leads unwittingly to the patient's injury this is more likely a case for the *civil court* (see below). Here the patient would be seeking compensation for his/her injury. If the carelessness leads to the patient's death, this is not the same as *(intentional) murder*. It is more likely the perpetrator would be charged with the lesser crime of *manslaughter* (Box 3.2).

If we kill someone deliberately we commit a *common law offence* of *murder*, punishable by imprisonment. Law gives patients/clients the right not to be hurt by health professionals. We should not sexually touch or molest our patients. We should not inflict any form of physical or emotional hurt on patients.

Global incidences of nurses hurting and killing patients: implications?

There are numerable global cases where health professionals such as nurses have deliberately ignored proper professional and legal standards and hurt, even killed, their patients, thus facing the common law offence of murder. For example, in the USA a nurse's aide, Mr Landon, murdered an elderly patient with an overdose of the drug lidocaine (*Hargreve v Landon*, 584 F. Supp. 302 [E.D. Va. 1984]). A registered nurse, Mr Angelo, was found guilty of murdering two patients by injecting them with the drug Pavulon. In the case of *Havrum v United States* 204 F.3d 815 (8th Cir. 2000) the court held that Nurse Williams had actually killed the *plaintiff's relative* (the *plaintiff* being the party bringing the action).

In the UK we have many instances of nurses being found guilty of either hurting or murdering their patients. Nurse Julia Levitt unlawfully killed a cancer patient (Kenneth Heaton, 79) by injecting him with an unauthorised sedative. It was reported that she stated that she gave the drug to help the patient to 'have a good night' (BBC News, 8 March 2006). The BBC News (18 April 2006) and *The Times* (15 February 2006) also reported the case of nurse Benjamin Green, 25, who was found guilty of killing two of his patients and of causing grievous bodily harm to 15 others, at Horton General Hospital, Oxfordshire. He injected the patients with unauthorised drugs, apparently to make himself the 'centre of attention', the BBC claimed.

Another infamous murder by a nurse is that of nurse Colin Norris, who was labelled 'angel of death' and jailed for life, with the court's recommendation to serve a minimum

---

BOX 3.2 The case of Dr Adomako

An anaesthetist, Dr Adomako (*R v Adomako* [1995] 1 AC 171; [1994] 3 All ER 79), was tried in the criminal court and convicted of *manslaughter*, when through his *gross negligence* he allowed a patient to die on the operating theatre table. He had failed to notice that the patient's life-saving endotracheal tube (connected to his oxygen supply) had become disconnected.

of 30 years, for murdering four elderly women patients (*Daily Telegraph*, 4 March 2008). Apparently, his motive was hate of elderly patients and 'arrogance'. So arrogant he was that he would predict which patient on his shift of duty would die next and when. Norris was reported to have made disparaging comments to patients such as 'I hope you suffer' and 'rot in hell' (*Daily Record*, 4 March 2008). This was worrying from every angle and from the perspective of any caring person – most of all from the perspective of any health professional.

From the perspective of a psychologist, Mr Norris's utterances were chilling and predictive. They should have raised suspicion. Nurses are not God and so cannot really accurately predict patients' time of death the way Colin Norris did. If you are strongly suspicious of the behaviour of any of your professional colleagues, in the sense that you feel (s)he is hurting, or could hurt, patients, you are legally and professional bound to report it to the authorities, for example your mentor, your tutor, your practice placement manager or someone higher up in the Trust you are working for. It is better to be cautious than to be sorry, after procrastinating and then coming on duty to discover that the colleague you had strongly suspected of hurting patients has actually killed one of them. (Consider student portfolio reflection exercise 3.2 in Box 3.3.) The NMC website even gives guidance to nurses on how they may

---

BOX 3.3 Student portfolio reflection exercise 3.2

You are working on the late shift with the ward manager and a fellow second-year student nurse. A poorly 82-year-old female patient, in a semi-conscious state, is being cared for in a side room off the main ward. The patient is very ill and the medical staff believe she could die within days. The patient is not for resuscitation. Nevertheless, you have been instructed to provide the patient with all basic nursing care, including maintaining her intravenous (IV) fluids intake. You notice that every time you leave the side room and return the patient's IV is turned off. You know for a fact that no other person but you and your fellow student nurse have been attending the patient, who is too ill to turn off the IV herself. On the last occasion you noticed the IV turned off, you restarted it. One hour later following your colleague's visit to the room, you noticed that the IV is off again. You asked sister and your colleague if they had switched off the IV and both said no. You said nothing else, but calmly went to the room and switched it on again. One hour later you asked your colleague if she had checked the patient in the last forty-five minutes. She said she did. You deliberately walked past the room to go to the loo just to observe if the IV was still flowing; it was not, so you restarted it. However, when the night staff arrived the ward manager told you and your fellow student you could both go home. You left the ward first, but hesitated outside the ward door. You noticed that on her way out the ward your colleague went into the side ward and quickly came out again. She caught up with you but then went her own way. You doubled back, peeked into the side ward and the patient's IV was turned off. The night staff are still on the main ward. You are sure the patient has not interfered with the IV. You strongly suspect, in fact you feel 99 per cent certain, your colleague is deliberately turning off the patient's IV. You also recall how two days ago she had remarked, 'I don't like elderly patients'; 'they take up too much time and are a waste of NHS resources'. You also recall how she had said jokingly, 'My boyfriend is cheating on me, and if I knew I would get away with it I would do away with him.' Consider how you would deal with both situations. Jot your thoughts down in the Nursing Practice and Decision Making section of your portfolio. Provide justification for your actions.

whistle-blow if they suspect or have evidence of any form of patient cruelty and abuse. See further information on whistle blowing below.

The answer to the issues in Box 3.3 will become clear as you read on and understand more about the law. You must also reflect on relevant professional guidelines within your nursing code of conduct. Reflect too on your own moral values and key ethical principles you have read up on, such as Beauchamp and Childress's (2008) *ethical principles*:

* beneficence;
* non-maleficence;
* autonomy;
* justice.

Always remember:

* You owe your *patients* a duty of care to provide the best-quality care, not to harm them or allow anyone else to do so.
* There are circumstances in which you may even owe a legal duty of care to a *third party*.
* Lord Atkin's powerful statement in the *Donoghue v Stevenson* case: 'Take reasonable care to avoid acts and omissions which you can reasonably foresee . . . likely to injure your neighbour'.

In a well-known American case (*Tarasoff v Regents of the University of California* [1976]) it was held by the courts that a positive legal duty can be owed by a health professional to a third party. In this case the harm that was done to a third party was considered by the court to have outweighed the need for confidentiality. Clearly, in the scenario above you do not owe a duty of confidentiality to your colleague. However, you owe your patient a duty to stop her coming to harm. If your suspicion is so strong, why have you failed to report the situation to the ward manager? You have a responsibility and an obligation to protect your patient, thereby helping the NMC with its legal obligation to protect the public. Even though you are a student you still have a professional duty to help uphold this legal obligation. It is also a moral and ethical one. You have mentors and tutors you can share your concerns with. Moreover, *whistle blowing* is encouraged by the NMC. Where nurses suspect patient abuse, or failure on the part of those informed about it to tackle it, they are within their rights, as well as having a professional, moral, legal and ethical obligation, to blow the whistle on it. In a Web press release on 5 November 2009, Caroline Williams, the NMC lead on whistle blowing policy development, said:

> Nurses and midwives have a code of conduct they must follow. Within that code they have a duty to manage risk which could mean speaking out against a colleague. As nurses and midwives work as part of a multidisciplinary team they will recognise the difficulty they may sometimes face if they have a concern about a colleague's actions or behaviour or the environment of care.
>
> Our goal is to provide nurses and midwives with clear information about the steps they should be taking when raising or escalating a concern while acting within that code.
>
> (http://www.nmc-uk.org/Press-and-media/News-archive/
> Nurses-and-midwives-to-receive-whistleblowing-guidance/)

The NMC has since consulted on and developed whistle-blowing policy guidelines for nurses and midwives. Please visit the NMC website at http://www.nmc-uk.org/publications or write to the Council for a copy of the policy document *Raising and Escalating Concerns: Guidance for Nurses and Midwives*, published in November 2010.

With respect to the American case I raised above, yes, healthcare professionals have been shown to owe a duty of care to a third party. I am not saying here that, with respect to the scenario case, you should become over suspicious about what your colleague had told you days before about her cheating boyfriend. However, by reflecting on the statement she had made to you days before about her boyfriend, and the fact that you now have a very strong suspicion that she is tampering with the patient care (IV fluid administration), you should be alerted to the necessity to speak to the ward manager about your concerns for the patient in the side room. It is better to be cautious than to be sorry. You have more grounds of certainty your colleague is turning off the patient's IV fluids than doubt that she is not. Act on your strong feelings. Speak to the ward manager or some other person in authority. Do not miss an opportunity that could save your patient's life. This scenario presents you with the opportunity to use a practical reflective model such as Gibbs's (1988) to reflect on the situation you are observing in the scenario above and to bring it to the attention of an authority figure in the Trust or your university.

In an American case, *Tarasoff v Regents of the University of California* (1976) 551 P(2d)334, the Supreme Court of California held that a mental health professional owed a duty of care not only to his/her patient, but also to an identifiable individual who was specifically being threatened by the patient.

This US decision is proving to be influencing jurisprudence outside the USA as well. Some legal authorities believe that it is unlikely an English court would have made the same decision as the California court. The fact, however, that the NMC (2008a) advises you to 'disclose information if you believe someone may be at risk of harm, in line with the law of the country in which you are practising' suggests that, if for example one of your patients tells you he will go out and murder a known third party and you believe this, then you should act, for example report it to a senior authority at work who may report it to the police. Now examine where you think your decision would lie in respect to the situation where you recalled your student nurse colleague telling you she would probably kill her cheating lover if she thought she would get away with it. What is your answer and why? Reflect on how you are now feeling about that situation.

A fuller version of the Tarasoff case

This case is important because the legal principles on which it was decided have at least persuasive influence on the UK jurisprudence. This was a case in which a male graduate student (Poddar, of Indian origin) at University of California at Berkeley received a 1968 New Year's Eve kiss from a fellow student, Tatiana Tarasoff. He interpreted this to mean love, a view not shared by Tarasoff; she conveyed this to Poddar. Resentment built up in Poddar, who started to stalk Tarasoff in revenge. Poddar underwent severe emotional crisis, and became depressed and weepy, with disjointed speech, neglecting his health, study and appearance. He had occasional meetings with Tarasoff but no love was on the horizon. Poddar confided his intention to kill Tarasoff to his psychologist, Dr Moore (at UC Berkeley Memorial Hospital). On Dr Moore's recommendation the campus police detained Poddar as a dangerous person, suffering from paranoid schizophrenia; he was committed to hospital. By now Tarasoff was abroad. Poddar was detained at first but released shortly after, as he presented as rational. He stopped seeing his psychologists. Neither Tarasoff (now back in the USA) nor her parents received any notice of the threat (doctor–patient confidential privilege). On 27 October 1969 Poddar made good the threat he had confided to the doctors, stabbing Tarasoff fatally. In a criminal case Poddar was found guilty of second-degree murder. He appealed against the conviction, which was overturned on the grounds that the jury was not properly informed. He was released on the condition that he left the USA and returned to his country, India. Tarasoff's parents sued the doctors and various other employees of UC Berkeley. The Supreme Court of California held that health professionals owe a duty not only to the patient but to a known party that the patient has threatened to harm.

In the NMC Code, under 'Advice and confidentiality' the NMC requires you to:

- disclose information if you believe someone is at risk of harm;
- collaborate positively with those in your care, patients/clients and colleagues you work with;
- not collude and conspire in things that are negative and could harm your patient;
- listen to your patients/clients and respond to their concerns.

Legal and professional standards of care to keep us out of trouble

The NMC Code tells us to provide a *high standard of care at all times*. Correspondingly, case law such as *Donovan v Stevenson* (1932) (the 'ginger beer and dead snail case') tells us that we have an obligatory, professional, legal 'neighbour' relationship with our patients: persons who are so closely and directly affected by (our) acts or omissions that we ought reasonably to always think about them (have them in 'contemplation') when we are planning their care or doing things with or for them. In other words we should always seek to provide them with the highest standard of care. If we fail to do this we could be called to account by negligence law. Thus we should do nothing to undermine established and obligatory standards of care.

As we have seen in a preceding chapter, the case law of *Bolam v Friern Barnet Hospital Management Committee* [1957] tells us that our standard of patient care must at least be equivalent to, not lower than, that prescribed or recommended by a competent and *responsible, reasonable and respectable* body of nursing opinion. That standard is set by the NMC, and backed up by strong research evidence. Moreover, as the *Bolitho* case has shown, the body of expert nursing opinion informing standards must flow logically and reasonably from the circumstances of the patient's situation and available *evidence*, so that *risks* can be weighed up, and the courses with least risk and danger to the patient followed.

Rolf, Jasper and Freshwater (2011) have made the case for 'reflective evidence' to be used to support 'research' evidence in informing caring standards. Such reflective knowledge, they argue, is derived from and marked by 'dispassionate and objective' observation. It is also derived from a critical review and analysis of what has happened, how it happened, how things could have been different if alternative approaches had been followed, and what needs to be followed in the future. The resultant reflective knowledge is seen as strong and valid evidence that can be used to support 'research' evidence that informs acceptable practice standards.

Law and interpersonal and communication skills

Looking above at the NMC's standard defined as 'communication and interpersonal skills', you may be thinking, just what could this possibly have to do with the law? There are many ways in which the law may inform *nurse–patient communications and interpersonal relationships*. For example, both the NMC Code and the law require nurses to respect patients' *autonomy*, informing them appropriately and gaining their *informed consent before treating them*. Be *truthful* when called to court to give evidence under oath, or risk perjuring yourself. Tell patients the *truth as a prelude* to gaining consent to treatment, or you obtain consent *fraudulently* and could be liable for *breach of your duty to inform*. You could also be liable for trespassing on the patient's person or for a criminal assault if you touch and treat patients without first informing them truthfully of the purpose of your touch and gaining their consent. Protect patient's confidential information and do not breach data protection legislation.

Evidence that good interpersonal communication reduces law suits

What is more, research has shown that health professionals who are able to effect high quality communications, by having and exercising excellent interpersonal skills, are able to foster effective nurse–patient relationships that are characterised by respectful, caring, honest and open caring attitudes, respect for cultural diversity, equity, fairness and sensitivity – all of which are capable of reducing the number of law suits brought by patients against healthcare staff (JCAHO, 2005; Marquis and Huston, 2008). Moreover, Smith (2005) claims that failed management and leadership communications styles increase patients' malpractice claims against healthcare professionals. Good management communications also reduce the number of legal tribunals dealing with healthcare workers' claims of unfair treatment by healthcare managers.

The NMC and the European Union (EU) Directive 2005/36/EC

The law of the EU lies at the root of the NMC's standards for pre-registration nursing and practice. The NMC points out that in setting standards for pre-registration nursing education and practice it operates within the European Union (EU) Directive 2005/36/EC of the European Parliament and the Council, *Recognition of professional qualifications*. Essentially, these (legal) Directives set out specific requirements for training general (adult) nurses in the EU, for example requirements on length of training, content, theory/practice ratio, nature of practice learning, range of experience, pre-requisite educational standards and specific outcomes for general nursing students. If you are undertaking the adult nursing branch and wish to do midwifery afterwards, on a short course route, non-direct entry midwifery, you need to have satisfied the EU requirements in your pre-registration adult training. So these Directives have more applications than one. As we shall see in other chapters of this book, law, both case law and statutes, pervades nursing and sets the legal framework within which sound nursing must be practised.

NMC competency domains and law

Whether you are aspiring to become a nurse in *general (adult)*, *learning disability*, *mental health* or *children's* nursing, the NMC (2010a, p. 13), states, within *Domain 1: Professional values*, that certain key competences must be achieved. Below I have picked out some of those that I believe the law can help the nurse to achieve:

* professionalism and integrity, and ability to work within recognised professional, ethical and legal frameworks;

- understanding and applying current legislation to all service users, paying particular attention to the protection of vulnerable people; for example the elderly, children, people with learning disability;
- respect for individual choices and diversity, being able to challenge inequality, discrimination and exclusion;
- partnership working, with service users, carers, others;
- professional accountable and responsibility;
- independent practice and recognition of professional limitation;
- respect for individual rights, confidentiality; safe record keeping in accordance with the law;
- capacity to share personal information with others when interests of safety and protection override confidentiality;
- appreciation of evidence to inform practice.

Additionally mental health nurses must have an in-depth understanding of mental health legislation.

I picked out the above as they offer the opportunity to use law to inform them.

Chapter summary and conclusion

The chapter first focused on the NMC competency requirement that nurses 'Act with professionalism and integrity and work within agreed professional, ethical and legal frameworks and processes to maintain and improve standards'. To do this it defined the concept of law and legal precedent and examined how law and legal standards are related to key NMC competency domains centred on 'professional values, communication and interpersonal skills'. The chapter cited relationships between ancient biblical laws and moral codes of conduct and law as we know it today, pointing out key instrumental and positive legal rules that nurses must abide by in order to give care within sound legal framework. We examined the notion of accountability under law, linking this to accountability in nursing, especially under the NMC (2008a) Code. The *Tarasoff* case also demonstrates that health care professionals may have a positive legal duty to protect third parties. Cases and instances were cited in which nurses and other health professionals of the past have failed to be properly accountable and responsible; thus they have deliberately hurt, even killed, their patients. We focused on a patient scenario that enables you to examine the possibility that not all those who have come into nursing have good intentions towards their patients. Moreover, you may be the nurse who discovers a colleague's ill intentions towards his/her patient. The scenario gave you a change to examine your professional obligation to protect your patient, working within the framework of sound ethics and law to do so. We concluded that nurses and other health professionals who work within the law and sound ethical principles are unlikely to go off the rails, forgetting their professional objective, and as a consequence hurting, even killing patients.

4   Introduction to the English legal system

Given that the previous chapters have exposed you to a 'friendly' and 'applied' understanding of law, its relationship to ethics, moral values and the NMC Code, and standards of professional education and practice in respect to patient care, let us now focus on what I consider to be the 'drier' notions of law. It is important for you to have an overview of the English legal system, including the courts, and how it could affect you and your practice as a student nurse and later as a registered practitioner.

Objectives of this chapter

After reading this chapter you should be able to:

- distinguish between different types and sources of law;
- explain the difference between statute and common law, primary and secondary legislation, civil and criminal law, and private and public law;
- explain the relationship between UK domestic law and European Community law;
- describe how a Bill becomes an Act of Parliament, providing examples that have implications for nursing practice;
- define 'crime', and use examples to illustrate how nurses and other health professionals have committed crimes against their patients;
- talk confidently about possible defences to crime;
- demonstrate understanding of the court system, and say how it may impact on nurses and nursing;
- describe how contract law may relate to you as a person and a nurse;
- use your developing professional portfolio to extend your legal knowledge and understanding.

There are three major and primary sources of law: legislative or statute law; common law; and European Union and human rights law.

Legislative or statute law

This is law made by Parliament: the House of Commons and the House of Lords, working together. It is 'legislative' because the two Houses of Parliament are legislative bodies that enact statutory law. *Legislative* law is *written law*. For a written piece of UK legislation to become an *Act of Parliament* it must receive *Royal Assent* (the Monarch's signature).

Reflective question

In the law section of your portfolio write the names of all the statutes/Acts of Parliament you have heard of; especially ones having influences on your role as a nurse.

Examples of legislative or statute law that you have probably already heard of are:

- The Disability Discrimination Act (DDA) 1995, which legislates against you discriminating against those of your patients with a disability.
- The Equality Act 2010, which has replaced most of the DDA. However the *disability equality duty* in the DDA still applies. The Equality Act aims to protect disabled people from discrimination and provides rights in areas of employment, education, access to goods, services, transport and so on; it also clearly defines 'disability'.
- The Human Rights Act 1998, which you have heard something about in earlier chapters and which we will return to in later chapters. Basically this Act grants us specific rights, from the right to life through to other fundamental rights such as freedom from discrimination and degrading treatment, right to be first tried before punished and so on.

Other examples of statute law you may have heard about and which will affect your practice include:

- the Mental Health Act 1983, which creates the conditions under which people may be detained in mental health facilities for observation and/or treatment (read Chapter 15);
- the Mental Capacity Act 2005, which is dealt with substantially later in this book;
- the Health and Safety at Work Act 1974;
- the Race Relations Act 1976 (Amended 2000);
- the Abortion Act 1967;
- the Data Protection Act, 1998;
- the National Health Service and Community Care Act 1990;
- the Access to Medical Report Act 1988;

All of these as you will see have implications for your role as a nurse. Please go on to complete the exercise in Box 4.1.

Secondary, delegated or subordinate legislation

Whereas primary legislation, Acts of Parliament, gives rise to Public Acts and Local or Private Acts, secondary (delegated or subordinate) legislation comprises things such as *Statutory Instruments* (SIs), which are a form of subordinate legislation made by or under powers granted to Ministers, Her Majesty in Council, a National Assembly such as the

---

BOX 4.1 Student portfolio reflection exercise 4.1

In an appropriate section of your portfolio write down all the other statute law you have heard about and which you think may influence your education and practice as a nurse. Then choose any three statutes and list the ways in which you think they influence your training, education and practice.

one in Wales, Northern Ireland or Scotland, or other bodies such as Local Authorities and public corporations. The statute granting delegated power is the *Statutory Instruments Act 1946*. These instruments allow smooth running of the parent Act they arise from. SIs must therefore be 'inside' the scope of those parent Acts, or they are 'faulty' and worthless in enabling the legislative changes they seek. The NMC itself was set up by a Statutory Order 2001 (SI 2002/253), which came into effect on 1 April 2002, and has since been modified many times since, for example by the European Qualifications (Health and Social Care Professions) Regulations 2007 and the Nursing and Midwifery (Amendment) Order 2008 (SI 2008/1485). These orders allow the NMC to make the necessary amendments to its structural and operations framework in order to carry out its work, under the principal order (the Nursing and Midwifery Order, 2001), which itself is derived from the parent Act, the Health Act 1999.

Parliament is constantly making new laws; although it is not possible to keep up with all the changes, it is necessary to try and keep up to date with those new or amended statutes having implications for your healthcare practice. For example in 2007 we saw a new Mental Health Act (MHA) 2007 (the 2007 Act) that amends the 1983 MHA, the Mental Capacity Act 2005 (MCA) and the Domestic, Crime and Victims Act, 2004. As mentioned above, the Equality Act (2010) has made many amendments to the Disability Discrimination Act 1995 whilst maintaining the *Disability Equality Duty* in the DDA.

Common law

The English common law is derived from judicial decisions in cases tried in the courts by judges. Hence the alternative term 'judge-made law' is sometimes used. Given that England has existed for a very, very long time, and has been inhabited by different peoples, such as the Britons, Romans, Saxons and Danes, its common law is very old and historically reflects the lifestyles of these peoples. It has evolved, reflecting the ways these people made decisions about how their societies lived and how they regulated social order and human interactions, how they settled disputes and maintained law and order. The common law still does this for us today. It is not written down as statutes are, or as say the US (written) Constitution is. The common law operates by a system known as *precedent*. Some court decisions are more important than others. This sets up a hierarchy known as '*legal* precedent'. In weighing up the material evidence of a case and applying legal rules and principles to it, in order to arrive at a legal decision, a court (judges) might follow the decision of an earlier court; this is called *precedent*.

Binding decisions

The UK Supreme Court (previously the House of Lords acting as an appellate court) is the highest UK court. Its legal rulings must be followed by all other English courts. Thus we say that decisions made by the UK Supreme Court are *binding* on all other English courts. The Supreme Court can change its earlier decision if necessary.

English courts and rulings in the European Court of Justice

As Britain is a member of the European Union, British Courts are subject to relevant *precedents* of the *European Court of Justice* (ECJ) at Strasbourg.

Please carry out exercise 4.2 in Box 4.2 before continuing. Hopefully you will have recalled the names of land mark cases such as the following.

BOX 4.2 Student portfolio reflection exercise 4.2

In your portfolio write down the names of any two UK common law cases you have heard of and say what you think the important precedents in those cases are. A few of these cases were indentified in earlier chapters.

Donoghue v Stevenson [1932] AC 562 (the 'ginger beer–snail' case)

See the section on negligence in Chapter 7. You will recall that this was the *common law* appeal case, decided by the House of Lords, in which Lord Atkin said:

> You must take reasonable care to avoid acts or omissions which you can reasonably foresee would be likely to injure your neighbour. Who then in law is my neighbour? [Answer] . . . persons who are so closely and directly affected by my act that I ought reasonably to have them in contemplation as being so affected when I am directing my mind to the acts or omissions which are called into question.

The case underlines the key principles and cornerstones that make up English negligence law today. In summary, on Sunday 26 August 1928, Mrs Donoghue, neé M'Alistair, went to a Paisley cafe with a friend who bought her a tumbler of ice-cream, over which the cafe owner poured a quantity of ginger beer from an opaque bottle. She drank from the tumbler. When her friend topped her up the remains of a partially decomposed snail dropped out of the bottle. Donoghue later complained of stomach ache and her doctor diagnosed gastro-enteritis and severe shock. She brought an action against the manufacturers of the drink, claiming £500 as damages for the injuries suffered from drinking the ginger beer. However, as the drinker, Mrs Donoghue, was not the purchaser no contractual relationship existed between her and the cafe owner. The question referred to the House of Lords was, in the circumstances, did the ginger beer manufacturer owe a duty of care to the ultimate consumer? The House of Lords decided that such a duty existed. To the nurse, Lord Atkin is saying, although your patient has no contractual relationship with you or the NHS Trust you work for, your patient/client is your 'neighbour' in law. So take care when planning and executing his/her care and treatment that your planned actions (or omissions) do not injure him/her.

Airedale NHS Trust v Bland [1993] AC 789

This is another landmark case in which the House of Lords held that a patient in a permanent vegetative state, being kept 'alive' by artificial means, including artificial feeding, could have these means of life support withdrawn *if* this was considered to be in the patient's *best interest*. Such action would not criminalise the medical staff who decided to withdraw the support. Withdrawing treatment in this 'permanent vegetative state' does not amount to euthanasia. In the eyes of the law this is not murder. The material evidence was that Tony Bland was crushed in an accident at the Hillsborough football disaster. It left him in a permanent vegetative state, unconscious and fed via a naso-gastric tube. His quality of life was regarded as non-existent. We will visit this case again in relation to consent to treatment and end-of-life decision making. The precedent of this case is that we can turn off life support to any patient in a permanent vegetative state (brain dead) with a hopeless prognosis and a non-existent quality of life.

With respect to the principle of *precedents* within the English common law, the only point I want to make here is the fact that, were similar patient care situations to occur now and in the future, provided the material evidences were similar, such medical decisions could be repeated without risk of criminal charges being brought, or made to stick. However, the best course of action is always to assess each patient on the individual circumstances of his/her case. Individuality in nursing care is paramount.

Gillick v West Norfolk and Wisbech AHA [1985] 2 All ER 545

This common law case is important to all nurses, irrespective of their nursing branch, but even more so to child branch nurses, especially in the area of *consent* issues. The legal point in this case was whether it was proper to give contraceptive advice to children under 16 years without parental consent. The House of Lords held that it was proper and legal to do so. Brief material evidence: Mrs Gillick, mother of five girls, was concerned about the legality of a Department of Health and Social Security (DHSS) circular that indicated that doctors could legally prescribe contraception for girls under 16 without parental consent. Mrs Gillick, by letter, asked that under no circumstances should medical staff at Norfolk Area Health Authority give contraceptive or abortion advice to her daughters under 16, without her permission. The health authority replied that such an undertaking would be entirely a matter for the doctor's clinical judgement. Mrs Gillick brought a High Court action against the Health Authority, seeking a declaration that the information in the circular was illegal and wrong and could adversely affect her daughters and her own ability to discharge her parental right. Mrs Gillick lost in the High Court, and then won in the Court of Appeal. The DHSS and the AHA appealed to the House of Lords, which ruled in their favour. Mrs Gillick had lost her case, permanently, as the House of Lords was then the final appellate Court in England. Today it is replaced by the UK Supreme Court.

Such a landmark common law case must be borne in mind by all nurses, doctors, physiotherapists, surgeons and other healthcare professionals, because the real issue is whether a child under 16 can consent to their treatment without parental consent. Clearly, the answer is yes. Future courts must respect this most critical *precedent* provided the material circumstances and the principles involved are similar. If the child under 16 is 'Gillick competent', in other words mentally competent to comprehend and understand the treatment, its effects and risks, then that child may consent to treatment regardless of parental objection. However, (s)he cannot refuse perceptibly good, valid treatment the parents want him/her to have, to get him/her well or to save his/her life.

As a nurse, however, having the child's best interest in mind, you should always aim to work with the child and her parents as a family unit, remembering that in most instances a parent is likely to have the child's best interest at heart. Moreover, sometimes children are inclined to take personal decisions which in the long term may not be in their best interest. Remember also that parents also have parental rights and responsibility, plus moral and legal obligations to act in their child's best interests. Sometimes a relative lack of knowledge, experience and maturity may make children decide things not necessarily in their best long-term interest, and so it is vital, where possible and appropriate, to work with the child and the family in the best interest of the child as the patient.

European Union and human rights law

This is the third primary source of UK law. However, as will become clear, both are tied into Parliamentary law. In 1972 (under the European Community Act 1972) Britain joined the

European Community and so it is today subject to EU law. EU law is therefore *supreme* and even the UK Supreme Court (formally the House of Lords) must respect *legal precedents* arising from the European Court of Justice (ECJ). In 1998 the British Parliament incorporated the Human Rights Act 1998 into British law, effective in the UK since October 2000. British subjects have final right of appeal on human rights issues to the European Court of Human Rights (ECHR). A more complete history is that in 1973 Britain signed the *Treaty of Rome* and became part of the *European Economic Community* (EEC). By joining the EEC, the British Parliament decided that laws of the EEC would automatically affect UK law. In 1993 a new Treaty of the European Union was passed, giving rise to the present body, the *European Union* (EU), which is made up of all the countries of the *European Community*. The European Communities Act 1972 ensures that *Regulations* and *Directives* enacted by the European Union's *Council* and *Commission* take effect in the UK. Laws that emanate from the *European Court of Justice,* based in Luxembourg, take *precedence* over UK law (*Van Gend en Loos v Netherlands Belastingens-administratie* [1963] CMLR 105 ECJ). The *Articles of the Human Rights Act 1998* and how they inform nursing, healthcare more generally and care of older people particularly are examined in Chapter 13.

How a UK Bill becomes law or an Act of Parliament

Statutes start their lives as *Bills* that are introduced in Parliament as either *government-sponsored Bills* or *Private Members' Bills* by MPs. An example of a *Private Member's Bill* gave rise to the Abortion Act 1967, introduced by a Liberal Party MP, the Hon. David Steel MP. There are also *Private Bills* introduced by, example, Local Authorities. At the start of every new Parliament, for example following a general election, the government introduces its planned legislative (law-making) programme, in which it outlines its legislation plans for the life of that Parliament. This planned programme is outlined in the Queen's Speech.

The amount of legislation the government is able to pass depends, inter alia, on its Parliamentary majority, time, support from opposition parties, cooperation and support from the House of Lords. As a rule the Lords is said to be 'objective', but this may not be necessarily so because Labour and Conservative peers in the Lords will tend to favour Labour government and Conservative government-sponsored Bills respectively. With large Parliamentary majorities, governments tend to get more Bills passed.

Private Members' Bills that do not have the support of the government stand little chance of becoming law. A piece of government-sponsored legislation is typically preceded by a *Green Paper* (Figure 4.1).

If the Lords recommend changes, the Bill is returned to the Commons. Otherwise the House of Lords approves the Bill. Although the government relies on the House of Lords supporting its Bills through Parliament, should it meet with entrenched opposition it can use the 'guillotine' procedure to overcome opposition from the Lords. As indicated above, a Bill becomes law only when it final receives the Royal Assent, the Monarch's seal, and now becomes an Act of Parliament, taking effect on the date according to its commencement order; for example the Human Rights Act was adopted by British law in 1998, but in effect only commenced in October 2000.

Amendments and repeal of statutes

In the same way that the British Parliament enacts a statute it can amend, repeal or expand it. Equally, Parliament can enact *Statutory Instruments* which create other sources of legislation. For example the *European Communities Act* 1972 is an Act enacted by the UK

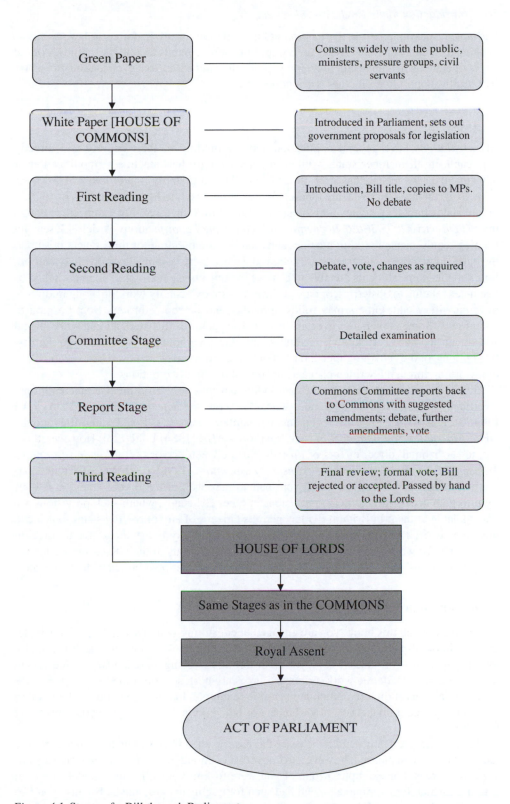

Figure 4.1 Stages of a Bill through Parliament.

Parliament making possible the incorporation of EU law into UK domestic law. As far as healthcare is concerned the Treaty on European Union demands that all the countries of the EU cooperate on human health prevention, protection and education, even lending preventative health support to each other when necessary.

EU regulations

EU *regulations* have general application and are binding in their entirety and directly applicable in all member states without the need for further enactment (modification or adjustment). This means that a UK court is duty bound to apply *regulations* to UK cases. *Directives*, on the other hand, are binding only as to the result to be achieved. It is up to individual states how they achieve the objectives linked to a directive. For example, although the *EU Directive 2005/36/EC Recognition of professional qualifications,* Article 13, sets out training requirements for adult nursing, and establishes a baseline for this branch, it is up to the NMC how those requirements are achieved. Hence there is some flexibility in operation; for example, some students are able to achieve the objectives, learning outcomes and competencies relating to obstetrics, or care of the newborn, by actually working along midwives in a midwifery unit. Others may follow a mother and newborn through from hospital to community. Some universities even create obstetric packages that students can work on and still obtain the necessary knowledge and competences without having to undergo the first two options, or the care of mother and newborn objectives can be achieved by a combination of a working through a written package and one of the first two options.

However, as Curzon (1998) notes, an individual may rely on a precise, unconditional ('vertical') *directive* against a member state (*Van Duyn v Home Office (No. 2)* [1975] 3 All ER 190). This applies to *directives* against state authorities such as Local Authorities and the NHS (*Marshall v Southampton and SW Hampshire AHA* [1986] ECR 723). However, there are no 'horizontal' direct effects of *directives* as between persons (*R v London Boroughs Transport Committee ex p Freight Transport Association* [1991] 1 WLR 828). An interesting point about EU directives which your patient may well bring to your attention is their right to gain access to healthcare provisions in other EU states, where such provisions are not available to them in Britain. EU law permits citizens of any of the EU states to achieve this objective. Therefore under EU regulations citizens of any EU state are free to travel to other states for work and healthcare. This point is contentious in the UK, as on account of long waiting lists some UK citizens have sought medical treatment in other Member States.

Secondary sources of law

As a nurse reading this book, you are engaged in consulting with a secondary legal source: this text book. Equally, when you pick up any other text book on law and healthcare, or a journal paper on legal issues in care, you are resorting to relying on secondary sources. As in referencing your academic work, primary sources are best, so from time to time please see an actual law report on a (common law) case for example. Equally, I would implore you to occasionally read primary Acts of Parliament or law reports that are kept in your university law library.

Read the facts of any landmark case, the case itself and the judgement made by the judges. You will be pleased, however, to know that even judges sometimes refer to secondary law sources. For example, if one of you were to find yourself a respondent in a civil action, in which for example a patient had sued for negligent care, maybe because you had not followed proper NMC standards or Trust policy guidelines, a judge might well ask an expert witness or your employer what the proper professional procedures were. The judge might also decide to consult the NMC Code to satisfy him-/herself that you had been correctly guided. Indeed, (s)he could request your university department to provide copies of your curriculum, training manuals or the like. The judge could even ask the NHS Trust that you are working for as a registered nurse to provide the court with a copy of your contract of employment to assess whether you had clear express terms as to your responsibilities, accountability and with respect to the standards of care expected of you.

Judges may also consult established, sound academic sources of law that have been written by competent legal authorities. Although a judge may not apply these writings as though they were the law per se, (s)he may well use them to check that (s)he is taking the right course of action. We saw in the preceding chapter that the Supreme Court of California held that psychologists treating mentally ill patients owed known third parties a duty of care to inform them that their patient had made a threat on the life of the third party. That was a US case, but it would not be beyond the bounds of possibility for an English judge to cite that case and be influenced by it.

Distinction between criminal law and civil law

So many nurses and doctors across the world have fallen foul of the criminal law, having committed serious crimes against their patients and in other capacities, that we ought to spend some time on this area of public law. Equally, so many civil litigation cases arise against the NHS each year, particularly regarding patients suing the NHS for negligence, that we also need to spend some time on civil litigation, although there is a separate chapter (Chapter 7) on negligence.

Criminal law is sometimes referred to as 'penal' law because one of its aims is to *punish criminals*: persons charged, tried and found guilty of crimes. Criminal law is therefore that body of statutory and common law that concerns itself with *crime* and the state punishment for it. The *state* defines the social behaviours defined as *crimes*. Crimes are harmful and disruptive to society and deserving of public prosecution in the criminal court. In spite of its ethos on penalty, criminal law has other objectives, for example:

- maintenance of public order;
- safety and protection of people;
- rehabilitation of criminals to society; thus
- stabilisation of the social order of a community and prevention of anarchy.

Elements of a crime

There are certain elements that *define* a crime and the prosecutor must prove 'beyond reasonable doubt' that these elements are present for the defendant to be found guilty. The three elements are:

1. The *act itself* (*actus reus*). This means that the event or the state of affairs, for example the murder or the shoplifting, has taken place. However, the event is not enough to convict beyond reasonable doubt. Although it was abundantly clear that nurse Allitt killed her patients – caused the *actus reus* – she would have been acquitted of murder if there were a reasonable possibility that the killing was accidental. It would not have been proved beyond reasonable doubt that she had the requisite mental element, the *intention to do the killing*.

2. This mental element of the crime is the *mens rea*, or *guilty mind*.
3. The third element is the 'attendant circumstances' (Pozgar, 2007, p. 54); all the related circumstances need to be considered, such as motive.

However, we must not forget that carelessness can be so 'gross', so great, so profound, that it becomes *gross negligence*, which is a crime, no longer just a civil case of negligence (*R v Adomako*). The *gross negligence* of the anaesthetist Dr Adomako in failing to realise the patient's endotracheal tube had become dislodged led to the patient's death. This was manslaughter, as it was not planned; not intentional. What on earth was Dr Adomako doing? Why he did not notice that the patient's life-sustaining (breathing or endotracheal) tube had become dislodged? Overseeing the effective working of the tube to maintain the patient's breathing during the operation was the anaesthetist's primary function. His carelessness was so gross that a criminal charge of manslaughter was brought against him; gross negligence by you the nurse can be a crime.

Distinction between criminal and civil law

One of the best distinctions made between criminal law and civil law comes from Pozgar (2007, p. 54), who wrote:

> Criminal law distinguishes crimes from civil wrongs such as tort or breach of contract. Criminal law has been seen as a system of regulating the behaviour of individuals and groups in relation to societal norms at large whereas civil law is aimed primarily at the relationship between private individuals and their rights and obligations under the law.

Nurses and doctors killing and falling foul of the criminal law

Although nurses and doctors are perhaps less likely to face a criminal prosecution than they are to face civil liability for negligence, I would remind you that history has shown criminal convictions amongst professionals from these groups. In the UK a State Enrolled Nurse, Beverley Allitt, was convicted of murdering four children, attempting to murder three others and causing grievous bodily harm to a number of other children. She was sentenced to life imprisonment. The issue of nurses being convicted for murdering patients is not unique to the UK. In a US case, *The People of the State of California v Diaz*, 834 P.2d 1171 [Cal 1992], a registered nurse was found guilty of murdering 12 of her patients, by deliberately and consciously injecting them with a rhythm-controlling drug, Lidocaine. She was sentenced to death, a conviction which on appeal was upheld by the State of California Supreme Court.

One of the most notorious crimes against patients in recent times is the UK case of Dr Harold Shipman, a GP, who in January 2000 was convicted of murdering 15 patients. He was suspected of murdering many more. Whilst serving his life sentence he committed suicide by hanging. Further details of the case appear in Chapter 3.

In the UK case *R v Cox* [1992] 12 BMLR 38, Dr Nigel Cox, a rheumatologist, was found guilty of attempted murder of a patient to whom he had given the drug potassium chloride, after repeated doses of heroin for pain relief had failed. He was sentenced to prison for one year, suspended for 12 months, which means that, although the conviction stood, he did not actually physically go to jail. Relating to the 'elements of a crime' outlined above, Dr Cox's case demonstrated that both the *actus reus* (the crime event itself – administration of the lethal potassium chloride to kill the patient) and the mental element or *mens rea* (the conscious and intentional administration of the lethal drug) were present. Dimond (2005) notes that Cox case contrasts with that of Dr Bodkin Adams, who, although he was charged with the murder of an elderly patient who probably died as a result of the analgesia he had prescribed for her, was found not guilty of murder. Why? He did not demonstrate the *mens rea* or the mental intention to kill the patient. The judge stated that the doctor was not guilty of murder if he prescribed the analgesia appropriately for relief of the patient's pain, but in the process the drug happened to shorten the patient's life. Critically, by implication, then, it is possible for a healthcare practitioner who seriously intended to commit murder to claim that instead (s)he had given the drug for therapeutic reasons, such as pain relief. My advice to you is, do not do it! Do not murder your patient or you will go to jail! By all means administer the analgesic to the patient to relieve pain. If it shortens his/her life, that was not your intention. More recently we have in the UK the case of a then nurse, Benjamin Green, aged 25, who used morphine-based pain killers, anaesthetics and muscle relaxants to murder two patients (*The Times*, 15 February 2006). There is also the case of a then staff nurse, Colin Norris, nicknamed the 'angel of death', who was jailed for life for the murder of four of his patients (*Daily Telegraph*, 4 March 2008).

Some relationships between criminal offences and civil law liability

Whereas criminal law reflects the state's definition of crime and the punishment accorded to it, *civil law* is that body of law that defines the private rights and responsibilities of individuals (Pozgar, 2007) and is concerned with the legal actions one person files against another in an attempt to seek a remedy or damages, usually money, when they consider they are wronged by that party. There is a close relationship between criminal and civil law. For example, a nurse who commits a crime against a patient, for example deliberately and intentionally hitting that patient (a criminal assault) may be prosecuted by the state and punished for this crime. But the patient may equally pursue a civil claim for damage (monetary compensation) against the nurse. So, although a civil liability would be actionable in the civil court, it could also have a criminal element actionable in the criminal court. A nurse who exceeds the speed limit, drives without due care and attention, and knocks down and hurts an individual may not only be prosecuted for a crime, driving recklessly without due care and attention, but also face a civil claim for damage. Torts and breach of contract suits are held in the civil court. Also you are *guilty* of a *crime,* but *liable* for a *civil wrong* (tort), such as negligence.

Defences to crime

There are a number of defences to crime and it is worth noting them here:

Absence of the elements of a crime

The accused must be acquitted if both the *actus reus* (the crime event/act itself) and the *mens rea* (intention) are missing, because the condition of *beyond reasonable doubt* is missing. Sometimes even where the defendant has caused the *actus reus* with the requisite *mens rea* there may still be defences; for example, the public hangman's homicides are legally justifiable. I said 'legally' since it is morally possible to argue that such killing is morally indefensible. Without a body it is more difficult (but not impossible) for the court to convict on a charge of murder. Even with the actual *actus reus* – the body itself – the accused may plead insanity or absence of the conscious intention to murder. The intent to murder must be proved beyond all reasonable doubt for a murder charge to stick. In the cases of Norris, Allitt, Shipman and others, the evidence of their murder crime was overwhelming: bodies in evidence; forensic evidence present; motives established; and so on.

Infancy

By statute law, *a child under 10 years* is *exempt* from *criminal responsibility* even though there may be clear evidence that (s)he caused the *actus reus* with *mens rea*. The child is said to be *doli incapax*.

It may be interesting to note that in one case (*Walters v Lunt* [1951] 2 All ER645) in which a husband and wife were charged with receiving from their seven-year-old son another child's tricycle, knowing it to have been stolen, the court held that they should be acquitted because the child *could not steal*; the tricycle was not stolen. Clever advocacy. Criminal responsibility begins on the child's tenth birthday.

Insanity

A person's insanity may be relevant in the criminal charges brought against him/her at two stages: before trial begins and during the trial. Before the trial, the plea of insanity is not a *defence*, because the trial has not yet commenced. If insanity is being used at the preliminary proceedings stage it is to *prevent* the accused being tried. After the trial has commenced, the defence may use insanity as a defence. Where the defendant at the custodial stage is committed for trial and, by virtue of two reports from at least two medical practitioners, the Home Secretary is satisfied that (s)he is suffering from a mental illness, the Home Secretary can order that the defendant be held in a hospital and not be tried. In making this decision the Home Secretary would take into account public interest, the necessity to hospitalise rather than try, as a trial may have an injurious effect on the defendant's mental state. When well enough, (s)he could still be brought to trial.

If a defendant is unable to understand the charge and the difference between pleas of guilty and not guilty, unable to challenge jurors, instruct counsel (barrister or defence solicitor), unable to concentrate and follow the trial, insanity could be pled for him/her. The situation of a plea of insanity is complex because in some cases even where a person has been certified insane he may still be able to stand trial, being able to plead and follow his trial. The defendant also has the right to be tried and society has an interest in fair play and justice. It is desirable that a person charged with an offence should, whenever possible, stand trial so that the question of whether or not (s)he committed the crime can be determined. It is in society's interest to know who committed the offence. In UK law persons are presumed to be sane unless the contrary is proved. For a plea of insanity to be effective, it must be beyond doubt that at the time of committing the *actus reus* the person was of unsound mind.

Diminished responsibility and provocation

The Homicide Act 1957, s. 2, makes it possible for a defendant to plead *diminished responsibility* and *provocation* as defences to murder. These defences are not available to any other crime. However, if successful that may mean not absolute acquittal, but a much less severe guilt of *manslaughter*. As in the case of *insanity*, it is for the defence to prove *diminished responsibility* or *provocation*. Smith (2000) points to the fact that *diminished responsibility* has been successfully pleaded in cases where it would have thought there is no chance of a defence of *insanity* succeeding; for example mercy killers or deserted spouses and disappointed lovers who killed while in a state of depression or chronic anxiety. The nature of the defence of *diminished responsibility* is apparent in Section 2 of the Homicide Act 1957, which states:

Where a person kills or is a party to the killing of another, he shall not be convicted of murder if he was suffering from such abnormality of mind . . . as substantially impaired his mental responsibility for his acts and omissions in doing or being a party to the killing . . . A person who but for this section would be liable, whether as principal or accessory, to be convicted of murder shall be liable instead to be convicted of manslaughter.

Self-defence

Under English law it is acceptable for a reasonable degree of force to be used to protect oneself or another person against an attack. No more force than is reasonably required should be used (proportionality). The question is: what is reasonable force? If you deliberately load your gun and intentionally wait to shoot your tormentor, for example the person who burgled your house four times before, and in fact shot him when he returned, this would be unreasonable (unlawful) force and you could be found guilty of murder. You had the *mens rea*. If, however, you unexpectedly encountered a burglar in your home, waving a gun or some other weapon, such as the family's kitchen knife, threateningly at you, and you felt strongly that this was a death threat to you and your family, and in a struggle to disarm him you actually killed him, with whatever previously unplanned means, then in all probability this is an excellent example of self-defence.

Mistake as a defence

It has been settled in *DPP v Morgan* [1976] AC 182; [1975] 2 All ER 347 that mistake is a defence to crime where it prevents the defendant from forming the necessary *mental element* (*mens rea*). Where the law requires *intention* or *recklessness* to be present with respect to the *actus reus* (the act itself, e.g. a rape), a *mistake*, whether reasonable or not, which precludes both states of mind (i.e. *intention* and *recklessness*) will do. The defendant had sex with the plaintiff, having formed the mistaken belief that she consented. The *intention to rape* or the *recklessness* (required in law to convict) was missing, so he was not guilty of rape. Mistake in criminal law is usually no excuse or defence, for as a rule knowledge that the act is forbidden forms no part of the *mens rea*.

Where the law requires only *negligence* to be present, then only a reasonable mistake will operate as a defence. For an *unreasonable* mistake (one that a reasonable person would not make) there is no excuse. A mistake that does not preclude the *mens rea*, or negligence if this is the issue, is no defence at all. In the case of Dr Adomako (the culpable anaesthetist who failed to notice that the life-saving endotracheal tube was undone) the House of Lords upheld the earlier Court of Appeal decision that the doctor was *grossly negligent* (*manslaughter*). Here, a criminal act (gross negligence) unintentionally cost the death of the patient. Plain negligence, for want of a better term, is a tort/civil wrong issue, but gross negligence is a crime. The tort element provides opportunity for the patient's relative to seek compensation for their relative's death. In the Adomako case the House of Lords established that the anaesthetist had breached his duty of care to the patient. The breach was so serious that the patient died, in which case the breach constituted *gross negligence*. 'Gross negligence' in this case means that the doctor showed marked indifference to the risk of serious injury or even death. This is a point nurses need to bear in mind. Take care that your actions or omissions cause the patient no harm; but take even more care to ensure you do not get yourself involved in gross negligence, or you could go to jail.

No diligent, committed and careful practitioner would deliberately hurt his/her patients. Yet Beverley Allitt, Colin Norris and Harold Shipman did. Manslaughter, besides being a crime, can also serve as the basis for a tort or civil wrong, for which the healthcare professional or his employer may have to pay compensation.

Duress and coercion as defences

Duress: threat and circumstances

The law recognises the defence of *duress by threats*. *Duress of circumstances* is also recognised by law. In the latter case the defendant commits the act alleged out of fear of losing his life, but this time no one is demanding (s)he do it (Cole [1994] Crim LR 582; Ali [1995] Crim LR 303). The accused commits the act because his/her life is threatened and doing the act is the only way out. Had it not been for the defence of duress the act would have been a crime. Duress is unlikely to be accepted as a valid defence to murder.

Coercion

At common law defence of *coercion* is reserved for a wife who commits certain crimes in the presence of, and under the coercion of, her husband. There is no consensus on the use of 'coercion' by judges, lawyers and legal writers. Coercion does not apply in cases of treason or murder.

Necessity

Necessity as a defence in English law is uncertain. The courts have never recognised a defence of necessity in broad terms. In theory a defence of necessity is, like duress, a situation in which the person is faced with two unpleasant alternatives, one in which (s)he would breach the criminal law, and the other some evil done to self or to others. If the evil to self outweighs the evil involved in the breach of the criminal law, it is argued that the person should have a defence in *necessity*. However, defence of *necessity* was recognised and applied by Lord Goff in the case of *Bournewood Community and Mental Health NHS Trust* [1998] 3All ER 289, as a way of justifying the detention a patient suffering from mental disorder where there was no statute to rely on. The *necessity* lies in the belief that the person was a very serious potential danger to himself and others. In the case of *Southwark London Borough v Williams* [1971] 2All ER 175 at 159, Lord Denning did not accept the defence of necessity of hunger as being an inevitable excuse for stealing. The court held that homelessness did not excuse even an orderly entry into empty houses owned by local authority. The court stated:

> If homelessness were once admitted as a defence to trespass, no one's house could be safe. Necessity would open a door which no man could shut.

There are civil cases in which *necessity* was allowed without the threat to life being identified; for example, in *Gillick v West Norfolk and Wisbech Area Health Authority* [1984] QB 581, one of the reasons given for the lawfulness of the contraceptive advice or treatment to a girl under 16, without parental consent, was that unless she received it her physical and mental health would suffer.

Superior orders as a defence

Under English law it is not a valid defence for the defendant to state that a crime was committed under the orders of a superior, be this military or civil. Both the House of Lords and the Privy Council approved the following statement from the Australian High Court:

> It is fundamental to our legal system that the executive has no power to authorise a breach of the law and that it is no excuse for an offender to say that he acted under the authority of a superior officer.
>
> *(A v Hayden (No. 2)* [1984] 156 CLR 532 at 540)

The fact that a war crime was committed in response to superior military orders does not remove the characteristic of 'crime' from it. The trial of Hitler's henchmen for war crimes following the Second World War is testament to this. More recently the trial of Saddam Hussein's generals for war crimes is an example in point. 'Following superior orders' is not enough. In his book *Introduction to the Study of the Law of the Constitution*, Dicey (1959, p. 303) wrote that a soldier may be 'liable to be shot by a court-martial if he disobeys an order and to be hanged by a judge and jury if he obeys it'. Reflect on this statement.

Implication of the superior order concept to nurses

There are a number of learning parallels for nurses with respect to civil law, for example in situations of claims of negligent practice. The defence of *superior orders* appears to be a myth. This should alert nurses to the dangers of following *'questionable' superior orders* without questioning. The days have long gone when nurses did things simply because the doctor ordered them to. Nurses have their professional registration and personal, professional, legal, employment and ethical liability and accountability, to consider when faced with questionable superior orders. The NMC maintains that registered nurses are responsible and accountable for their own individual practice. Registered nurses cannot use the defence of 'my superior instructed me to do that'. Not even student nurses can claim that their superior ordered them to do this, if they knew what they were doing was wrong. If in doubt, question the order. This can only raise the standard of nursing care given to your patient. Patients are entitled to the same high standard of care from students as they are from qualified nurses. This is not to say they will get it, as clearly students are less skilled than experienced, qualified nurses. However this does not stop a patient from wanting the highest care irrespective of the professional care giver.

Impossibility as a defence

The defence of *impossibility* is nebulous. However, where the law imposes a duty to act, it has sometimes been held that, through no fault of the defendant, it was impossible for him to act. For example, in *Harding v Price* [1948] 1 KB 695; [1948] 1 All ER 283, a driver is not liable for failure to report an accident if he did not know the accident had occurred. In *Lim Chin Aik v R* [1963] AC 160; [1963] 1 All ER 223, a person is not liable for failure to leave a particular place if he did not know of the order requiring him to do so. In a New Zealand case, *Finau v Department of Labour* [1984] 2 NZLR 396, it was held that failure to leave a country following revocation of permit is not an offence if because of the advanced state of her pregnancy no airline would carry the defendant. Yet in *Davey v Towle* [1973]

RTR 314, it is not an excuse when a driver fails to produce a test certificate even though it was impossible for him to do so given that the owner of the vehicle was unwilling or unable to produce it. There appears to be inconsistency in the law with respect to *the principle of impossibility* as a defence. Hence it may be concluded that no general defence of *impossibility* is recognised. The most that may be claimed, justifiably, is that there may be instances when this defence may hold.

Contract law and its implications for you as a nurse

Contract law is part of civil law. A civil action may be brought under contract, for example for breach of contract, such as if the landlord breached his contract by asking you to share the room you rent from him for yourself with another student, for a second rent to him, after you had signed a contract to be the sole occupier of that room. A breach of contract can lead to actions for compensation or specific performance of that contract. Contract law deals with legally enforceable agreements and promises between parties, and so they are *legally binding on the parties*.

Contracts are usually bilateral but may be *unilateral*; for example one party promises to do something (e.g. give a reward in return for an act from another person). Whoever finds my gold chain will get £20! This would constitute a unilateral contract that is binding on the promiser.

Simple contracts may be *written*, *oral* or implied from *conduct*, for instance a handshake, or from words. Imagine that a landlord allows you to start occupying the room you are renting with the express intention of giving you the contract for signature in a day or so. He was rather busy at the time but you shook hands as an implied agreement that the room was yours for the academic year. Moreover, in the presence of your witness the landlord had espoused the broad terms of the contract, such as the length of tenure and rent payable. This sounds as good as a written agreement. But not really! Even with a witness, your unwritten contract could be vulnerable because in a dispute it could be your word against his, especially if your witnessing friend decided not to stand up for you. It is always best to have a written tenancy agreement signed by you, your landlord and your witness.

For a valid contract the parties must:

*   reach agreement of *offer* and *acceptance;*
*   agree to be legally bound;
*   have provided valuable *considerations*: your money for his promise and delivery of your living accommodation.

In terms of offer and acceptance, suppose for example you go to a job interview for a staff nurse post and you are offered the job unconditionally, by letter. You write back to accept the post. In effect then the contract is in place.

However, if having agreed the terms of the contract following the interview and having now received the confirmation letter you now decide you want the contract terms changed, then you have now made a *counter offer* which could invalidate the original offer and you have no job! You cannot now hold the person who offered you the job to be legally bound by the agreement. Maybe as a kind gesture your potential employer may decide to negotiate new terms with you (one does not in law have to). By doing so the employer varies the terms of his/her own contract and this puts you in a slightly better position. Do not forget, however, that when you *counter offered* you in effect cancelled the original contract. In this case the employer is not legally obligated to you in terms of the job you just turned down.

Is a sales advertisement a contract?

Offering something for sale through an advertisement does not constitute a contract. The advertiser does not have to sell you the car advertised for sale. The advert in law is only *an invitation to treat*. Similarly the advertisement of a staff nurse job in the *Nursing Times* is an *invitation to treat*. Until you apply, are interviewed and get offered the job it is not yours. Equally, the offer of the job to you does not bind you to the potential employer; you can if you wish turn down the employer's offer. It might of course not help your cause in future if that employer, having interviewed six others for the job, turned them down and offered it to you instead and you then turned the offer down. The employer probably spent a fortune on advertisement, interviewing and the like. Turning the offer down by letter weeks afterwards, before starting the job, after verbally accepting the post does not make for good interpersonal relationships! After all, the NMC insists on good communication and interpersonal relationships between the nurse and her patient. Such skills and competences will also help you in your business and collegiate relationships with your peers and employers.

An invitation to treat

Picking up the goods and taking it to the counter does not mean the shop keeper is legally bound to sell it to you. In taking the goods to the counter you are offering to purchase it. If the shop keeper takes your money he agrees to sell you the goods and the contract is in place.

A good example of *an invitation to treat* was in Box 4.3 when I approached the first shop assistant and asked the price of the plate. Once she had accepted my money, put it in her till and given me my receipt, the situation had gone from 'an invitation to treat' to a legitimate and bona fide contract: the exchange of my £3 for the goods – my precious Victorian bread plate!

To satisfy your curiosity, you may be interested to know that I did not accept the money back and I refused to return the plate to the woman. In fact I challenged her to call the police, reminding her of my right in law. I had not stolen the plate. I had a legal right to it as evidenced by my receipt, evidence of purchase. Receipts are always a sound evidence of purchase, so always hold on to yours. Needless to say, the lady soon saw sense, although not until after she had heard me outline my legal case and my right to the plate. On reflection I was rather glad I had studied law, because at the point of the controversy I had had no fewer than two law degrees, including a postgraduate Master's degree in law. Hopefully this incident has demonstrated to you how important it is to know your rights in law. It is equally important to know your legal position when caring for patients. Know the legal principles that you must follow whether you are nursing a patient or buying a Victorian bread plate from your local charity shop! Knowing the aspects of law relating to your daily activities within the nurse–patient caring relationship or your more social and everyday business interactions does give you confidence in your interrelationships, and knowledge and competence to operate professionally within a sound legal framework.

An invitation to tender

A good example of *an invitation to tender* would be if a NHS Trust puts out a tender for people to offer to contract for its cleaning services. An invitation to tender does not constitute a bona fide offer to contract. To be effective a contract must be accepted *unconditionally without* a *counter offer*. Your tender has got to be accepted by the trust for you to secure the cleaning contract.

BOX 4.3 A personal reflection on contract law affecting my rights: my purchase of an antique Victorian bread plate from a second-hand shop

Some years ago I went into a second-hand shop and saw what I thought was an expensive Victorian bread plate. I fell in love with it, picked it up and asked the shop assistant how much it was. She replied, '£3'. I paid her the £3. She gave me the plate, which I placed on the counter on top of a bag containing other purchases I had made at a shop I had gone to minutes before. I was alert to another shop attendant coming into the shop from what appeared to be a room at the back of the shop, where the staff appeared to sort the old stuff people delivered to the charity shop. This second shop attendant asked the assistant who had sold me the Victorian bread plate whose it was. The assistant told her 'it belongs to that man over there', pointing to me. The second shop attendant reacted rather angrily, telling her fellow shop attendant that the plate was not for sale; it was due to go to the auction, where it would fetch a lot of money. On hearing this I quickly picked up my purchase and continued to look round the shop, appearing not to be listening to the conversation. The angry shop assistant approached me, demanded I gave the plate back to her, further stating that it was not for sale. She had £3 in her hand and tried to give it to me, at the same time reaching out for my plate. I refused to take back the money, holding onto my purchase. In fact I pushed my receipt for the plate deeper into my wallet! The lady became more angry and threatened to call the police, all the time trying to hand me back the £3 on insisting on being given back the plate. I insisted it was mine and held on to it.

Under the law of contract what do you consider to have been my position and if you were me what would you have done under the circumstances described above?

NHS contract of employment under threat and fraud

If the contract is made under threat or duress it is invalid. It may also be invalidated by mistakes, errors and fraud. If at the point of pursuing a contract of employment as a staff nurse your potential NHS Trust employer asks if you have a criminal record and you deny it, when in truth you have, then if he later finds out he can dismiss you. So a fraud or a lie on your job application form may later cost you your job. You cannot justifiably threaten a person to sign any contract. Equally, if you lie on your UCAS form to get onto your nursing degree programme, although you may succeed in passing the course you may find that you are denied registration by your professional body when you come to apply for such a registration. Be honest all the way and it will serve you and your career well.

Your contractual obligations to your NHS employer

When discussing negligence in this book (Chapter 7) the point is made that NHS patients cannot sue in contract as they have no contract with the NHS. They can however sue in the *tort* (civil wrong) of negligence under what Lord Atkin, in *Donohue v Stevenson* (1932), described as the *neighbour principle*, as well as the principles of *foreseeability* and *proximity*. You must remember, however, that to be employed as a registered nurse you will have signed a *contract of employment*. Your obligation in signing such a contract is your promise to form legal *neighbour* relationships between yourself and your employer. You contract with him to the benefit of your patients; to anticipate and reasonably foresee any problems you may cause them, manage their difficulties as you share this very near (or *proximate*) professional relationship with them. You have a contract not with the patient, but with the employer. The employer can discipline, even sack you, if you fail to come up to the expectations of the express terms of that contract. Moreover, you have made a promise to take *reasonable care* in delivering *safe care*, *minimising risks* and so on. If you then, in the course of your duty as a nurse, deliver unsafe care, negligently or deliberately, your employer has the legal right to call you to account under contract.

Family law

Family law is a subspecies of civil law. It deals with legal relationships within families and includes disputes about child upbringing, divorce and, to some extent, domestic violence. The guarded phrase 'to some extent' is used, because domestic violence, like any form of violence against the person, can be subject to criminal law.

If as a children's nurse you suspect or can prove that a parent is abusing his/her child, this is a matter for the police and the criminal court, and so you have a legal as well as a professional, moral and ethical obligation to report the matter to your seniors, who are obliged to report the abuse to the legal authorities. If parents decide, for whatever reason, to divorce and the question of who secures child custody becomes a legal issue, under family law the Family Court could be asked to sort out the dispute and custody of the children concerned. Things such as visitation rights come under the auspice of the family court.

Nurses, particularly children's nurses and health visitors, may find themselves at the centre of children-focused disputes, especially in matters relating to consent to treatment, such as life-saving surgery for young children. There may be parental disagreement about the appropriateness of controversial and life-saving treatment, perhaps one parent wanting the child to have the treatment whilst the other may not. Perhaps both parents are refusing to consent to life-saving treatment. In such cases the High Court may, on recommendation from the medical staff, decide on the proper course of action to save the child's life. The family court would be seeking to make judgements in the child's 'best interest'. The health professional always acts in the patient's best interest.

Lower down the hierarchy of the court system, less important civil cases are dealt with by county courts, with appeals to the Court of Appeal. Magistrates also have some civil jurisdiction in matrimonial matters, guardianship, adoption and the maintenance of illegitimate children. In matrimonial cases in the Family Division of the High Court, the person who brings the action seeking dissolution of marriage is called the *petitioner* and the person from whom the divorce is sought is the *respondent*. If the action succeeds it results in decrees of divorce. The Family Division of the High Court hears appeals from the Magistrates' Courts.

Public law versus private law

You may at times read about the two legal distinctions of *public law* and *private law*. Public law includes the criminal law, but is also concerned with the *constitutional* and *administrative* rules that regulate and administer public bodies such as the courts, Local Authorities, the NHS, the police and the civil service. Constitutional law regulates and controls government, for example decisions about who can be MPs and who has the right to vote on. Public law also gives powers to individuals to challenge public authorities on how they decide to deliver public services. The individual may feel the way these public bodies deliver services interferes with his/her civil liberties or freedoms. Moreover, the operation of these bodies may be claimed to be beyond or outside the power that statutes afford, or that the body has wrongly exercised the discretion allowed it under law. Thus a person may seek a *judicial review* of the public body's operation and decision making. This means that the citizen can ask the court to determine whether the body has acted legally. The court cannot directly correct the public body's decision or substitute its own decision, but it can declare the practice of the body illegal.

The simplest way to understand a judicial review is to view it as a control that is exercised by the court over procedures and conduct of statutory and other subordinate bodies, for example the NHS, which may result in grant of what are known as *prerogative orders*, otherwise called *declarations*. (Sometimes instead of 'prerogative orders' the term 'prerogative writs' is used.) These *prerogative orders* or *writs* will state the rights of the persons who sought the judicial review. Judicial reviews are concerned not so much with the decision of the body challenged, but with the manner of the decision making.

What are the possible declarations that the court may make as a part of its judicial review? Various remedies are available; for example, a court may issue a *prerogative order* or *prerogative writ* of *'certiorari'*, to quash an improper decision, such as a criminal conviction. (It will be remembered that criminal law is a type of public law.) See, for example, the case *R v Bolton Magistrates ex p Scally* [1991] 2 WLR 239. Another of these special orders/writs is the *order of mandamus* that may require a public body to carry out its statutory duties. Another of these special writs is the writ of *habeas corpus ad subjiciendum*, 'the great prerogative writ of liberty' which commands a person to produce the detainee, with details of the day and cause of his/her caption and detention, and be ready to do what is directed by the court. The Queen's Bench Division of the High Court has jurisdiction to issue such a writ. The application and/or the demands of the writ take precedence over other business of the court. The term 'habeas corpus' literally means 'you have a body'.

The purpose of seeking a *judicial review* may be to have a point of law straightened out, for example where there is doubt and confusion as to just what is the law on a particular issue. In the *Gillick* case described above, this was precisely what Mrs Gillick sought, a declaration from the High Court that it was illegal for the doctors employed by West Norfolk and Wisbech AHA to give contraceptive or abortion advice to her daughters under 16, without her (parental) consent.

Also read the case of *R v Cambridge Health Authority ex parte B (A Minor)* [1995] 23 BMLR 1 CA; [1995] 2 All ER 129. In this case the parent of a 10-year-old girl with acute myeloid leukaemia, who was refused a second course of chemotherapy and bone marrow transplant, petitioned the High Court to rule the health authority (HA)'s decision illegal. The High Court upheld the parent's application for a judicial review. The HA appealed to the Court of Appeal, which held that the HA's decision was the right one, as further operations would not be in the child's best interest and resources had to be considered.

In another case (*In re Walker's application*, *The Times*, 26 November 1987) Mrs Walker's baby's heart operation was postponed by Birmingham Health Authority. Her application to the court for judicial review of the HA's decision was refused. Her appeal was also turned down by the Court of Appeal. The Court held that it was not for it to replace the HA's decision with one of its own with respect to resource allocation. The court would not interfere unless the HA had failed to carry out its public duties, or there had been illegality in the HA's distribution of its funds.

Court decisions about use of NHS resources

The court is reluctant to uphold applications for judicial reviews against HAs and NHS Trusts in respect to resource allocation. Resource management is for the HA or the NHS Trust, and central resource allocation a matter for the government. However, in a recent case (*R (Watts) v Bedford Primary Care Trust and Another*, *The Times Law Report*, 3 October

2003) the High Court held that the NHS should pay for the patient to be treated abroad where the treatment was immediately available and the patient had waited significantly long for NHS treatment. This suggests that if NHS Trusts cannot treat patients on their list they could be asked to fund their treatment abroad.

Private law is that division of law that deals with and regulates legal relationships between private individuals and organisations. It is concerned principally with duties and rights of individuals that the state is not immediately and directly concerned with, for example where one individual seeks compensation against a healthcare professional or the professional's employer, or where, under contract law, one party seeks monetary compensation for breaches, or seeks specific performance of contract. *Contract* and *tort law* are types of *private law*, as is the law relating to property, for example legal rights to property. *Family law*, which deals with *marriage*, *divorce* and *responsibility for children* also fits under *private law*, as does the law relating to state, housing and employment and welfare benefits and rights.

Please complete student portfolio reflection exercises 4.2 (Figure 4.2) and 4.3 (Box 4.4). If you need more space use your portfolio. Answers to exercise 4.2 may be found in Table 4.1 at the end of the chapter.

Should a nurse commit a crime, for example steal from a patient or indeed the hospital, in all probability (s)he would be *reported* to the police. The police would *investigate* the matter, for example talk to both parties to establish facts. The nurse may be asked to voluntarily accompany the officer to the police station for questioning even though (s)he may not be formally arrested. On the other hand (s)he may be arrested and taken to the police station. The nurse is entitled to a caution if the police suspect him/her of the offence, and certainly before they start to gather evidence that could be laid before a court. The caution is fairly standard and must indicate to the nurse that (s)he does not have to say anything but it may harm his/her defence if she does not mention when questioned something which (s)he later relies on in court. The nurse must be cautioned that anything (s)he says may be given in evidence.

The police are expected to follow guidelines for questioning and detention as laid out in a code of practice under the Criminal Evidence Act 1984, s. 60(1) (a) and S 60(1), revised in 2003. If the police believe they have enough evidence to successfully prosecute, they may charge the nurse with theft, issuing him/her with a second caution and with a written account of the offence (s)he is charged with. Once (s)he knows (s)he is a suspect and being questioned as such, (s)he is best advised to seek legal representation. Following arrest the nurse is entitled to seek and obtain *bail* pending further detailed evidence gathering and attendance at court. A bail is the release of the person following detention, on security or accepting specified conditions for that release. The police will usually formulate their report relating to the allegation and submit it to the *Crown Prosecution Service* (CPS), headed by the *Director of Public Prosecutions* (DPP), who will decide whether or not to proceed to trial. The nurse is the *defendant*. Thus in the law books and law report, if this were a very important case to be decided high up in the court hierarchy, for example the Court of Appeal or the Supreme Court, you may see a case set out as *R v Bloggs*, where 'R' stands for *Regina* (the Queen, or *Rex*, if a king is on the throne), 'v' for versus, and Bloggs the defendant's surname. As the case of theft, however, is a fairly everyday affair it would in most cases be tried in the Crown Court, the court of first instance for this type of crime. It could also be tried in a magistrates' court. Irrespective of the court it is tried in it will usually be listed in the court's order of cases as *R v Bloggs* (Bloggs being the surname of the accused – the nurse).

For the purposes of his/her trial and defence in court, it would be in the nurse's best interest to have a defence barrister as advocate. That barrister is briefed by the nurse's solicitor who has given the nurse initial legal advice. (The crown prosecutors – solicitors or barristers

Questions	Civil law	Criminal law
1. Main purpose(s)?		
2. Who brings the case? (Clue: think of Bloggs v Bloggs)		
3. Legal title/name of person who brings the case?		
4. Legal descriptor of person against whom case brought?		
5. Standard of proof required?		
6. If found culpable we say the person is?		
7. Legal sanction against the culpable person?		
8. Name all the courts (hierarchically) that could take part in the trial; including appeals. Working from left to right name the highest court first		
9. Name the person(s) making the decision in the courts		
10. State the powers available to the courts		
11. If this is a Scottish case with which court in the UK does final appeal rest?		

Figure 4.2 Quiz to test your understanding of differences between criminal law and civil law in England and Wales.

– advise the police on criminal offences.) As stated above, the case would be heard by a *criminal court* such the Crown Court or magistrates' court, but certainly not by a civil court. [Civil courts handle issues such as breach of contract and negligence cases. It is worth saying here that some criminal offences may turn out to be both criminal acts and torts or

---

BOX 4.4 Student portfolio reflection exercise 4.3

A criminal law case scenario

A patient newly admitted via the accident and emergency (A&E) department alleges that a nurse in the unit has stolen his gold ring. (This scenario is based on an actual case witnessed by the writer whilst working as a student nurse in A&E.) What do you suppose would happen? Use your law portfolio to help you analyse the situation and come up with an answer that you can justify.

---

civil wrongs. For example, if a nurse deliberately harms a patient in his/her care, not only could the appropriate criminal charges be brought by the police, but the patient (or family) may also bring a claim for damage (monetary compensation) against the nurse or his/her employers.] You may recall that, in the Dr Adomaka case, his negligence, which would normally be tried in the civil court, was so 'gross' that he was tried in the Crown Court for alleged manslaughter, a criminal offence.

In the alleged murder of his then ex-wife, Nicole Brown Simpson, and her friend Ronald Goldman, in the USA in 1994, O. J. Simpson first faced criminal trial (from 29 January to 3 October 1995) for the alleged murders. On 3 October, he was acquitted – found not guilty of murder by a jury. He later (in 1998) faced a civil trial for wrongful death, brought by Mr Goldman's family, seeking compensation for the death of their son. Equally, the Brown estate brought a civil action against Simpson in a 'survivor suit', a trial lasting four months, which was decided in favour of Brown and O. J. Simpson's two children, as well as in favour of the victims' families. Some $12.5 million was awarded to Brown and Simpson's children and some $33.5 million to the victims' families.

In the case of the alleged theft by the nurse reported in the scenario above, if found guilty the nurse may be forced to pay a fine, and/or face imprisonment, or (s)he could face a suspended jail sentence; this is a sentence ordered not to take effect immediately, and must cover a specified period. In such a case, the nurse will be reported to the NMC, which will conduct its own investigation and take professional disciplinary action as appropriate. The employer may also take disciplinary action against the nurse as a *contracted* employee. This could result in the nurse being sacked. Should the NMC remove the convicted nurse from its register (s)he cannot practise nursing. If the nurse is not found guilty then (s)he walks free from the court. Stealing from your patient is both serious crime and gross professional misconduct for which you may face discontinuation of your training as a student or, if qualified, registered with the NMC and employed as a nurse, loss of registration status as well as loss of your employment.

In terms of very *serious* criminal cases against healthcare professionals, for example in the cases of Shipman and nurses Norris and Allitt (who all killed a number of their patients) the Crown Court, not magistrates' courts, tries the cases. The court administers the trial and decides punishment. Let us now look at a civil action against a registered nurse, for example for a negligent conduct that harmed a patient in his/her care.

In the scenario in Box 4.5 the civil court is trying to establish whether the nurse (Brown) is *liable* for negligence. In this (civil) trial the term 'guilty' is *not* used. In the criminal court Beverley Allitt, Colin Norris and Benjamin Green were found guilty of murdering patients. The present civil case for negligence is not a police case; it is a civil case in which the patient seeks *compensation or damage* (money) from the nurse or, more usually in the real world, from the nurse's employer, under *vicarious liability*.

BOX 4.5 Student portfolio reflection exercise 4.4

A civil law case scenario: negligence (naturally in the civil court), plus other civil actions

Lets us say that a nurse is accused by a patient of hurting him/her through *negligent* practice. That is not intentional or wilful *hurt*. Here a poor standard of care caused the injury. The nurse would be tried in a *civil court*, for example the High Court, where (s)he would be the *defendant*. The patient who brings the case is the *claimant*, (called the *plaintiff* before April 1999). The nurse in this case is not a criminal since (s)he did not wilfully and intentionally hurt his/her patient. The case would be listed to reflect one private individual suing another; thus we may see, for example, *Bloggs v Brown*, where Bloggs is the patient and Brown the defending nurse. Read the main text to gain an understanding of some fundamental legal issues in this case. Use your law portfolio to record your learning.

Primary v vicarious liability

It might be the nurse's employer who is sued. The patient may sue the nurse direct under *primary liability,* but is more likely to sue the nurse's employer under *vicarious liability* (the employer for the negligence of its employee). Economically, patients are financially more assured suing the employer, for example an NHS Trust with a more assured financial capacity to pay compensation. The NMC strongly recommends that nurses have suitable indemnity insurance as they could be sued directly. Moreover, where the nurse's employer pays out under vicarious liability, that employer could seek an indemnity against the nurse in order to recover the financial loss. What is the implication? Make sure you have proper indemnity insurance cover, for example by joining a professional union such as the RCN or UNISON.

Professional and employment actions against the nurse

In the civil case described above, the nurse may also face the wrath of his/her employer who may discipline her for professional ineptitude within the terms of the *contract of employment*. Equally, the nurse may be reported to the NMC for professionally failing to deliver care competently. As in the criminal case discussed earlier, a nurse facing a claim of negligent practice in the civil court is best advised to be represented by a competent barrister.

Tort law/action

A suit of negligence against a nurse will be brought under the civil law (tort law) of negligence. A *tort* is a *civil* wrong, not a criminal wrong. A civil wrong by a nurse may be where (s)he unintentionally wrongly applies a splint that causes the patient a pressure sore. It could be where the healthcare professional carries out an operation on the patient without gaining his/her consent. This is known as a *battery* or *trespass to the person*. In a case of battery or trespass a claimant only needs to show that (s)he was touched without his/her consent. Proof of injury is irrelevant. If the case is brought in negligence, the claimant must prove that that the healthcare professional, having owed him/her a duty of care, breached that duty and the consequence of this is that (s)he has been *injured*. If the action, the negligence, was so great (e.g. a doctor or nurse had carried out an operation on a patient without his/her consent) this could bring about a criminal charge that would most certainly be tried in the criminal court.

Civil action for breach of confidence

A civil action for breach of confidence could be brought against a nurse. In the New Zealand case *Furniss v Fitchett* [1958] NZLR 396, the defendant doctor had disclosed, in writing, confidential medical information about his patient (the plaintiff) to her husband without her permission. (The husband and his wife were both patients of the doctor.) The husband used the information against his wife in a separation proceeding. The patient successfully sued the doctor for breach of confidence. The court held that the defendant ought to have reasonably foreseen that the disclosure could have come to the plaintiff's attention and injured her health. The doctor had breached his duty of care to the plaintiff. The same situation could arise if a nurse disclosed to a third party confidential information about a patient. It matters not that the person receiving the information is a relative, however close, such as a husband to his wife. The reality in law is that it is entirely up to the competent adult patient to decide if (s)he wishes confidential medical information to be disclosed to a third party.

Civil actions for other torts (civil wrongs)

There are other forms of civil wrongs that could be mentioned here, although the tort of greatest significance to nurses is negligence, which will be dealt with more fully in Chapter 7. The forms of civil action that could be brought are:

- defamation – libelling or slandering (written and spoken respectively);
- trespass to land (trespass to persons already mentioned);
- false imprisonment, for example detaining patients against their will (e.g. stopping an informal patient – not detained under the Mental Health Act – from leaving hospital);
- wrongful interference;
- nuisance;
- malicious prosecution;
- breach of statutory duty;
- interference with interest in trade or business.

Civil actions for breach of contract

Although a civil action could be brought under contract law for a breach of contract, the *law of contract* lies outside the *tort system*. It is unlikely a patient would bring an action against a nurse for a breach of contract, because most UK nurses work for the NHS, and NHS patients do not have contracts with the NHS. If a patient did have a contract with the NHS or private doctor or physiotherapist for treatment, then should they harm the patient through carelessness or negligent practice there would technically be nothing to prevent the patient from suing in contract, for a breach of contract. The express or hidden contract terms would demand care at an acceptable high standard. Therefore a failure to deliver care at the level and standards expressed in such a contract could be the basis of a law suit in contract, but as stated NHS patients do not hold contracts with the NHS and so are likely to sue in the tort of negligence. A suite in contract would be similarly for monetary compensation.

The courts

The UK Court system can be divided into two main divisions: civil courts and criminal courts. In order of hierarchical importance the two court systems are outlined in Figure 4.3; the most superior court in either grouping is at the top of the diagram, the most subordinate court at the bottom. In the criminal court grouping the magistrate's court comes at the bottom, whereas on the civil justice side the county court and the magistrate's court are at the bottom. There are some differences between Scottish law and English law, hence certain differences in the court system, and I will point out some of these differences later.

The UK Supreme Court

In October 2009 the UK Supreme Court replaced the House of Lords as the highest UK domestic appellate court. The members of this court (justices of the Supreme Court) are distinguished judges, 12 members who sit in benches of up to nine judges. Like the House of Lords before it, the Supreme Court is an appellate court which hears appeals from the Court of Appeal, which has a membership of 32 Lord Justices of Appeal. Whether we are dealing with criminal or civil appeals, the Supreme Court now hears those appeals. However, because the UK is now part of the European Union, the *European Court of Justice* (ECJ), based in Luxembourg, is the final appellate court, where appeals from the Supreme Court lie. Decisions of the ECJ are binding on English courts (European Communities Act 1972).

The criminal court system	The civil court system
o The European Court of Human Rights (Strasbourg)	o The European Court of Justice (Luxembourg) and European Court of Human Rights (Strasbourg)
o The UK Supreme Court replaced the House of Lords as the most senior UK domestic appellate court in October 2009	o The UK Supreme Court replaced the House of Lords as the most senior UK domestic appellate court in October 2009
o Court of Appeal (Criminal Division)	o Court of Appeal (Civil Division)
o High Court (Queen's Bench Division)	o High Court (Chancery Division; Queen's Bench Division; Family Division) [Divisional Court]
o Crown Court	o County court and Magistrate's court
o Magistrate's court	

Figure 4.3 The English court system (highest court at top).

English courts must take note of the rulings of the ECJ. If an English court finds a particular UK statute in conflict with European law, it must hold European law supreme (*Van Gend en Loos v Netherlands Belastingens-administratie* [1963] CMLR 105 ECJ). If there is uncertainty about how a European *directive* applies in English law then a reference can be made to the ECJ under *Article 17*, seeking an opinion.

In civil cases the UK Supreme Court hears appeals from the Court of Appeal (CA), with leave of that court. The CA and all courts below it are bound by the rulings of the UK Supreme Court, which in turn must abide by the ruling of the ECJ.

In criminal cases the Supreme Court hears appeals from the Criminal Division of the Court of Appeal, on *indictable* (serious criminal) offences. The CA must certify that a point of law of general public importance is involved. The Supreme Court also hears appeals from the Civil Divisional of the CA on civil matters. There is no appeal from the Criminal Division of the CA to the Supreme Court on acquittals.

As an *appellate court*, although *judicial* decisions from the Supreme Court are legally binding on all UK courts below it, it does not, however, bind itself and can change a previous ruling. Its decisions may be overruled by legislation enacted by Parliament and by statutes of the European Union or by decision of the ECJ.

Court of Appeal

This court has two Divisions, the Criminal Division, which hears appeals from the Crown Court, and the Civil Division, which hears appeals from the High Court, tribunals and county courts (Figure 4.4).

The CA is a very important and busy appeals court. It deals with more appeal cases than the Supreme Court for obvious reasons. Its decisions bind all the courts below it; in turn it is bound by decisions of the Supreme Court. As the CA hears both civil and criminal appeals, it has a *Criminal* and a *Civil Division*. From the CA a further appeal lies (in important cases, with leave) to the *Supreme Court*. The CA must certify that the point of law is of general public importance, with both courts agreeing that it is worth the Supreme Court hearing the appeal.

The Criminal Division of the CA hears appeals against convictions and sentence. Appeals from the Crown Court in criminal cases come to the Criminal Division of the CA. The appeal may be on a point of law or against a sentence, but only the defendant can appeal, not the Crown. If the appeal against conviction is successful the CA will *quash* the conviction. Having quashed a conviction the CA can substitute a conviction for another offence that a jury could have convicted on.

The UK Court of Appeal	
Civil Division Hears appeals from High Court, tribunals and county courts	**Criminal Division** Hears appeals from the Crown Court

Figure 4.4 The Court of Appeal.

The Civil Division of the CA hears civil appeals mainly from the High Court and the county court. It tends to follow its previous rulings, which bind lower courts.

The High Court

The High Court has 92 Justices or Puisne Judges and comprises three divisions: the *Queen's Bench Division*, the *Chancery Division* and the *Family Division*. Each Division has the authority to act as a court of *first instance* – hearing a case for the first time. Each Division is also an appellate court. High Court work usually involves one judge sitting alone and decisions of the court are binding on lower courts.

The Queen's Bench Division administers the common law, relating, for example, to civil cases, such as nursing negligence cases. With respect to both criminal and civil law, a magistrate's court could be unable to resolve a point of law and may ask the Divisional Court of the Queen's Bench, on the basis of *a case stated*, to resolve the matter. Appeal lies with the Divisional Court from the Crown Court where the latter has received an appeal from the magistrate's court. A further appeal may lie from the Divisional Court to the CA on a point of law. The prosecution or the defence can lodge that appeal.

The Chancery Division handles mainly equity cases. Equity is a branch of law, dealing with 'natural justice'. Williams and Smith (2006) note that in the Middle Ages common law courts sometimes failed to give redress in certain cases. Disappointed litigants would petition the King for extraordinary relief. The King set up the Court of Chancery to deal with such cases. The present-day Chancery Division still operates some of those rules, settling disputes, relating to trusts and wills. If a patient writes a will but there are a number of words that are unclear in a strict legal sense, equity may give legal interpretation thereto. In summary Chancery deals with financial and property cases.

Civil cases from the High Court may be appealed to the CA (Civil Division), or may 'leap-frog' to the Supreme Court (Figure 4.5). As a court of first instance the High Court will hear major civil disputes such as medical and nursing negligence claims.

The Family Division of the High Court deals with family law, including matrimonial cases, adoption, family proceedings and care of children, including disputed medical treatment. It can order family maintenance out of a deceased's estate. As an appellate court it hears appeals from magistrates' courts, county courts and the Crown Court.

Crown Court

The Crown Court mainly handles criminal proceedings. It tries most indictable (serious) criminal cases: rape, murder, manslaughter and so on. As well as being a court of first instance the Crown Court hears appeals from magistrates' courts. Its trials are by a jury of 12 men and women, presided over by a judge. Sometimes justices of the peace sit with a recorder or circuit judge, voting on sentence. However, it is the professional judge/recorder who rules on legal trials procedures. You may have heard of the *Old Bailey*, sometimes the 'Bailey'. This is the Central Criminal Court or the Crown Court sitting in the City of London, off Ludgate Hill. The court is bound by decisions of the superior courts. Any member of the public may listen to a criminal trial at the Crown Court. As a student you may wish to visit a Crown Court hearing. You may also want to ask your tutor to set up a visit of your cohort to a coroner's court, which is usually happy to receive students to observe its proceedings.

Appeals from the Crown Court in criminal trials lie with the CA (Criminal Division). The appeal may be on a point of law or of fact or against sentence. Only the defendant can appeal. Successful appeals from the Crown Court against a conviction leads to the

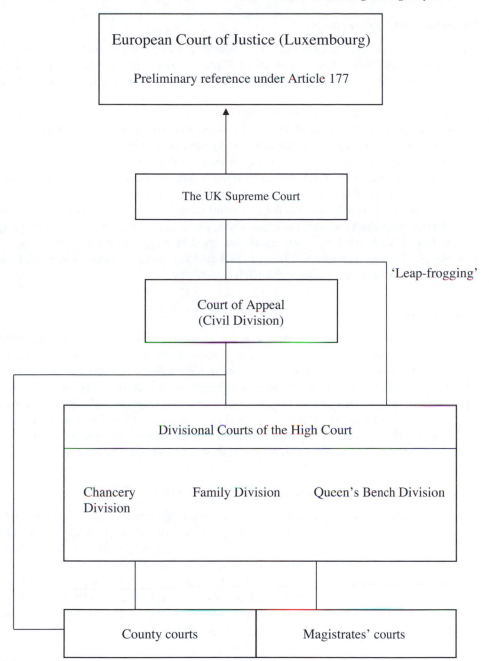

Figure 4.5 System of civil judicature in England and Wales.

conviction being quashed or the lower court's decision being overturned; the higher court can of course substitute a conviction for some other offence for which the jury could have convicted.

Appeals from the magistrates' courts in criminal convictions lie with the Crown Court. Sometimes magistrates, on a point of law, bypass the Crown Court to the Divisional Court of the Queen's Bench Division for a decision (see Figure 4.5).

Magistrates' and county courts

Magistrates' courts deal with the majority (about 98 per cent) of criminal cases; the other 2 per cent are tried in the Crown Courts, or dismissed by the magistrates at the *committal proceedings*. Magistrates decide the fact, the law and the sentence for the least serious criminal cases, the *summary offences*. In the more serious criminal cases (*indictable cases*) the magistrates will act under *committal proceedings* to decide whether there is sufficient evidence for a Crown Court trial. If the criminal offers a plea of guilty to a summary offence, the magistrates will sentence; if a plea is not guilty the magistrates will try the case.

The magistrates also have some civil jurisdiction – matrimonial matters, adoption, child guardianship, maintenance of illegitimate children. There are many magistrates' and county courts in England and Wales, but there are many more magistrates' than county courts.

County courts are at the lowest in the civil court hierarchy. They hear civil claims, especially actions in contract and tort. For example, they hear cases for the recovery of property, such as land. Usually trials in county courts are heard by judges, rarely by a jury. Appeals from the county court on matters of law, fact and evidence go to the Court of Appeal. If the appeal is about bankruptcy it goes to the High Court.

Coroners' courts

A coroner's court is presided over by a coroner, appointed under the Coroners Act 1988, from barristers, solicitors or registered medical practitioners of at least five years' experience. It holds inquests into the death of persons dying suddenly, unnaturally and accidentally. Its jurisdiction is fact finding, for example the cause of death. A coroner may order a post-mortem to establish cause of death. An inquest into someone's death is not a trial, just a fact-finding inquiry to establish cause and circumstances of a sudden, unexplained or suspicious death or suicide. The inquest presents a good learning opportunity for medical, nursing and even law students. If you get the chance to attend one, please take it.

Personal reflection on my only visit as a student nurse to the coroner's court

My first and only coroner's court attendance as a witness goes back to when I was a student working on an admission ward for acutely disturbed and violent psychiatric patients. One of these patients had for no apparent reason punched a fellow patient who fell suddenly to the wooden floor, hit his head, vomited, inhaled and choked on his vomit. He was dead within minutes despite the efforts of myself and the emergency resuscitation team to save him. The coroner's inquest declared 'death by misadventure'. Educationally the visit was eye-opening. See if you tutor will arrange a visit for your class to the coroner's court; then reflect on your visit using your developing portfolio of learning.

The European Court of Justice (ECJ)

Enough has been said above about the ECJ, which adjudicates on European Community matters affecting all member states. The only other point I will make here about the ECJ is that it is not to be confused with the *European Court of Human Rights* based in Strasbourg.

European Court of Human Rights (ECHR)

This is the judicial body of the *Council of Europe* based in Strasbourg. The Council of Europe is to be distinguished from the European Union, whose judicial body is the ECJ based in Luxembourg. The ECHR hears cases alleging breaches of basic human rights and fundamental freedoms from citizens of countries who are signatories to the Convention on Human Rights. Citizens of any country that is a signatory to the Convention on Human Rights may seek redress from the ECHR, if they feel their country in any way abuses their basic human rights and fundamental freedoms. In 1950 Britain signed the Convention and this gave British citizens rights to seek redress from the ECHR, but they had to take their case direct to the Court based in Strasbourg.

The European Convention protects rights and freedoms such as right to life, freedom from torture and slavery, right to liberty and fair trial, freedom of thought and religion. However, before the year 2000 access to the Court by British citizens was limited by availability of personal funds, and a long waiting period of up to five years. Since the Human Rights Act was adopted by British law, British citizens no longer have to depend on the European Court of Human Rights for hearing of their human rights issues but can now go direct to the British courts using the Human Rights Act 1998, which became active in the UK in October 2000.

Brief commentary on the Scottish legal system: differences from England and Wales

There are a number of differences between English law and Scots law, even though both judiciary systems are based on the division between criminal law and civil law.

Criminal cases in Scotland

With respect to the criminal law there is no appeal to the UK Supreme Court (formerly the House of Lords) in Scottish criminal cases unless they involve a human rights issue. In Scotland the highest criminal court is the *High Court of Judiciary*. The court serves the dual function of acting as a court of *first instance* and acting as an appellate court. The *Sheriff Court* tries the most serious *summary* cases (those involving a summons and tried without a jury) as well as the least serious *indictable* cases. In these indictable cases the Sheriff sits with a jury. In the Scottish criminal court the person who brings the case against the accused/defendant is a 'local' prosecutor called the *Procurator Fiscal*, quite a contrast to England and Wales, where the Crown Prosecutor/Crown Prosecution Service brings the case.

In Scotland the lowest criminal court is the *District Criminal Court*, which is presided over by a magistrate. These District Courts, like magistrates' courts in England and Wales, deal with a wide variety of summary cases, petty crimes and minor offences. Under the Children (Scotland) Act 1995, children under 16 years old who are alleged to have committed a crime, and who for whatever reason may be in need of compulsory detention, are tried in specialist courts that are in addition to the District Courts.

Civil cases in Scotland

Unlike the situation in Scottish criminal cases (except those with a human rights issue), the UK Supreme Court is the final appellate court in the UK for Scottish civil cases. The UK Supreme Court decisions bind all lower Scottish civil courts. For the purposes of Scottish civil cases, below the UK Supreme Court is the *Court of Session*, made up of an *Inner House* and an *Outer House*. The Outer House operates as a court of first instance, hearing new cases. Occasionally the Outer House operates with a jury. The *Inner House* deals mainly with appeals. The lowest civil court in Scotland is the *Sheriff Court*, which is the equivalent of the English county court. It deals with a large number of civil cases.

Table 4.1 Answers to the quiz given in Student portfolio reflective exercise 4.2

Questions	Civil law	Criminal law
1. Main purpose(s)?	Upholds rights of individuals; regulates legal relationships between people, e.g. in families (family law). Regulates legal agreements and promises, e.g. contract law; provides compensation for civil wrongs, e.g. negligence, defamation, trespass. Awards injunctions	Maintains law and order, protects society, defines crimes and therefore society's limits of acceptable human behaviour. Punishes and rehabilitates criminals
2. Who originates/brings the case? (Clue: think of Bloggs v Bloggs)	The person(s) whose rights are affected	The state, through the Crown Prosecution Service
3. Legal title/name of person who brings the case?	'Claimant' ('plaintiff' before April 1999)	The prosecutor in the name of the Crown. (Hence *R v Bloggs*.)
4. Legal descriptor of person against whom case brought?	The defendant/respondent	The defendant
5. Standard of proof required?	On the balance of probabilities	Beyond reasonable doubt
6. If found culpable we say the person is?	Liable (if not culpable we say 'not liable')	Guilty (if not culpable we say 'not guilty', and person acquitted)
7. Legal sanction against the culpable person?	Pays compensation, sometimes forbidden to do certain things, specific performance of e.g. contract, etc.	Punishment, e.g. fine, imprisonment, community service, probation, mental hospital, suspended sentence, guardianship order
8. Name all the courts (hierarchically) that could take part in the trial, including appeals. Working from left to right name the highest court first	European Court of Justice (Luxembourg) – UK Supreme Court – Court of Appeal – High Court with Chancery, Family and Queen's Bench Divisions – County Courts and, to lesser degree, Magistrates' Courts in certain family proceedings	European Court of Justice (Luxembourg) and European Court of Human Rights (Strasbourg) – UK Supreme Court – Court of Appeal – High Court (Criminal Division: Queen's Bench) – Crown Court – Magistrates' Court
9. Name the person(s) making the decision in the courts	Judge or a panel of judges, occasionally a jury	Magistrates or a jury under guidance of a judge
10. State the powers available to the courts	From injunction to damage, otherwise called compensation	From absolute discharge, through conditional discharge, bindover, fine and compensation, probation, community service, suspended sentence, hospital order, to imprisonment, e.g. life
11. If this is a Scottish case with which court in the UK does final appeal rest?	UK Supreme Court (formerly House of Lords)	High Court of Judiciary (Scotland)

Chapter summary

This chapter underpins the legal issues covered in this book. In this chapter we examined types and sources of English law, distinguishing between statute and common law, primary and secondary legislation, civil and criminal law, private and public law, and the relationship of English law to EU law. All the way through the chapter we have examined the implications of the various aspects of law for nursing care, focusing on certain key common law cases such as *Donoghue v Stevenson*, *Airedale NHS Trust v Bland* and *Gillick v Norfolk AHA* as important examples of case law impacting on nursing. We also examined how a Bill becomes an Act of Parliament. We examined what is meant by crime, elements of a crime, and defences to crime, and have linked these elements to situations where health professionals have engaged in criminal and negligent practices to the disadvantage of their patients. In examining defences to crime, we stressed the critically of nurses not being able to rely on the notion of *following superior orders* as defences to criminal or negligent nursing practice.

We looked at contract law in relation to definition and explanations, application in private life and in relation to your contract of employment as a nurse. The chapter gave you an opportunity to analyse two patient scenarios, one relating to the crime of theft, the other to negligent nursing practice. We looked at the English court hierarchy and how it may affect us as nurses; for example, references were made to nurses and other health professionals being able to take advantage of visiting the Crown Court or the coroner's court in relation to their learning and development as a health professional. In relation to public versus private law, we examined the case of *R v Cambridge Health Authority ex parte B* (A Minor) [1995], where the child's parents had failed to force the health authority to treat their 10-year-old daughter suffering from leukaemia. The case was discussed in relation to the management of scarce NHS resources. Many opportunities were presented throughout the chapter for personal reflection and portfolio development, drawing on legal knowledge.

5 Consent
Legal, ethical and professional issues

Objectives of this chapter

After reading this chapter you should be able to:

*   demonstrate understanding of consent – definition, meanings, informed consent, nursing practice implications;
*   describe types/forms of consent in clinical practice – strengths and limitations;
*   discuss consent and mental capacity in adults and children, mentioning patients detained under the Mental Health Act;
*   use law to discuss grounds for refusal of consent to treatment and implications for treatment and nursing care;
*   critically evaluate the links between consent under nurses' PCC, case law, contract of employment and ethics;
*   describe how the Mental Capacity Act 2005 relates to consent.

Introduction

Certain key *legal principles* and the *ethics of autonomy* lie at the root of the necessity to always obtain patients *informed* consent to treatment. 'Informed' means the patient has been given the right type of information on which to base his/her consent. Informed consent is a prerequisite for any medical intervention (WHO, 1994). The aim of this chapter is to examine *consent* in terms of its ethical, legal and professional dimensions, relating the discussion to the relevant NMC standards for pre-registration nursing education and competencies domains. Links will be made between the Mental Capacity Act 2005 and the nature of patient consenting or refusing to consent to treatment. Every nurse needs to secure patients' consent before treating them. Consent may be for investigations, observations, treatment or even participation in research. Consent can also be for sharing the patient's information with other health professionals who have a need to know.

Patients have the right to consent to, or to refuse to consent to, treatment, investigations or participation in research, even if refusal to consent to treatment is to the patient's peril. Yet, sadly, research by Aveyard (2005, p. 19) has found that registered nurses with at least one year's post-registration experience revealed that they have not always obtained patients' consent prior to giving nursing care. Furthermore, refusal of care 'was often ignored' and nurses 'were often unsure how to proceed with care when the patient was unable to consent'. This is a sad state of affairs that helps to justify inclusion of this chapter in the present book.

Patients do not have a right to demand treatment, but have an undisputed right to expect that health professionals will obtain their consent prior to treatment (Aveyard, 2005). Indeed the BMA (2002) makes the point that not only patients have right to consent and refusal, but doctors and other health professionals too where the latter consider requested treatments as 'clinically inappropriate' (p. 4). But why should nurses bother about consent? What are the implications of failing to obtain patients' consent? The answer to these questions lies in the ethical, legal and professional obligations a nurse has towards a patient and these will be explained in this chapter.

Definition and meanings of consent

Definitions and meaning of 'consent' are at best 'ambiguous' (Gillon, 2003, p. 113). In the most simplistic everyday sense, *consent* means *agreement, acceptance* or *assent*. But to simply *agree* or *assent* to something does not satisfy the notion of *informed consent* in clinical practice. There must be genuine agreement to consent, for example to nursing care and medical treatment. Consent must show that the patient consenting is:

- properly informed (What is to be done? How? Why? Risks?);
- mentally competent;
- not subject to undue influence, coercion or threat but consenting freely.

Informed consent

Unless otherwise indicated (e.g. if the patient is unconscious) the nurse is expected to provide sufficiently appropriate information to the patient (e.g. the nature of the treatment, risks involved, nature of the observations and investigations to be done). The nurse must ensure the patient understands the information; if (s)he does not, then the consent obtained is not *informed* and is therefore fraudulent.

When the appropriate pre-consenting information is provided and understood by the patient the resultant consenting act is an *informed* one. If the consent is not properly informed it is invalid because the patient who is 'consenting' would not have been aware of what (s)he had consented to. For consent to be valid it must be given *voluntarily* in an *uncoerced and non-threatening manner* by a mentally competent patient. Where the patient is incompetent but has in place a valid *Lasting Power of Attorney (LPA)*, consent to or refusal of treatment may be given by the donee of that power on the patient's behalf, according to the strict terms of the LPA and the patient's best interest. (More is said below about an LPA in Chapter 13). 'Consent' given under *threat, duress or persuasion* is not *autonomous* consent. Indeed, O'Neil (2003) takes the view that *informed consent* is designed to prevent deceit and coercion.

Mental competence and autonomy in consent

The information given to the person to inform his/her consenting decision must be understood (Hope *et al.*, 2003; Lidz *et al.*, 1986). To be valid the consent must also come from a *mentally competent patient* exercising his/her right to autonomy. Within healthcare practice, *informed consent* can best be defined summarily as a conscious, active (rather than passive) autonomous decision on the part of the competent consenting person.

The Mental Capacity Act (MCA) 2005, Section 2(1), makes clear that as a health professional you should assume patients aged 16 or older are competent to make decisions about their care, unless evidence suggests otherwise, and that their consent in matters of their care is essential (*R v Sullivan* [1984] AC 156, 170–1). *Mental capacity* within the terms of the MCA means ability to make a decision. The MCA takes the view that where capacity is lacking then care is given in the patient's *best interest*. Moreover, the MCA S. 2(1) states that a person 'lacks capacity in relation to a matter if at the material time he is unable to make a decision for himself in relation to the matter' due to 'impairment' or 'disturbance in the functioning of the mind or brain'. Furthermore, S. 3(1) of the MCA indicates that for a person to be regarded as unable to make decisions he must be unable to:

- grasp and understand the information pertaining to the decision;
- retain the necessary information;
- use the information in the decision making;
- communicate the decision so it can be understood.

A person is not to be regarded as unable to understand the information that informs his decision making if he is able to grasp it in a manner appropriate to his situation. For example, if the nurse can make his/her patient who is suffering from some brain dysfunction, for example a degree of learning disability, understand what is expected of him/her, using simple language, drawings and/or diagrams, then this will be satisfactory to the principles within the Code relating to the MCA. Every reasonable practical step must be taken to help the person to understand the information necessary for his/her decision-making. The MCA Code of practice further states that a person must not be regarded as unable to decide simply 'because he makes an unwise decision'. In spite of these facts the MCA Code of Practice lists below possible conditions that may lead to impairment, disturbance and mal functioning of the brain. For a nurse it is important to bear in mind that it is also possible that any of these conditions or a combination of them may have a propensity to lead to the patient's lack of capacity to make competent decisions:

- long-term effects of brain damage;
- effects of mental illness;
- severe learning disability;
- degrees of dementia;
- mental/physical conditions inducing confusion, unconsciousness;
- delirium states and altered consciousness from brain damage;
- alcoholic and drug-induced intoxication or drunkenness.

One should not assume that because one's patients may be suffering from any of the conditions above they have lost the capacity to decide or give consent to treatment. For example, people with mental illness do not necessarily lack capacity. By the same token people with a severe mental illness may experience a temporary, or even permanent, loss of capacity to make decisions about their treatment. In the case of *Re C (Adult: Refusal of treatment)* [1994] 1 WLR 290, a patient C, at Broadmoor, was suffering from paranoid schizophrenia. He developed gangrene of his foot following an injury. He refused to let doctors amputate his foot even though he accepted that the doctors believed he would die if he did not have surgery. At court when doctors tried to get the court to give authority to remove the man's gangrenous leg, Judge Thorpe said the doctors should not be allowed to amputate his foot without his consent, because in spite of his mental illness he:

- understood the condition and treatment offered;
- was able to retain the information;
- was able to weigh up the information in arriving at his refusal;
- in his own way, believed the information and used it to arrive at a clear choice – not to have the surgery which would have amputated his foot.

Personal cultural and religious values impinging on legal decision making

Another dimension in the *Re C* case was the patient's strong cultural and religious belief that he and God would get him through the illness without the need for surgery. Apparently he was proved correct as it was later reported that he recovered without surgery. It seems his religious faith and other factors too had worked for him. This point serves to show the criticality of accepting that your patient is not just a person with legal rights; (s)he also has personal, cultural and religious beliefs on which (s)he may well base his/her consent to treatment or live his/her life otherwise. Nevertheless the court was there to ensure C's right to refuse treatment, thereby preserving for him a climate that allowed him to hold on to his religious and cultural values and beliefs.

Many of your patients have deeply held rational values and beliefs which need to be respected. Simply because your patient may be labelled 'mentally ill' does not mean they have lost their right to autonomous consent or refusal of treatment. A decision that may appear irrational to you as a nurse may make good and rational sense to a patient, within the context of his personal and cultural values, beliefs, morals, ethical values and religion. In spite of a patient experiencing some mental or mind disturbance (s)he may still be able to make decisions about his/her health and care. It will be a matter of degree of mental impairment. All patients must be properly assessed as to their capacity to consent. Opportunity needs to be afforded the patient to help him/her understand information necessary to give consent in matters of his/her treatment. Under the legal ruling in the common law case of *Re C*, an adult who has mental impairment or disability of mind can still possess capacity, however irrational and impaired his/her reasoning seems to be. Under the MCA 2005 a person without mental impairment or disability of mind cannot be regarded as lacking capacity.

Refusing to consent on religious grounds: case of Jehovah's Witnesses

Patients who object to treatment on religious grounds, for example Jehovah's Witnesses refusing to have blood transfusion, must not be deemed to lack capacity to decide. Having said this, in the case of *Re T* (1992) Refusal of blood transfusion (see further details below) the court authorised a life-saving blood transfusion, previously refused by a young pregnant woman. Why? The judge took the view that the young woman, a Jehovah's Witness, was not in a fit state (did not have capacity) to make a valid decision of refusal at the time she did. In fact her devout Jehovah's Witness mother had overborne her mind in persuading her to refuse the transfusion. In this sense it could be argued that her decision was not her own rational decision. Her mother had overborne her will. Had the court been satisfied that this young woman had made her mind up in the absence of undue pressure from her mother, its ruling that she should have the blood transfusion might have been different. The message for healthcare professionals dealing with the issue of patient's consent to treatment is to ensure that when the patient makes the decision (s)he is in a fit state of mind to do so; not under undue influence, pressure or coercion. In other words (s)he has capacity and has made his/her decision freely. Consent has to be freely given to be recognised in law.

However, contrast the above case with that of *Re E (A Minor: wardship: medical treatment)* [1993] 1 FLR 386. In this case a boy of 15 years 9 months, suffering from leukaemia, required a blood transfusion. This was refused by him and his parents, devout Jehovah's Witnesses. However, the court made the youth a ward of court so that he could receive the transfusion. In this case a number of critical issues influenced the court's decision: the judge decided the boy was sensible enough to make decisions regarding his own well-being; however, he lacked full understanding of the blood transfusion; the child's health was paramount and had to take priority.

A similar ruling was made by the High Court in the case of *Re S (A Minor: consent to medical treatment)* [1994] 2 FLR 1065. In this case a girl, of 15.5 years, suffering from thalassaemia, had decided to discontinue having monthly blood transfusion, after she and her mother had started to attend the preaching of Jehovah's Witnesses. The court ruled that her blood transfusions were to continue in the girl's *best interest*, because she lacked *Gillick competence* to decide for herself what was best for her. (The Gillick case is explained in Chapter 4.) In the case of the 15.5-year-old *(Re S)*, the judge did not think the girl was emotionally mature enough to make the decision to discontinue her life-saving blood transfusions.

These two cases do offer some grounds to question the consistency of the court's rationale and how these decisions stand alongside the present MCA 2005 principles. Why? In the case of *Re E* the judge appeared to agree that the boy at 15 years 9 months was intelligent enough to make decisions regarding his well-being. Yet the court ruled that the boy should have the transfusion. The judge may well have thought that, in spite of his intelligence, under the 'Gillick'/'Fraser' competence principle he lacked the necessary emotional maturity and full understanding of what was involved in a blood transfusion. The current MCA 2005, in setting out the grounds for determining capacity, emphasised the situation in respect to those aged 16 and over only; a point that may prevent confusion and clashes between past common law cases and future cases using the MCA.

In the case of *Re B (Consent to Treatment: Capacity)* [2002] 1 FLR 1090 the court made the point that healthcare professionals:

> must not allow their emotional reaction to or strong disagreement with the decision of the patient to cloud their judgement in answering the primary question whether the patient has the mental capacity to make the decision.

So, regardless of how the healthcare professional personally feels about the patient's final decision to accept or refuse treatment, one should try to remember that so long as the patent is competent (has capacity) (s)he has the legal and autonomous right to decide for him-/ herself, even if to the health professional the patient's reasoned decision seems illogical, irrational or foolish.

Advanced decisions and lasting power of attorney under the MCA 2005

As a health professional you should note that under the MCA 2005, ss. 24–25, mentally competent adults (18 years and older) can make *advanced decisions (living wills) to refuse treatment* at some point in the future should they lose capacity to so decide for themselves. Only the Mental Health Act 1983 can override such advanced decisions. The person must be at least 18 and competent to make a living will. The decision is only negative, not positive; in other words it can only refuse, not order specific treatment. Where the advanced decision refuses life-saving treatment it must be in writing, signed by the patient and witnessed.

Invalidity of advanced decisions

Section 25 of the MCA 2005 explains that the living will may become invalid if the person still having capacity withdraws the will, or has set up an LPA that cancels the advanced decision. In the case of *HE v A Hospital NHS Trust* [2003] EWHC 1017 (FAM) a Jehovah's Witness had previously made a living will to the effect that under no circumstances should she be given a blood transfusion even if this meant her death. She later needed a blood transfusion, which the court agreed she could have since evidence at that stage indicated that she was no longer a Jehovah's Witness; she was in fact engaged to be married to a Muslim. Hence the court suspended or cancelled the advanced decision. Where life is threatened and the status of an advanced decision in doubt the court will usually come down in favour of life support being given (Herring, 2008).

Lasting power of attorney

In the case of *Re F (Mental Patient: Sterilisation)* [1989] 2 All ER 545, the House of Lords had made it clear that no one had the power to consent on behalf of an incompetent patient. Nevertheless, there may be instances where an individual would wish another to make medical decisions about their treatment, if they became incapacitated. A person when mentally competent can donate power to another party to consent or refuse to consent to medical treatment on their behalf at some time in future should they lack capacity. The donated power is called a *lasting power of attorney (LPA)* and must be registered with the Office of Public Guardian. The competent person donating the power is the *donor*, and the recipient of the power the *donee*; both must be 18 years old or over. More than one donee may be appointed, and, unless the LPA says otherwise, both must act jointly [MCA 2005, s. 9(5)]. If the donees genuinely believe they are making the correct decision (i.e. in the patient's best interest) and the court subsequently thinks otherwise, they will not face legal action in either tort or criminal law [MCA 2005, s. 4(9)]. Under s. 11(8) the LPA has no power to authorise or stop the carrying out of life-sustaining treatment unless the instrument makes specific provision in this regard. Donees must be seen to operate on the critical maxim of *the patient's best interest*.

LPAs can be for decision making relating to health, welfare and the management of property. If your patient lacks capacity you should find out whether an LPA or an advanced decision is in place. (It is also possible that some patients' files/notes may contain the older *enduring power of attorney*, made before 1 October 2007. What is important about these older powers is that they delegate power to donees only in cases of property and affairs, whereas the newer power, the LPA, also covers power in respect of personal welfare, including right to consent or refuse consent to treatment on the donor's behalf.) From 1 October 2007 no new *enduring power of attorney* could be set up, but those in existence then can remain. The person holing an LPA must be consulted and his/her consent obtained regarding consent to or refusal of treatment where the donor has lost capacity.

Court of Protection and deputy

Where there is no existing LPA and the patient's mental capacity is lost, the Court of Protection is there to appoint a suitable deputy to act on the patient's behalf, making decisions about health and other welfare issues relating to the patient. Only under such strict legal standards can such consent to treatment on behalf of another be given. Normally, there is no consent by proxy for a competent adult, and this is where the principle of acting *in the patient's best interest* comes in, in an emergency unconscious state for instance, where urgent medical care is needed.

Advanced decisions may be verbal but must be evidenced or aurally evidenced by others. In other words other people should be able to attest to the fact that that was indeed the patient's wish; they had heard him/her say so. Under the MCA 2005, for legal or authenticated certainty, an advanced decision involving refusal of life-saving treatment must be in writing, signed by the person or his deputy in his presence, witnessed by a third party and clearly stating that such a decision stands regardless of any risk to the patient's life in future.

Ethical component of consent

Autonomy

Beauchamp and Childress (2008) have argued that human beings are *autonomous*, having a right to self-determination. Ethically, every nurse must respect a competent patient's autonomy: his/her right to self-determination, right to decide, right to consent to or refuse treatment. Besides, this makes for a good nurse–patient relationship, since it presents a sound basis for the trust necessary to facilitate good patient care outcomes. An autonomous person is capable of self-decision. Autonomy is about freedom, liberty and right to self-decisions. It is the capacity to determine what happens to one's body when one becomes a patient: who touches one's body, when, how, for what reason and where. According to Beauchamp and Childress (2001), autonomy is about freedom to act 'freely in accordance with a self-chosen plan' (p. 58). The NMC Code stipulates the centrality of nurses respecting their patient's right to autonomous decision making, and the nurses' obligation to act in the patient's best interest where (s)he has lost the capacity to act him-/herself.

Temporary or permanent lack of competence

What about the individual who lacks autonomy and mental competence temporarily or indeed permanently? Even the autonomous, self-determined person may at times lack mental capacity and may therefore be temporarily unable to give/refuse or even withdraw consent. This can be for a number of reasons, such as illness, unconsciousness, a drunken state, learning difficulty or transient mental confusion. Some of our clients/patients may have been declared legally and mentally incompetent to take personal decisions and to give consent. Some may have had their right to give or refuse to consent to treatment taken away from them, for example by the Mental Health Act (MHA) 1983 as amended by the MHA 2007. Section IV of the Act explains exceptional circumstances under which consent to treatment may not be a prerequisite. Under the MHA 1983 (as amended by the 2007 Act) detained patients can be given medical treatment for mental illness against their will only in accordance with Section IV of the Act. As a nurse you should always act within the law, ensuring you do so in your patient's best interest. (Chapter 15 covers the Mental Health Act 1983 as amended by the MHA 2007.)

It is possible therefore that nurses may be required to care for people who lack mental capacity. As a nurse you need to care for incompetent people to the highest standard possible, just as you would care for and advocate for mentally competent patients, since the mentally incompetent person has no lesser right to treatment and care than the mentally competent individual. Moreover, the mentally incompetent person is even more vulnerable and requires the strong advocacy of the healthcare professional. Ethically then, the nurse's moral and professional duty to respect the person's autonomy to give or refuse to give consent to nursing care and treatment is centred around people's right to *autonomy* and their entitlement to self-determination. No healthcare professional has a paternalistic right to override a patient's autonomy and *self-determination* unless the MHA permits compulsory detainment for treatment. Even so under the new 2007 MHA a detained patient having capacity cannot be forced to have electroconvulsive therapy.

A realistic scenario: how would you deal with it?

What about a situation where a patient says, nurse, I respect the fact that there are several care options, so could you please decide for me? (For example, should I choose radiotherapy for my prostate cancer or should I choose surgery?) What is happening here? Is the patient giving away his autonomy to choose? Such a patient respects the fact that he controls the right to decide but is perhaps attempting to pass over the decision making to the nurse. The first point to make about this situation is that the nurse is not there to decide for the patient. (S)he is there to explain the care options, and where (s)he feels the patient needs extra clarification provide it. In all probability the doctors would have already explained the choices. However, sometimes patients ask nurses to clarify the situation regarding choices available to them. This is acceptable if the nurse has the necessary knowledge. The NMC says you should work within the remit of your competence. What the patient needs is someone prepared to listen to his anxiety and concerns, perhaps re-emphasising the benefits and risks that the doctor has already explained. This approach is really doubly ensuring that the patient is provided enough information for him to exercise autonomy of choice and consent. No one but the mentally competent patient can ultimately decide for him-/herself. Consent is an active rather than a passive act, in which the patient exercises responsibility, autonomy and competence in decision making and gives permission/consent to health professionals to carry out the care available.

Do health professionals always do the right thing in respect to patients' consent?

Although we have said here that nurses and other healthcare professionals owe it to their patients to respect their autonomy, right and freedom to give or refuse consent, history has shown that this clear professional objective has not always been the focus of some nurses or even doctors. For example, research by Aveyard (2005) has shown that registered nurses have not always sought patients' consent, adhered to their refusal of treatment or shown certainty in how to proceed when patients demonstrate inability to consent. Failure to do the right thing in relation to obtaining patients' consent is not confined to the UK or just a recent issue. In the well-known *Tuskegee experiments* in the USA in the 1940s, it was a nurse, Eunice Rivers, who was instrumental in recruiting 399 African-American men to participate in the unethical and horrid research which set out to observe the natural and untreated progress of syphilis in the African-American men's bodies, even though by the 1940s penicillin was available to treat syphilis. The chances are that had the men been correctly informed of the objective of the study they would not have consented to it. In the UK, Beverley Allitt's, Colin Norris's and Harold Shipman's patients too did not consent to dying at their hands. Yet they did!

Nazi atrocities and the Nuremberg Code in relation to patient consent in research

The atrocious Nazi Holocaust in Europe in the period 1933 to 1945 saw some of the most extreme cruelty to humanity, to ordinary citizens, to prisoners of war and to Jews particularly, by medical men, for example the infamous 'Angel of Death', Dr Josef Mengele. The Jews reported to have died at his hands gave no consent to the horrific experiments he carried out on them. Such cruelty was carried out in the name of medical research. The Nuremberg trials not only revealed such atrocities, but led to the famous Nuremberg Code of ethics, followed by the Declaration of Helsinki in 1964 and 1975, setting the standard against which medical research with human subjects would in future be judged. Accordingly, today human participants in medical research must suffer no harm. All participants must be fully *informed* of the nature of the research, including any risks involved, and their *consent sought*.

Other legal components of consent

Here I want to focus on consent in relation to the law around *negligence* and *trespass to the person*, often referred to as *battery*, as well as further focusing on *mental competence* or *capacity*. A number of statutes are relevant to consent. For example, the Children Act 1989 sets out some fundamental principles with respect to consent and minors. The Family Law Reform Act (FLRA) 1969, s. 8(1), and the MCA 2005 make it possible for competent children aged 16 and 17 years to consent to treatment even if parents object. Section 8(1) of the FLRA states: 'and where a minor [16–17 years] has by virtue of this section given an effective consent to any treatment it shall not be necessary to obtain any consent for it from his parent or guardian'.

As the MHA 2007 (see Chapter 15) demonstrates, competent 16- and 17-year-olds can consent to their own 'informal' admission to a mental health hospital notwithstanding parental objection. Moreover, under the 2007 MHA, s. 131 (2)–(5), parents can no longer consent to the 'informal' admission to hospital of their mentally competent child, if the child does not consent, although they can consent in respect to their incapacitated child of any age. This new 2007 MHA provision replaces the common law rule by which a parent could have given consent to treatment (that could have included admission and treatment in a psychiatric hospital) notwithstanding the refusal of the 16- or 17-year-old to consent (read *Re C (Detention: Medical Treatment)* [1997] 2 FLR 180 and paragraph 11.50). To reiterate, under the 2007 MHA that amended the 1983 MHA no person with capacity can be forced against their will to have electro-convulsive treatment (ECT) even if such a person has been formally detained under the MHA. See Chapter 15 for further information on this. As we have seen, the Mental Health Act 1983 (as amended by the Mental Health Act 2007) and the Mental Capacity Act 2005 both play an important part in relation to people consenting or not consenting to treatment.

We will look at the common law (judge-made law) in respect to *battery* and *negligence*. At common law all mentally competent individuals have a right to give or withhold consent, even where refusal of consent to treatment could lead to the individual's death. The reason for refusal of treatment can be good, bad or no reason at all (*Re MB (Adult: refusal to medical treatment)* [1997] 2 FLR 426; *St George's Healthcare NHS Trust v. S* [1998] 3 All ER 673). Maliciously touching a person without his/her consent can constitute a *criminal* offence actionable under the criminal law, or where there was no criminal intent a touch without consent constitutes a *battery* (trespass to the person), actionable under the law of tort. The person who did the touching is sued for *trespass to the person*, being the more correct legal term. Where the touching is malicious, for example a sexual assault, or has other intent to harm the person, the matter is a *criminal* offence. To summarise, then, touching patients without consent is a battery (trespass to the person). Touching maliciously as in a sexual assault is a criminal offence. A careless touch that causes the patient harm can be sued for under the law of negligence. There is a distinction between 'battery' and 'negligence'. In the tort of battery the patient did not give consent to touching and no harm or injury needs to be demonstrated or proved by the person touched. 'Battery' simply means touch; the person touched simply just has to prove that (s)he was touched without his consent; touching without consent is enough for a suit of battery.

In negligence the patient gave consent to the touch, but in the process of the treatment the health professional carelessly injured the patient. The health professional may also be sued in negligence if he had failed prior to the treatment to provide sufficient information to the patient, or has misrepresented the facts in relation to the treatment or the risks involved. In negligence the question is whether the nurse acted in accordance with an acceptable body of nursing opinion in providing sufficient information to the patient, whereas in battery it is a question of whether the patient gave permission (consented) to be touched. To reiterate, the patient in the tort of battery does not need to prove harm; just that (s)he was touched without his/her consent.

To succeed in negligence the patient must show that owing to inadequate information he went ahead and had the treatment which has demonstrably harmed him/her.

Breach of duty

In negligence the patient has to prove that the health professional *owed him/her a duty of care*, *breached it* and *demonstrably injured* him/her. As a nurse you have a legal duty to provide your patient with adequate care, including adequate information to inform his/her decision making regarding consent. In battery the patient needs only to show that (s)he was touched without his/her consent; no harm needs to be proved.

Where the person fears from hearing threatening words that (s)he will be touched without his/her consent this constitutes an *assault*. As indicated above, sexual touching (without consent) is a criminal act, so the male nurse who on reflection took a vaginal swab from the patient without the patient's consent and furthermore without being medically requested to do so committed a criminal act on the patient. He was dismissed from his job as a staff nurse and reported to the then General Nursing Council for professional misconduct.

Remember then, that in *negligence* the patient must prove duty is owed and broken, and harm manifests. The origins of the legal precedent of battery go back to the 1914 judgement in an American case, *Schloendorff v Society of New York Hospital*, in which the presiding judge (J. Cardozo) said: 'every human being of adult years and sound mind has a right to determine what shall be done with his own body; and a surgeon who performed an operation without the patient's consent commits an assault'. English law adopted this US principle.

Negligence and consent

It must be noted that having gained the patient's consent to treat him/her does not prevent a case of *negligence* from being brought if there were failure on the part of the clinician to provide the patient with the necessary information, or to treat him/her carefully so that no unreasonable harm came to the patient. However, in relation to *consent*, it is imperative for the healthcare professional to supply the patient with the necessary information for informed choice/consent. If a nurse fails to provide the prerequisite information, despite having the patient's subsequent 'permission' to carry out the intervention, (s)he can be sued in negligence for *failure to properly inform*. Furthermore, consent without the necessary pre-information is 'fraudulent consent'.

How much information is required for consent to be valid?

In *Chatterton v Gerson* (1981) Judge Bristow said: 'once the patient is informed in broad terms of the nature of the procedure which is intended, and gives her consent, that consent is real, and the cause of the action on which to base a claim for failure to go into risks and implications is negligence, not trespass' (in other words, negligence and not battery). Here is an example: a patient is to have a colonoscopy (looking into the colon by means of a light source passed up via the rectum) to investigate the presence of blood in the patient's stool. The doctor informs the patient that this procedure is confined to just looking into the colon; it is not for treatment interventions. In this case the patient cannot sue the doctor for battery since she was informed of the procedure of a colonoscopy and consented to it. However, the doctor has given no information to the patient about possible risks of the procedure; equally, he had not told the patient in advance that further intervention would be carried out during the investigation. However, whilst carrying out the investigation the doctor finds some polyps which he regards as precancerous and removes them. In the process he perforates the patient's colonic walls such that she bleeds heavily and develops peritonitis (painful information of the peritoneal lining of the gut). Here the doctor could be sued in negligence for failure to inform the patient of the additional interventions he would pursue (trespass on the patient's person) and of the risks associated with the procedure (negligence). He may face a charge of criminal negligence for removing part of the patient's body without her permission. As a nurse you must obtain the patient's permission for all the treatment given. Do not take it for granted that because the patient held up her arm the last time to have her blood pressure taken, you still have that consent tomorrow. Ask for that consent and get it before you proceed.

Failure to inform

One of the best authorities in case law for evidence that a health professional can be sued in negligence for failure to inform is the case of *Sidaway v Bethlem Royal Hospital Governors* (1985). Mrs Sidaway had persistent neck and shoulder pain. Her surgeon advised her to have a spinal operation to relieve her pain. He told her the operation could disturb a nerve root and what could result from this, but failed to mention the possibility of damage to her spinal cord. Although the risk of damage was less than 1 per cent, any resulting injury could be mild to very severe. Mrs Sidaway consented to the operation, which was carried out with due care and skill. However, during the operation her spinal cord was damaged and she became severely disabled.

She sued the surgeon and the hospital governors, alleging the surgeon's breach of duty owed to her to warn her of all possible risks linked to this operation. She argued that her consent to have the operation in the first place was not an informed one. Mrs Sidaway lost in the court of first instance and at the Court of Appeal also. The case was appealed to the House of Lords, where it finally failed. The Lords held that the liability in respect to a surgeon's duty to inform his patients of risks was the same test as that in diagnosis and treatment. In other words, the *Bolam test* applied. This test says that, if a doctor's practice is in accordance with and to the same standard as a respectable and responsible body of medical opinion operating at the time, then he will not be liable. At that time Mrs Sidaway's surgeon's non-disclosure of risk of damage to her spinal cord accorded with the neurosurgical opinion and practice of the day. Thus the surgeon was not liable.

A word of warning to nurses

It may in future be considered by the court that it is out of step for clinicians (nurses included) to be simply following what other clinicians of the day are doing, without further questioning and checking for the latest and most up-to-date research evidence (evidence-based practice). Nurses must constantly strive to emulate the best practice, based on the most up-to-date available research evidence, such as NICE guidelines, such that when a patient consents to a procedure, (s)he is in fact consenting to the most up-to-date science and art of nursing and medical practice. Besides, as the *Bolitho v City & Hackney HA* case shows, the bodily of qualified nursing opinion relied on must have a 'logical basis', all risks and benefits being weighed up and care discharged only on the best available evidence.

Forms of consent

Consent may be implicit or explicit, oral or written (BMA, 2002; Aveyard, 2005). The law respects the three types of consent used in medical and nursing practice: *written, verbal* and *implied. Written consent* represents the strongest evidence that consent was given. Consent for invasive procedures involving risks must be given in writing. It is difficult to state categorically at what level of risk health professionals should inform patients, as courts are reluctant to state precise figures of risk to be disclosed. In the Sidaway case Lord Bridge suggested that a doctor would need very good reason not to inform his patient of a 10 per cent risk of stroke. Hope and colleagues (2003) note that doctors need to disclose lower probabilities of serious risks.

Patients need information on the nature of the event, the problems, risks and benefits of the procedure. *Information must be understood. It is not good enough to just talk at the patient, believing (s)he understands. Merely signing a 'consent-for-operation form' is not enough.* Information must be given sensitively, clearly, with care, using appropriate language and vocabulary, relevant to the capacity of the person, to facilitate understanding. When speaking to a person whose level of intelligence is low and uptake of information slow, the information giver needs to take these factors into account. As long as the person receiving the information has the requisite mental and legal capacity to understand and consent, then the most appropriate means of communication should be used. It may be appropriate to use audiovisual aids to facilitate understanding when giving information to patients with learning disability, hearing, sight and speech defects. The overriding objective is that the patient understands the information so that his/her subsequent consent is *informed.*

One recalls detecting that the information doctors claimed to have given to patients prior to signing consent for operation has not always been understood. Hence it is a good practice for nurses to ensure that patients fully understand what has been said to them and what they understand they have signed up to. If a nurse believes a patient has not understood what the doctor said, (s)he has a professional, legal, moral and ethical responsibility and obligation to ask the doctor to properly inform the patient. This team approach reflects holism; an approach that puts the patient at the centre of care and accords respect to the ethical notions of beneficence and non-maleficence within the framework of the multidisciplinary team. Forms relating to written consent may be found on the DOH website.

Consent by word of mouth

Consent by word of mouth is valid under English law. Dimond (2008, p. 141) points out that many of the less risky treatments are carried out without formal signature. The real problem with verbal consent is the possibility that the patient could deny having consented, unless the nurse had a witness that the information had been given. I always remind nurses that, should they have any reason to believe a verbal consent could be questioned, they should get another nurse to evidence oral consent, for example where patients express a wish to discharge themselves against nursing and medical advice, and are perhaps refusing to sign a piece of paper indicating their self-discharge. Where one considers that self-discharge is potentially dangerous to the patient, but the voluntary patient insists on such discharge, it is best to get him/her to sign a self-discharge form. If there is not a standard form, then ask the patient to write his/her intention on a sheet of paper and sign to the effect that (s)he has discharged him-/herself against medical advice. If the patient refuses to sign a *discharge against medical advice form*, it is best to get a colleague to witness that you had advised the patient against self-discharge. Best of all, write accurate nursing notes about the event, sign it and get your colleague to witness and countersign your entry.

Implied consent

Implied consent means that the person indicates consent by action, not writing or by speech. It needs to be clear that a particular action represents consent. Implied consent may be from a patient/client who cannot speak or write, but whose action nevertheless indicates consent; it can be from a person with none of these limitations. Some of the (implied) actions are obvious, for example a patient opens his mouth to receive a thermometer, or rolls up her sleeve to indicate willingness to receive an injection or to have her blood pressure taken, or smiles to indicate consent, or nods the head to indicate consent. In implied consent no words are uttered, no form signed, but from experience it is clear that the patient is consenting. In implied consent by a mentally competent person, it is important for nurses to provide the patient with the necessary information that informs the consent. Implied consent has certain weaknesses: it may not be clear that the patient is consenting or what to; the wrong conclusion about the implied consent may be drawn. Putting an arm forward may be for a vaccination, but it could also be for having one's blood pressure and pulse recorded. To avoid confusion smart nurses always tell the patients precisely what they want them to do, the behaviour required, to make it clear they are consenting, and to what. In the case *O'Brien v Cunard Steamship Co.* [1891] 28 NE 266 (an Australian case), a passenger on a ship who held out his arm to indicate willingness to accept a vaccine lost his case claiming battery.

Who can give consent and what is the position of children?

If a child with capacity or without capacity is unconscious medical emergency medical care may be given to him/her in his/her 'best interest'. In the case of a child of any age lacking capacity those with parental responsibility may consent to treatment on his/her behalf. No relative, friend or health professional can give consent to treatment on behalf of a competent adult, or a competent 16- or 17-year-old child. Consent by proxy is not allowed.

With respect to minors under 16 years, a child who has capacity under what is called 'Gillick' or 'Fraser' competence can consent to treatment notwithstanding parental objection. It is expected that parents will always act in their children's best interest. However, in reality this is not always the case and is precisely for such reasons that we have law such as the Children Act 1989 as amended in parts by the Children Act 2004 protecting children's rights. Hope and colleagues (2003) have pointed out that the Children Act 1989 holds the general principles that children must be protected. Children are real persons and although they may not have full power of autonomy they should nevertheless be listened to and their concerns considered.

Under the Children Act 1989 as amended by the Children Act 2004, parents have *parental responsibility* in the following order:

- mother of the child;
- father if married to mother at time of insemination or birth;
- father not married to mother at time of insemination or birth but who acquires parental responsibility by a later marriage, or by written agreement with the mother, by a court order (e.g. residence and parental responsibility orders), or if following the mother's death father is appointed the child's guardian.

For further information on 'parental responsibility' see Chapter 14, which deals with the protection of children.

Parents with parental responsibility can consent to treatment on behalf of minors under 16 who are not 'Gillick' competent. Parents having parental responsibility may also consent for their child under 18 who lacks capacity. One parent can give consent. Moreover, one parent does not have to confer with the other for consent to be valid.

It must be borne in mind that people may acquire parental responsibility in ways other than those outlined above; for example, by adoption where the 'blood' parent(s) has/have relinquished parental responsibility and the adopted parents have taken on this responsibility through court proceedings. It may be where parents with parental responsibility appoint guardians to look after their children after their death. It may be in a case where a person has acquired a residence order for the child usually through the court, for example where grandparents have taken over the residential care of the child, where the mother is incapable or unable to care for the child. A person may also gain parental responsibility by being granted an emergency protection order. Parental responsibility is a complex thing; a nurse could find him-/herself obtaining consent from people who acquired parental responsibility in different ways.

Statutes, common law, children and consent

The Mental Capacity Act 2005 presumes that 16-year-olds have capacity to consent unless otherwise indicated. Under the Family Law Reform Act 1969, 16- and 17-year-olds in England and Wales are presumed to have the capacity to consent to medical treatment unless there are grounds to the contrary. Consent obtained this way is as good as that of a competent adult. Children under 16 years of age are deemed not to have the capacity to consent unless they have acquired such capacity by being 'Gillick' or 'Fraser' competent. Under *Gillick competence* [arising out of the (common law) case of *Gillick v West Norfolk and Wisbech AHA and the DHSS* (1985)], where healthcare professionals make a judgement that a child under 16 years old has the requisite capacity, by virtue of possessing the requisite maturity, intelligence, understanding and knowledge to understand the purpose of the treatment and the effects and side effects of such treatment, (s)he can consent to treatment without parental approval. (The *Gillick* case is summarised in Chapter 3.) This competence is sometimes referred to as *Fraser competence,* after the Judge, Lord Justice Fraser, one of the Law Lords who decided the case.

With respect to children under 18, the law (e.g. the Family Law Reform Act and the Mental Capacity Act 2005) asserts that unless otherwise proven those of 16 and 17 years of age have capacity to consent to their own treatment. Equally, the law accepts that children of any age who lack capacity can have decisions made for them by their parents or legal guardians. It seems that the law is prepared to grant increasing freedom, right and autonomy to minors in relation to acknowledging their ability to be heard with respect to consent to medical treatment. The health and welfare of the child is paramount and this can lead to an override of parental objection to treatment where that treatment would prevent harm to the child. The general direction of the law is that neither parental nor the child's decision should make a child be exposed to injury or dangers.

Treating patients without consent under the Mental Health Act (MHA)

Under the MHA 1983 (revised by the MHA 2007) there are circumstances in which formally admitted patients with a mental disorder may be treated against their will. For example, under the MHA a nurse could administer medication to a patient with a mental disorder if (s)he were formally admitted to hospital for treatment and his/her condition warranted the medication. Under the Mental Capacity Act (MCA) 2005, a person who lacks the prerequisite mental capacity may have actions taken by healthcare professionals in his/her best interest. 'Informal' patients in mental healthcare facilities can consent to their own treatment if they have capacity, but if they lack capacity and therefore are unable to consent they can be treated under the MCA 2005. Under this Act the Court of Protection or appointed deputy under the Act can act on behalf of the patient. If the patient has in place a valued lasting power of attorney that (s)he as the donor of the power agreed to and signed when (s)he had capacity, that authority stands, but can only rule out a particular treatment. It cannot compel the medical staff to give a specified treatment. Under the MCA 2005 a donee of the power, who has a 'power of attorney' to make decisions (including healthcare ones) on behalf of the donor, must do so in the donor's *best interest. A court of law can override a donee's decision where it considers that such a decision is not in the interest of the donor.*

Right to refuse treatment

In English common law, mentally competent patients have a right to refuse consent to treatment even if medical opinion supports the fact that by not consenting to treatment the patient will die. Outside the Mental Health Act 1983, as amended by the MHA 2007, a mentally competent patient cannot be forced to accept treatment. This principle was also borne out in the case of *Re MB* (1997):

A pregnant woman suffering a needle phobia refused a pre-Caesarean section injection. The High Court held that her phobia rendered her mentally incapable to decide not to have the operation. The Court of Appeal concurred with the High Court, but emphasised that had the lady been competent she could have refused the operation.

A mentally competent adult can refuse treatment even if (s)he is 'mentally ill'. Being mentally ill does not automatically deprive the person of capacity. Here is a longer summary of *Re C (An Adult: Refusal of Medical Treatment)* (1994), referred to above.

A 68-year-old male patient suffering from paranoid schizophrenia was detained in Broadmoor Hospital. He developed gangrene on one foot and the doctors tried to persuade him to have it amputated to save his life. He refused to consent to this and successfully petitioned the court to issue an injunction to stop the hospital from amputating his foot without his consent. He accepted and believed what the doctors told him would happen to him if he refused to have the foot amputated. However, although he was somewhat paranoid, he shared the belief that he and God would help him through his illness, and so decided not to have the leg amputated. He won the case in the Court because the hospital was unable to establish that he lacked adequate understanding of his problem and the medical treatment proposed. The court believed that he possessed mental capacity as (a) he was able to understand and retain relevant treatment information; (b) he believed the information; (c) he had arrived at a clear conclusion, good or bad.

The message to the nurse is this: simply because a patient is mentally ill does not mean (s)he has lost capacity to consent or refuse to consent. Another important principle related to consent is this: *when a patient refuses treatment you must be sure that (s)he has the necessary capacity to make such a decision and had not been subjected to undue influences of another.* This was established in *Re T* (1992) – Refusal of blood transfusion: see below.

In *Re T*, a pregnant woman who was injured in a road traffic accident needed a life-saving blood transfusion following a Caesarean operation. Prior to her operation she told the medical staff that she would not accept a blood transfusion; she signed a form to that effect. Her mother was a Jehovah's Witness and influenced her into refusing the transfusion. The patient's co-habitee, the father of her child, applied to the court for permission for the medical staff to give her the transfusion. The court ruled that the blood could be given as the evidence showed that at the time she decided not to have the transfusion she did not have the necessary capacity to make a valid decision; her mind had been overborne by her mother.

What is important here is not that the court had by proxy consented for a mentally competent adult. The reality is that at the time of making the decision this adult was not in a fit state of mind to do so. Her competence was distorted; so in her and her child's best interest she was given the blood to save her life.

In as much as the decision of some mentally competent patients to refuse treatment may not sit comfortably with the nursing and medical objective of saving life where it is possible to do so, the competent person's wishes must be respected. A mentally competent patient may deliberately go on a hunger strike, refusing food and water as well as other life-saving measures, such as an operation or a blood transfusion. A heath professional may in good faith and with a caring professional attitude try to persuade the patient otherwise. However, the health professional cannot force the competent patient to eat, drink or accept other medical interventions. The law relating to consent by competent children, weighed against what appears, contentiously, to be a decline in parental power to veto children's decision, is discussed in an interesting paper by Cave (2009).

Nurses' NMC Code of conduct and consent

It has already been established in this book that the NMC Code is not a body of laws, but professional guiding principles designed to guide nurses' professional conduct and protect the patient. However, as was stated in the introduction to the book, one of the objectives of writing it is to map relevant aspects of the NMC Code onto relevant law and ethics. There are many senses in which the Code directly and indirectly addresses *consent/informed consent* issues. The Code stipulates that as a nurse you are personally accountable for actions and omissions in your practice. The concept of consent comes in here, since every nurse has the responsibility to ensure that they respect the patient's right to autonomous consenting or refusal of consent. If nurses fail to recognise this obligation they could find themselves paternalistically eroding the patients' right to consent or refuse to consent.

The Code also demands that nurses ensure they gain consent before beginning to treat patients, respecting and supporting patients' right to 'accept or decline treatment and care'. Nurses are obliged to 'uphold people's rights to be fully involved in decisions about their care' and be aware of legislation relating to mental capacity. Within this, nurses must ensure that those in their care, particularly the most vulnerable, who lack capacity, are placed *at the centre of care* and are safeguarded. The code demands that when nurses treat people who lack capacity, for example unconscious patients, they do so in the patients' best interest.

Linking consent to the professional, ethical and legal notion of confidentiality, the NMC Code requires nurses to gain patients' consent to reveal or share their confidential information with other health professionals, but only on the basis of their need to know. In other words those with whom the patient's information is shared must be part of the caring team administering care to the patient. On admission the patient needs to know this and his/her agreement to this needs to be secured. By the same token, the NMC Code advocates disclosure of information if a nurse is satisfied that non-disclosure may put third parties at risk of harm. In doing so you must work within the law of the country where you are practising.

Box 5.1 contains a case study. In analysing the issues within the scenario, please follow your own problem-based learning (PBL) model or the one used with you by your tutors. If you have never used a PBL approach before, I suggest that as an integral group you address yourselves to the following:

1. Who will act as the leader/coordinator/facilitator for your group in getting the group to work through the scenario issues?

**BOX 5.1 Student portfolio reflection exercise 5.1: using a problem-
based learning approach in a group of your peers**

Case study

You are a staff nurse on ward 5. John, a 40-year-old gay man with HIV, is one of your
patients. Although his parents and his gay lover visit him regularly, the parents do not
know that he is gay or has HIV. The parents also do not know who the male visitor is
as John has not 'come out' or discussed his situation with his parents. John tells you
he has been a married man with one eight-year-old daughter and he is thinking of
going back to his wife, from whom he has lived apart for the last four years, and who
does not know he is bisexual and is HIV positive. She turns up on the ward to visit
him and popped into the office, asking you why John is in the ward and what progress
he is making. That day prior to her visit to your office, the latest laboratory reports
on John's HIV status, together with the latest clinical manifestations, show that John
now has AIDS. You now begin to think that this is one of the reasons perhaps why
in the last few days John has been able to get around the ward only with the help of
a wheelchair. His parents and lover are also seeking information from you and the
medical staff about John's future health and his care. It is apparent that he wants to
have a bisexual relationship with his wife and lover.

How to proceed with Student portfolio reflection exercise 5.1

Organise a small group of your peers of student nurses within the classroom, with or
without your tutor present. Introduce the scenario and invite your colleagues to work
with you on it, using a problem-based learning (PBL) approach. Identify and analyse
the issues and problems in the scenario and resolve them.

---

2. Who will be the scribe and write down on the PBL activity work sheet the group's
    responses at each stage of this exercise?
3. The whole group brainstorm and address the question: what does the scenario tell us?
    In other words, what do we already know from reading this scenario? The scribe notes
    the responses ensuring (s)he captures everyone's responses. All views are important;
    everyone's views respected and noted.
4. Under the guidance of the group leader the group addresses itself to the question: what
    further thoughts does the group have about the issues within the scenario? (These are
    hypothetical views worth noting/writing down. The scribe puts them in a separate
    column from the first group of responses.) Hypothetical phase in the PBL.
5. What further critical issues lie within this scenario that we need to address? The scribe
    notes these.
6. What further issues and problems may emerge that may need to be tackled and resolved?
    The scribe notes these.
7. Have we made the necessary links with any learning outcomes we have identified for
    this scenario/trigger, or with learning outcomes linked to our modules and relevant
    NMC competencies domain? If yes, what links? The scribe notes these.
8. The facilitator/coordinator invites the group to recap and proceed. (S)he asks: are we
    sure we have identified and analysed all key legal and ethical issues (e.g. consent;
    confidentiality; ethics of autonomy; statute and case law; universal precaution against

spread of infection; NMC code of conduct and clinical competence issues)? You will have thought of many other critical professional, ethical, moral and legal issues. What are these other issues?

9. In the light of what is generated above, what do we as a group of students need to go away and *learn/research* for a follow-up feedback session (in order to deal with the issues/solve problems arising from our analysis of the scenario issues)? What resources and solutions do we already have? What do we need?

10. How should we proceed to divide up the work? Who is going away to research what? What further resources do we need? How do we propose to feed back? When? Where? How?

Remember that you will need to make reference to specific legal, ethical and other appropriate knowledge/subject areas/theories/frameworks to justify your answers or feedback at the next session. Perhaps all agree to prepare a one- or two-page hand-out of your feedback for each member of the group. Such a hand-out must contain key points to discuss and a full reference list to inform each student's research.

Portfolio reflection and entry

Following your feedback session, each student goes away to critically reflect on and write up their learning in their developing law, ethics and professional issues portfolio.

Summary and conclusion

This chapter:

- covered consent, including definitions, meanings and types of consent;
- examined weaknesses in consent and informed consent formats – oral, written and implied;
- discussed legal, ethical and professional dimensions of consent and implications for nursing practice;
- addressed consent in relation to mental capacity/competence – consent in adults, children and patients detained under the MHA 1983 (2007);
- analysed conditions under which persons may refuse to consent to treatment and the implications of these for health professionals;
- examined the concept and legal instruments of advanced decisions (living wills) and Lasting Power of Attorney in relation to consent;
- gave opportunity to students to analyse legal, ethical, moral and professional issues through a patient-focused scenario; using portfolio to further their learning.

It is concluded that consent as a concept and a process is designed to respect people's right to self-determination and autonomy. It has many facets to it. When practised correctly – professionally, legally and ethically – informed consent principles enhance the nurse–patient relationship and promote patient care outcomes. There are important links between the legal, ethical, employment of contract and professional dimensions of informed consent and what the NMC Code recommends in relation to nurses and consent issues in patient care.

6 Confidentiality
Legal, ethical and professional dimensions

Objectives of this chapter

After reading this chapter you should be able to:

*   demonstrate understanding of confidentiality – legal, ethical and professional dimensions;
*   discuss whether confidentiality is an absolute or relative moral obligation and the implications;
*   advance legal, ethical and professional arguments to justify confidentiality as well as what may justifiably militate against confidentiality in nursing practice;
*   outline principles of the Data Protection Act and discuss implications for nursing patients;
*   identify statutes having bearings on confidentiality. What are the links?
*   compare and contrast the NMC and GMC guidelines on confidentiality and discuss how they can help the nurse.

Introduction

Patients' rights to *privacy*, *autonomy*, *self-determination*, *justice*, *dignity* and *security* all lie at the root of the necessity to maintain their confidentiality. Essentially, confidentiality in nursing and the wider healthcare practice is about respecting patients' secrets. 'Secrets' in this context means information the patient gives *privately* to a healthcare professional, and which (s)he does not wish to be divulged without his/her permission. The nurse's professional (confidential) relationship with the patient by necessity offers an implied promise to keep secret the information entrusted. Infringement of the patient's right to confidentiality occurs when the professional to whom the information was confided fails to protect it or discloses it to a third party without the patient's consent. The NMC (2008a) Code states that, as a nurse, 'you must respect people's right to confidentiality' and 'ensure people are informed about how and why information is shared by those who will be providing their care'. Yet in the same paragraph the Code states: 'You must disclose information if you believe someone may be at risk of harm'. Are these two statements conceptually contradictory? To answer this question let's look at absolutism in confidentiality.

Is nursing confidentiality an absolute obligation?

The NMC's two seemingly contradictory statements above suggest that in nursing practice confidentiality is not an absolute requirement. This is because if on the one hand we are expected to hold as secret what a patient tells us in confidence about himself (and we should to preserve patients' right to privacy and maintain the foundations for patient–professional trusting relationships) and on the other we are free to disclose it to colleagues, and furthermore to others if we believe third parties may be at 'risk', then we would seem to be taking on a *contradictory* moral position. This is a real moral dilemma, because we must abide by the law and also we have an obligation to protect the wider public and known third parties within it who may be at risk of harm from patients themselves, or be at risk if patient information given in confidence is not revealed.

Further analysis of confidentiality in healthcare shows that traditionally rules of confidentiality have long been present in codes of medical ethics. The BMA (2005) in an online paper 'Confidentiality as part of the bigger picture' (20 June 2005) points out that health professionals are responsible to patients for the health information they hold, even though when patients provide information they 'imply consent to some sharing with other healthcare professionals'. The BMA states, however, that there should be no use of the information the patient provides us in our professional work for matters other than for the purpose of the clinical care of the patient concerned. However, like the NMC the BMA points out three exceptions to the view of confidentiality as an absolute requirement:

- where the patient has given consent to disclosure;
- where the law requires disclosure; and
- in the interest of an overriding public need for disclosure.

Havard (1985) points out that in France, for example, medical confidentiality is so strict that it is enshrined in law as an *absolute* medical privilege which no one can override. Yet Gillon (2003) points out that in practice doctors do not respect confidentiality as an 'absolute requirement'. It is perhaps for this reason that Siegler (1982) refers to confidentiality in medicine as a 'decrepit concept'. Beauchamp and Childress (2001) further explain that the reasoning behind Siegler's point is the idea that the traditional view that doctors and patients had about confidentiality as an absolute obligation has long been eroded and compromised by modern medical practice.

From the various sources on confidentiality consulted, it is possible to summarise the complex exceptions to confidentiality as an absolute concept:

- The patient or his/her legal adviser (e.g. someone holding an LPA) may give consent to disclose confidentiality.
- When other health professionals are participating in the patient's care and need the information to care for the patient. This must be seen as in the best interest of the patient.
- When the medical staff believes a close relative/close friend needs to know about the patient's situation but it is medically undesirable to gain the patient's consent. This is a difficult one and I personally have a problem accepting this view without questioning. If the patient is not mentally competent then I think there is no real problem here, but if I were competent and even put on the critical list of impending death, I would still want to know what is happening. Even if I were going to die next week from terminal cancer, which news would no doubt distress me, I would still want to be told. I do not think I would be alone in this regard. (Reflective question: how would you feel about professionals deciding not to tell you something about your situation simply for fear of upsetting you too much, and telling your relatives instead?)
- Court orders such as subpoenas and civil procedure rules, for example when a judge directs a health professional to disclose confidential medical information.
- Statutory duty to disclose, for example

- – Public Health (Control of Disease) Act 1984, in *notifiable disease* or *food poisoning*;
- – Public Health (Infectious Disease) Regulations 1988 – health professionals must notify local authorities of identity, gender and address of persons suspected of having a notifiable diseases, including food poisoning;
- – Abortion Regulations 1991 – a doctor carrying out a termination of pregnancy must notify the Chief Medical Officer, giving a reference number and the date of birth and postcode of the woman concerned;
- – Birth & Deaths Registration Act 1953 – notification of births and deaths;
- – Road Traffic Act 1988;
- – Prevention of Terrorism (Temporary Provisions) Act 1988;
- – the Terrorism Act 2000 says that all citizens, including health professionals, must inform the police as soon as possible of information that may help prevent terrorism, apprehending and prosecution of terrorists;
- – Misuse of Drugs Acts;
- – the Information Sharing Index (England) Regulations 2007 (Contact Point) – health professionals must provide basic identifying information to local authorities for children up to age 18.
- Public interest can override a duty of confidentiality.

The GMC's 2009 guidance on confidentiality issued to doctors is well worth reading for two reasons: (a) its comprehensive nature and (b) because it can act as good guide to any of the other clinical professions (nursing, dentistry, physiotherapy etc.). It can be found online at http://www.gmc-uk.org/guidance/ethical_guidance/confidentiality.asp. Compare it with the NMC's guidelines on confidentiality issues for the benefit of nurses, which can be found online at http://www.nmc-uk.org/Nurses-and-midwives/Advice-by-topic/A/Advice/Confidentiality/. It is also worth reading the Department of Health Guidance on Confidentiality and the Law, found online at http://www.dh.gov.uk/en/Publicationsandstatistics/Publications/PublicationsPolicyAndGuidance/Browsable/DH_5133529. The NHS Confidentiality Code of Conduct provides useful reading, and can be found online at http://www.dh.gov.uk/en/Managingyourorganisation/Informationpolicy/Patientconfidentialityandcaldicottguardians/DH_4100550.

From the analysis so far it seems reasonable to state that, although the UK medical and nursing bodies value confidentiality as a very strong professional and moral obligation, both bodies seem to assert that there are sometimes justifiable exceptions to the rule, and thus confidentiality in healthcare is not an *absolute* moral obligation.

Difference between 'permitting' and 'requiring' disclosure

Whereas the above laws require disclosure there are some statutes that permit, rather than require, disclosure; examples of those merely permitting are the Data Protection Act 1998, the Crime and Disorder Act 1998 and the Children Act 1989. In the case of a statute permitting disclosure, for example to the police, local authority, social services, Multi-Agency Protection Panels and government bodies, the health professional may disclose only when the patient has given consent or there is an overriding public interest (BMA, 2010).

Justification for confidentiality

Why is it so important to respect patients' confidentiality? There are a number of philosophical, ethical and pragmatic considerations that justify confidentiality. These are:

- consequentialism, or consequence-based arguments;
- respect for autonomy and rights to privacy arguments;
- virtue ethics arguments;
- fidelity, implicit and explicit promise;
- legal – common law and contract law (e.g. contract of employment) statutory duties;
- professional registration/PCC duties;
- ethics of beneficence, non-maleficence, justice.

Consequentialism as a justification for confidentiality

The duty and importance of confidentiality have been supported by well-reasoned arguments (e.g. Beauchamp and Childress, 2001; Hope *et al.*, 2003). One of the most commonly proposed philosophical and ethical arguments supporting confidentiality is the ethic of *consequentialism*. The arguments suggest that if patients' confidentiality is not maintained there will be serious consequences for patient and society as a whole. Patients' relationships with healthcare professionals are based on trust. Patients/clients need to trust the healthcare professional if they are going to feel confident to tell their personal health/illness stories to health professionals, and grant them access to their bodies for clinical observation, examination and various tests required for accurate diagnoses and treatments. If patients feel that their trust and confidence are likely to be broken, they will feel inhibited to tell their stories. Some patients will not tell their story at all, withholding potentially critical information that could have facilitated diagnosis and treatment. Such a situation is not likely to benefit the patient.

Furthermore, patients suffering from serious personality and mental health problems and from traditionally self-perceived 'embarrassing' and stigmatised diseases (e.g. sexually transmitted diseases, HIV/AIDS, tuberculosis) may be so apprehensive, embarrassed and fearful that their secrets will be betrayed, that they may not seek medical and nursing help. This would only compound their problem. The worsening of their illness may lead to their being a problem and a danger to themselves and the wider community. For example if patients feels a nurse will disclose to friends and relatives the fact that they have epilepsy, TB, HIV/AIDS, STDs and other illnesses considered to be stigmatising, they may keep these problems to themselves and suffer the consequences. A patient with epilepsy may fear that, if he tells his doctor, she may betray him to the vehicle licensing centre. Thus he does not seek treatment, and continues to drive with his epilepsy, one day having a fit at the wheel that causes his death and perhaps that of others. Here then lies a dilemma. The patient knows he has a problem to tell the health professional, but fears undue disclosure, so keeps the matter a secret, yet knows that unless he tells the health professional he could die untreated and risk exposing others to the consequences of his illness. An example of a real moral dilemma.

Beauchamp and Childress (2001) argue that consequentialism (results or consequence of an action) supports *exceptions* to confidentiality. If nurses were to follow rules that allow them to breach confidentiality and warn an intended victim of their client's threatened violence, this would benefit all the parties. Such a rule might have made the therapist in the case of *Tarasoff v Regents of the University of California* (1976) 551 P (2d) 334, described earlier in this book, inform the young lady she was about to be killed by her spurned lover. The consequentialist argument supports breach of confidentiality in such a case.

On the other hand, the consequentialist argument states that if patients fear betrayal of their secrets, by a therapist overriding the obligation to be confidential, then the fiduciary relationship between patient and therapist would be eroded. The patient would not want to trust the therapist. Thus (s)he would not disclose to the therapist valuable information crucial to his/her accurate diagnosis and treatment, or the fact that (s)he is thinking of hurting someone. Thus, violence on the street could increase as very ill and potentially dangerous patients may not seek help which might reveal their violent fantasies.

Although consequentialism supports the need for some rules of confidentiality, consequentialists disagree among themselves which rule to follow and about the rule's scope and weighting. Hence the arguments about rules are hinged on *empirical* claims as to which rule is preferred for the benefit of society. For instance, with respect to the *legal exceptions to confidentiality* (public health legislation to report infectious and contagious disease, statutory requirements to report child abuse and gunshot wounds, etc.) there is no empirical evidence that such requirements have 'reduced prospective patients' willingness to seek treatment and to cooperate with physicians or significantly impaired the physician–patient relationship' (Beauchamp and Childress, 2001, p. 307). Thus it may be concluded that consequentialists' justification for the value of confidentiality is as strong as it is for not making confidentiality an *absolute* moral, legal and professional obligation.

Deontological grounds for the duty of confidentiality

Deontologists believe that moral rules, motives and intentions are the all-important ingredients by which the moral worth of an action is judged. Deontologists believe that fundamental rules, duty and obligations must be followed to promote good outcomes, although, unlike utilitarianism, the deontological outcomes/consequences are not as important as the quality of the rules, motives, intentions and acts that produce the consequences.

For deontologists, there are certain acts that are right or wrong in themselves. This is because of the sorts of acts they are, not because of the consequences they produce. The value of confidentiality may be justified on deontological grounds, such as our beliefs that patients have *privacy* and *autonomy* rights, and we have a duty to respect these principles. Privacy and autonomy are intrinsic values and rights, the freedom to make self-decisions and determine one's destiny. Autonomy is about self-governance, independent reasoning and choice; it is about freedom of will and a capacity to determine one's behaviour. By accepting these values within autonomy, we are subscribing to the view that what the patient wants for him-/herself, for instance the right to privacy, should be respected. In this respect, then, an autonomous person must have his/her privacy and confidentiality respected. Note that these arguments have nothing to do with consequences, just the quality of the actions involved. Even if the patient is unaware of the breach of confidentiality it is still a breach that should not have happened.

Beauchamp and Childress (2001) argue that breach of confidentiality is particularly important when it exposes patients to dangers, discrimination, loneliness, segregation, loss of friends, loss of employment, physical, emotional and psychological devastation. These consequences are important, but for deontologists it is not as important as the values inherent in the exercise of privacy and autonomy in supporting the rules of confidentiality. A nurse who supports deontological ethics values the patient's intrinsic right to autonomy and privacy regardless of consequences. Autonomy aside, privacy is such an important human need that Article 8 of the Human Rights Act 1998 confirms its supremacy. If a nurse breaches the patient's right to privacy for self and family (s)he could be sued for such a breach. This helps to show the strength of deontological belief in maintaining the integrity of confidentiality.

Virtue-based ethics as justification for confidentiality

According to Aristotle *virtue ethics* defines the right act as that which a virtuous person does in the circumstances prevailing. A virtuous person is seen as imbued with, and exhibits, virtuous characteristics. Thus a virtuous nurse or doctor is endowed with virtues such as honesty, kindness, being caring, respectful and truthful, trustworthy, respecting his/her patient's right to confidentiality. The virtue-based ethical theorist would argue that it is the possession of virtues that directs the right behaviour, not what it is right to do in the situation. By this line of reasoning and analysis, any nurse who breaches patients' confidences demonstrates a serious lapse of virtue, for example honesty and fidelity. The argument of virtue ethics justifying confidentiality then puts the burden onto the behaviour of the healthcare professional, not on the patient's right to autonomy, privacy and confidentiality.

Fidelity, implicit and explicit promise

The *fidelity*, *implicit* and *explicit promise*-based arguments as justification for confidentiality have been advanced by others (e.g. Beauchamp and Childress, 2001; Hope *et al.*, 2003). These arguments are centred on the view that the relationship between the patient and the healthcare professional contains an *implied contract* and therefore a *promise* from the professional to hold in confidence that which the patient confides in him/her. The nurse's obligation to honour the patient's reasonable expectation of privacy and confidentiality is a way to state the 'general obligation of fidelity' (Beauchamp and Childress, 2001, p. 308).

Legal justifications for confidentiality

Tort of negligence in common law

In looking at factors that support confidentiality in healthcare, no healthcare professional can afford to neglect the fact that the English common law gives protection to people's right to have their confidentiality respected. Should a nurse betray a patient's confidence in such a way that the patient is damaged by the betrayal, that patient would be entitled to sue for compensation in the tort of negligence. There is a New Zealand case, *Furniss v Fitchett* [1958] NZLR 396, in which a doctor had divulged a woman's medical history to her husband without her permission. The husband successfully used the information against his wife in a custody battle. On realising the medical betrayal, and the damage done to her as a consequence, the woman sued the doctor (her psychiatrist) under negligence law and won. Under common law, then, there is an expectation that patients have a right to have their privacy protected even from their next of kin. If patients have their privacy disrespected by undue disclosure it could expose them to injury, loss and unfair discrimination, which under statute such as the Data Protection Act 1998, the Human Rights Act 1998 and the Disability Discrimination Act 1995 are illegal. Nurses need to work within the framework of the law.

Patients can exercise their right to refuse to have their medical records disclosed to third parties, for example relatives, the press, insurance companies, or even their employer. In the case of *Nicholson v Halton General Hospital NHS Trust* (1999), a patient refused to allow her medical records to be disclosed to her employer even though the records might have thrown some light on the case between her and her employer. The material evidence of the case appears in Box 6.1. The Court of Appeal upheld the employer's appeal for an 'unless' order, but ruled that the patient (claimant) could *not* be forced to give up her right to confidentiality. So, in essence, the employer was not allowed to see the patient's medical evidence without her consent. But equally, the patient's case could not proceed without the information.

> **BOX 6.1 The case of *Nicholson v Halton General Hospital NHS Trust*
> (*Current Law*, 46, November 1999)**
>
> The patient as the claimant brought legal proceedings against her employer (the
> defendant) claiming she developed radial tunnel syndrome of her (R) wrist because
> her employer was negligent in requiring her to perform repetitive movements at work.
> She had undergone remedial operation and the employer wanted to know why and
> the nature of the condition. She refused the employer access to her medical notes and
> refused also to have the employer's legal team discuss her case with her consultant.
> The employer sought to declare that 'unless' she produced the evidence sought her
> case would not go ahead. The trial court refused the 'unless' order. The court of appeal
> ruled in favour of the 'unless order' but indicated that the employer could not look at
> the patient's record without her permission. Hence her confidentiality remained intact,
> even it it impaired her case.

Contract law and patients' confidentiality

Contract law is also a source of the legal obligation to keep patients' confidences protected.
For example, although NHS patients have no contract with NHS doctors and nurses, those
patients who are seen in private medical practices can in fact enforce their legal right to
confidentiality and can sue for breach of confidence under contract law. More important for
student nurses is this: when you qualify and register with the NMC you are entitled to seek
a post with an employer, for example an NHS Trust. You will be required to sign a contract
of employment. Such a contract is likely to force you to maintain the confidence of the
patients you care for in that employment and even after you leave that employment. If you
fail to maintain confidentiality you could be dismissed; also the patient whose confidence
you breach can sue you in the tort of negligence.

Statute law

A number of statutes seek to protect the patient's right to confidentiality, including:

* Article 8 of the Human Rights Act 1998 (right to private family life);
* the Data Protection Act (DPA) 1998 (protects unauthorised disclosure of personal data).
  For key principles of the DPA see Box 6.2.

Under common law the English court has been known to give life-time anonymity to
protect people's confidentiality. In a previous case in which a toddler, Jamie Bulger, was
murdered by two under-aged boys a court injunction prevented a newspaper from revealing
the two boys' identities (*Venables v News Group Newspapers Ltd* [2001] Fam 430).
   In the age of computerised patient records there is some fear that hackers could make
confidentiality difficult to preserve. For this reason NHS Trusts owe it to their patients to
keep computerised patient records safely and proof against hackers.
   Pragmatically, the DPA 1998 requires that data subjects be:

1. told if personal data are being processed;
2. told of the data source;
3. provided with a copy of the data description;

BOX 6.2 Key principles of the Data Protection Act 1998

There are eight key principles applying to computer and manually kept records, including patients' medical notes. In summary, the principles are intended to ensure personal data are accurate, relevant, processed fairly and lawfully, kept only for the purposes for which the user is registered, not disclosed to unauthorised persons and not kept for longer than is necessary for the intended purpose. Personal data must be updated as appropriate and processed only in line with the rights of the *data subject* – this being the person to whom the data apply, for example patients, clients and participants who agree to participate in research. Appropriate technical and organisational measures will be taken against unauthorised and illegal processing, accidental loss, damage or destruction of these records. Personal records will not be sent outside the European Union unless the country or territory can guarantee adequate protection for the rights and freedoms of data subjects in relation to the processing of those records.

---

4. informed of the persons to whom the data may be disclosed;
5. given the opportunity to correct incorrect data held on them, and to seek compensation for harm suffered on account of inaccurate data.

To access personal data, data subjects must submit written requests to the appropriate individual or institution and a response must be received within 40 days. If appropriate the applicant must be told if there are grounds for withholding the information requested. Grounds for withholding information may be: where release of the data may seriously harm the data subject or others; where the request for the data comes from a person who is not the data subject, but the data subject had specifically requested their data be not released to other persons; where the release would identify another person who had not consented to be identified in this way.

Confidentiality and the ethics of beneficence, non-maleficence and justice

Essentially, we have an ethical and professional obligation not to harm our patients (non-maleficence) and to strive to ensure that what we do for or with them, and any advocacy role we carry out on their behalf, are in their best interest; in other words they should benefit from the nurse–patient interaction (*beneficence*). We should treat them fairly and equitably and not discriminate against our patients (the ethical principle of *justice*). If we betray patients' confidence we fall short of these professional, moral and ethical standards, for which we may be disciplined or at worst have our professional registration taken from us. As a student nurse please strive to attain the highest standards in moral, ethical, legal and professional behaviour; operate within your professional body's code of conduct, competencies and guidance regarding confidentiality in relation to patient care. Always remember too your patients' autonomous right to have their privacy and dignity maintained.

Law, sexually transmitted diseases and confidentiality: nursing implications

Nursing patients with sexually transmitted diseases can present nurses with a challenge in respect to the maintenance of confidentiality. The National Health Service (Venereal Diseases) Regulations 1974, Section 1, No. 29 (as amended by S1 1982 No. 288) ensures the confidentiality of information in relation to sexually transmitted diseases. This legal power ensures that authorities that collect information in respect to people treated for sexually transmitted diseases keep the information confidential. However, there are two exceptions to this requirement. First, disclosures can be made to a medical practitioner in respect of the person being treated for the disease; second, disclosure is possible for the purpose of such treatment and prevention.

HIV/AIDS

People suffering from HIV and AIDS are entitled to the same legal protection as any other patient in respect to consent, confidentiality and professional responsibility. Under the Public Health Act (Infectious Diseases) regulations 1985, a local authority has power to apply to a justice of the peace to remove a person suffering from AIDS to be detained in a hospital. These regulations also give power to a justice of the peace to require persons believed to be suffering from AIDS to be medically examined. Finally, these regulations also empower authorities to make decisions regarding disposal of the body of people with AIDS.

Nurses sometimes ask whether a prospective employer can insist upon a prospective employee being screened for AIDS before employment. Dimond (2008) argues that this is possible, given the fact that an employer wants the most suitable and competent employee for the job. An employer cannot insist that an employee reveal a criminal offence if that conviction is spent under the Rehabilitation of Offenders Act (ROA) 1974. However, NHS Trust and most other health services posts are excluded from the provisions of the ROA. The AIDS Control Act 1987 requires district health authorities to report to the regional health authorities and they in turn to the Secretary of State for Health the information in relation to:

- number of AIDS cases and timing of diagnosis;
- AIDS facilities provided;
- number of staff providing such facilities;
- planned provisions covering the next 12 months.

HIV is not strictly speaking a *notifiable disease*, like AIDS, cholera, the plague, smallpox, typhus, acute encephalitis and poliomyelitis, diphtheria, dysentery, measles, mumps, meningitis, rabies, meningococcal septicaemia, malaria, ophthalmia neonatorum, paratyphoid fever, rubella, scarlet fever, tetanus, tuberculosis, typhoid fever, viral haemorrhagic fever, viral hepatitis, whooping cough and so on. Notifiable diseases must be reported to the local authority under the Public Health (Control of Disease) Act 1984 and the Public Health (Infectious Diseases) Regulations 1988.

Not even the police have a right to the medical records of a patient suffering from HIV/ AIDS unless the person is suspected of committing a serious crime. If the coroner requests the record of a dead patient it will usually be complied with. If an insurance company requests the record of a dead person it will not be released if the person had before his/her death formally requested that such a record not be released. If there is no such request from the deceased, the release of the information to the insurance company will be made only if the dead person's legal representative consents to such a release. This principle applies in the case of the death of any patient.

If an employee's (e.g. a nurse's) mental and physical capacity to do the job is an issue, the employer can request the employee to submit for an independent medical examination. However, as Dimond (2008) points out, there are no legal powers available to the employer to insist on, or order the employee to submit to, a medical examination.

Nurses' professional registration: NMC Code and confidentiality

A nurse's professional registration carries the obligation of the registered nurse to respect patients' confidentiality. Professionalism is about accepting the responsibilities and accountability embedded within the 'professional' relationship; this is certainly the case with all healthcare professionals, not just nurses. Professionalism in respect to nursing means respecting patients' autonomy and right to privacy. It is not surprising therefore that the NMC Code stipulates that nurses 'must respect people's right to confidentiality', ensuring patients are assured how and why information about them is shared with other team members. The Code further states, however, that nurses can legally disclose information to prevent harm to others at known risk.

Compared with the GMC guidance on confidentiality given to doctors, the amount of guidance the NMC gives to nurses on confidentiality is sparse. It is worth looking at the GMC's guidance to doctors for two reasons: (a) nurses and doctors have to work together and it is a good thing for the one to understand the other's perspective on confidentiality; (b) nurses may well benefit from the more detailed GMC (2009) guidance on confidentiality, which is such a complex area. For the GMC guidance go to: http://www.gmc-uk.org/guidance/ethical_guidance/confidentiality.asp. I have used both NMC and some of the GMC guidance on confidentiality to help me deal with the issues within the scenario in exercise 6.1 (Box 6.3; see also Box 6.4).

The following are additional guidelines on confidentiality gleaned from NMC, HPC and GMC guidelines and are worth reading to firm up your understanding of circumstances where confidentiality must be observed and when and where the principle can be challenged. Whilst reading through these additional guidelines, decide for yourself if any of these principles about confidentiality could be used to further inform the scenario issues in Box 6.3. Please note that the following guidelines are intended for qualified practitioners such as registered nurses and doctors. So as a student you need to adapt them to your role as a student, being conscious always to operate within your sphere of authority, competence and experience, always remembering your obligation to be guided by qualified, competent professionals, and always referring any doubts you have to your mentor or your tutor, who

---

BOX 6.3 Student portfolio reflection exercise 6.1

A 23-year-old unmarried Muslim lady, Abibi, is admitted to the medical ward with severe abdominal pain, normal temperature, pallor, profuse sweating and hypotension. She is also suffering from blood loss PV. She is accompanied by her best friend, a Muslim lady, also 23 years old. They have been best friends from childhood, through school and university. The doctor examined her with a student nurse and the patient's female friend present. Neither the nurse nor the doctor had asked the patient if it was all right to have her friend and student nurse present during her examination and history taking. She was diagnosed with an ectopic pregnancy. The nursing staff was told to prepare Abibi for theatre. Her mother and father arrived in the hospital whilst she was in theatre, wanting to know what was going on with their daughter. When told by nurses and their daughter's friend that their daughter was in theatre having an operation for an ectopic pregnancy, her father walked out the ward, but her mother collapsed on the floor, weeping, and saying their daughter had disgraced the family and must die for it.

What are the issues here?

BOX 6.4 Some of the issues within the Box 6.3 scenario

It is hoped that your portfolio analysis will throw up some of the following:

Abibi's rights to confidentiality: principles of confidentiality and some necessary procedures

All patients (Abibi included) have a right to expect that information about them will be handled sensitively and held in confidence by nursing and medical staff. Abibi was in a very vulnerable situation on admission, in severe pain, which can cloud any patient's consciousness and ability to think clearly and to be in charge of his/her personal situation. The doctor and the nurse had a responsibility to protect her right to confidentiality. To do this one of the first things they should have done was to ask her if she was happy to have her friend present during her examination. Confidentiality is central to trust between the patient and health professional, in this case between Abibi and the doctor and student nurse present. Without assurances about confidentiality, patients may be reluctant to give health professionals information they need to provide good care.

The carelessness of the staff in failing to find out from Abibi if she was happy for her friend (even if her best friend, who accompanied her to hospital at this very difficult time) to be present led to her friend knowing about her medical condition without her consent. Clearly, confidentiality had been breached. The patient had been seriously let down by the medical and nursing staff – twice in fact: (a) by her friend being allowed to remain in the room whilst she was supplying her history and when she was being medically examined, without asking her if this was all right; (b) by having her medical details told to her parents without her consent. No one, however close to an adult mentally competent person, has a right to be told that person's medical history without the patient's express consent. Article 8 of the Human Rights Act 1998 gives the person the right to private and family life. The Data Protection Act protects patients' data from being disclosed to unauthorised persons without the patient's permission.

If medical and nursing staff are asked by a third party (as in the case here where both Abibi's parents wanted to know the reason for her admission) to provide information about patients they must:

- seek patient's consent to disclose the information;
- observe the requirements of common law and statute, including data protection law;
- keep disclosure to the minimum necessary.

For example, rather than telling the parents the reason Abibi had gone to theatre they could simply explain that details about the patient cannot be given to them without her consent as she is an adult, mentally competent person. It is against the law and Trust care protocols to release information on any patient to any third party without the patient's consent, even if the third party are close relatives, as Abibi's parents are. However, some reassurance could be given to the parents that the patient was in good medical hands and being given the best care. They could be encouraged to return home and visit later when the patient had returned to the ward.

Following surgery and full return to consciousness, and possibly on the patient's return to the ward, she should be told of her parents' visit and informed of what had happened, that is about the unfortunate disclosure and her parents' reaction. She should be asked whether she wanted them to be informed of her return from theatre. Under the circumstances she needs to be asked whether she feels she needs any special security put in place for her by the Trust. For example, does she wish the local police to be informed of the threat to her life by her mother? She should be asked whether she wants to contact her parents. If she wanted to and did not have a mobile phone she could be offered the opportunity to use the ward telephone. The staff should under the present set of circumstances bear in mind the fact that the patient's life could be in danger and the Trust has a responsibility to protect the patient given the threat made.

In the *Tarasoff* case the Supreme Court of California held that health professionals have a legal responsibility to protect the life of a third party. In the present case the patient, Abibi, has an even stronger case and need for Trust protection given that she is under the care of the Trust and her parents have issued a threat to kill her. Muslim societies tend to regard sex before marriage, and especially pregnancy outside marriage, as a serious breach of religious and cultural and family norms of behaviour; a form of dishonour of the family. Muslim young people have been known to be killed under such circumstances as those described here. The NMC requires nurses to assess risks involved in the care of people and those related to them and to do everything possible to protect patients and others from known threats. The present threat fits this NMC requirement.

Abibi has a right to have her autonomy and right to confidentiality and privacy respected under the Human Rights Act 1998, Article 8 – a right to private family life. Every health professional has a legal, ethical and professional duty of care to protect patients' confidence. They should manage patient information sensitively, working within data protection legislation, such as the Data Protection Act 1998. Keeping their patients' confidences and promoting their autonomy and right to privacy and confidentiality are essential tenets of nursing and medical practice.

Cultural understanding, multiculturalism and cultural competence in care

Nursing requires nurses to be culturally aware. In Britain multicultural care is crucial because Britain is a rich mix of people of different religious and cultural persuasions. Understanding cultural values, religious values and beliefs of patients is crucial in nursing and medical care. We have patients who follow Western and Eastern philosophical values and traditions and we owe it to our patients to understand their ethical and moral cultural and religious values that may impinge on their care. Abibi's situation was one requiring extreme care and sensitive nursing and medical management. This is even more crucial where nursing staff had erred in illegally and unprofessionally disclosing confidential information to both Abibi's best friend and her parents. There is no excuse or justification for the disclosure. Indeed, Saha and colleagues (2008) argue that cultural competence is at the heart of *patient-centred care*, which according to Gerteis and colleagues (1993) has seven critical dimensions that could be applied to Abibi's care:

1   respect for patients' values, preferences and needs;
2   (intelligent and sensitive) coordination and integration of care;
3   effective information, communication and education;
4   patients' physical comfort;
5   emotional support and alleviation of patients' fear and anxiety;
6   appropriate involvement of friends and relatives; and
7   transition and community.

As a student pick out from Gerteis and colleagues' seven dimension of patient-centred care those dimensions that you feel were not in accord with the care Abibi received.

Disciplinary action is most likely to be taken against the nurses for the disclosure to Abibi's parents. A major professional blunder of this kind may even result in the nurses who behaved so unprofessionally being reported to the NMC for professional misconduct.

Protect patients' information from unauthorised and improper disclosure at all times

Do not discuss patients where you can be overheard, or leave patients' records where they can be seen by other patients, unauthorised staff or public. Ensure your consultations with patients are private. Remember that much improper disclosure is unintentional. Yet Abibi's case was discussed with her friend present and disclosed to her parents without her consent. Often nurses carelessly expose patients' records at the foot of their bed, perhaps not realising that other patients and visitors are reading them. A patient could be even sensitive about someone getting to know his/her age. Some female patients in particular tend to be rather sensitive about others knowing their age.

Patients have a right to information about their care; so share such information with them but in private, ensuring they understand. The GMC recommends that healthcare professionals inform patients *of the need to share their personal information with members of the care team* but clearly on the basis of the need for those other health professionals to know. Patients also need to know how information may be used to protect public health, undertake research and audits, teach or train clinical staff and students, and plan NHS services. Having said this, the GMC recommends that we should respect patients' objection to sharing their information, unless this would put others at risk of serious injury or death. Most important of all, we as health professionals should work within the law. However, in Abibi's case there was no justification to disclose to her friend and parents.

In disclosing information about patients respect their confidentiality. This principle was ignored as far as Abibi is concerned. Ensure the patient knows what will be disclosed and to whom. Ensure those who receive the information know that it is to be treated confidentially. In circumstances of emergency where a patient cannot be informed about sharing, pass the information promptly to those providing the patient's care.

The GMC argues that disclosure of information for clinical audit is essential, to provide good care. As nurses you could explain to patients who ask and wish to know that data about them can be used for clinical audit. Where the patient objects, you must explain the benefit of the audit to their care. The BMA (2005) advises that 'legally and ethically health professionals are responsible to patients for confidentiality of health information they hold'. Moreover, there should be no use or disclosure of information patients provide in connection with their care except in relation to their care and treatment. The only exceptions to this principle are:

- where there is patient consent;
- where the law requires disclosure; or
- where there is overriding public interest to disclose.

None of the above three exceptions applies in the Abibi case.

Express consent is usually needed before disclosure of identifiable information for purposes of research, epidemiology, financial audit or administration. Obtain the patient's informed consent; assure him/her of reasons for disclosure, amount and nature of information to be disclosed, to whom it will be given. Where patients withhold consent, disclosure can only take place if it is permitted by law, or can be justified in the public interest. Keep a record of the patient's decision and whether and why you have disclosed.

will be more than happy to give you guidance. Sometimes your professional organisation or trade union representative (e.g. the RCN or UNISON) will be happy to guide you regarding any doubt you have about how to handle information you perceive to be confidential but which you feel should be disclosed to a proper authority. The NMC guidelines on *whistle blowing* are also a good source of professional guidance that impacts on the principles underlying confidentiality. Read these additional confidentiality guidelines below:

1. *Disclosure in connection with judicial or other statutory proceedings:* always disclose in line with statutory requirements, for example notification of a known or suspected communicable disease. Inform patients about this but their consent is not necessary.
2. *Disclose information if ordered by a judge or officer of the court.* However, the GMC makes the point that the health professional should object to the judge or presiding officer if compelled to disclose what appear to you to be irrelevant matters, for example relating to relatives or partners of the patient, not parties to the proceedings. Here again judges are wise to the law and are perhaps unlikely to invite unnecessary disclosures.
3. *Do not disclose personal information to a third party such as a solicitor, police or officer of a court without the patient's express consent, unless this is required by statute law,* such as the Public Health (Control of Disease) Act 1984 and Public Health (Infectious Disease) Regulations 1988; Abortion Regulations 1991, whereby doctors must notify CMOs where they have terminated pregnancies; Road Traffic Act 1988; Terrorism Act 2000; disclosure to police, social services and partner organisations under, for example the Data Protection Act 1998, Children Act 1989, Crime & Disorder Act 1998; disclosures of, say, health records in legal proceedings under the Data Protection & Access to Health Records Act 1990.
4. *Personal information may be released to a statutory professional regulatory body (e.g. GMC, NMC or HPC) for investigation into a health professional's fitness to practise;* where practicable, seek the patient's permission to disclose identifiable information.
5. *Disclosure in the public interest:* personal information may be disclosed in public interest without the patient's consent, where benefits to individuals or society of the

disclosure outweigh the public and patient's interest in keeping the information confidential. Where you decide to disclose in this way, you must weigh the possible harm to the patient, and the overall trust between you as the healthcare professional and the patient, against the benefits of the disclosure.

6. *Disclosing personal information without the patient's consent may be justified*, for example where failure to do so could put people at serious risk. Where others are at serious risk that outweighs patients' privacy and confidentiality interest, you should still seek the consent to disclose. The patient should be informed that the information will be disclosed. Circumstances around which this may arise are, for example:

   a. Where disclosure may assist in preventing, detecting, and prosecuting serious crimes, for example against the person, such as abuse of children.

   b. Where a colleague who is also a patient is putting patients at risk as a result of illness. If in doubt whether to disclosure consult with a senior or more experienced colleague or seek advice from a professional organisation. Patients' safety comes first at all times.

   c. Where a patient continues to drive against medical advice and it is clearly dangerous to him-/herself and the public to do so, the Driver and Vehicle Licensing Agency' (DVLA) medical advisor should be informed.

   d. Where, for example, (as in *Tarasoff v Regents of the University of California* (1976) 551 P(2d) 334) the patient informs you (s)he seriously intends to kill another party known to you, you are obliged to inform the proper authority so that the intended victim can be protected if at all possible.

7. *Disclosure in the case of children and others who lack competency to give consent:*

   a. The competency of children 16 and 17 years old to consent to their medical treatment, under the Family Law Reform Act 1969, and children below 16 who are *Gillick competent* to consent to treatment has already been covered in the chapter on consent (Chapter 5).

   b. There will however, be situations, even problems where children and others who lack competency ask you not to disclose information about their condition. It is advisable to persuade them to allow an appropriate person to be informed/involved. If they refuse and you are convinced it is essential, in their medical interest, to inform, you should disclose relevant information to an appropriate person or authority. You should tell the patient before disclosing, and, where appropriate, seek and carefully consider the views of an advocate or carer. Document the discussions with the patient and your reasons for disclosing in his/her notes.

   c. If you believe a patient to be a victim of neglect or physical, sexual or emotional abuse and that the patient cannot give or withhold consent to disclosure, you must give information promptly to an appropriate responsible person or statutory agency, where you believe that the information is in the patient's best interests.

   d. If you believe that (c) above is not in the best interests of an abused or neglected patient, you should discuss the issues with an experienced colleague. If you decide not to disclose, you must be prepared to justify your decision.

8. *Disclosure after a patient's death*: health professionals have an obligation to keep patients' personal information confidential after their death. Although under certain circumstances disclosure after death may be permitted, if the patient had asked for information to be remained confidential, his/her views should be respected. Where there is no such request from the patient, the health professional should consider requests for disclosure taking into account:

   a. whether disclosure may distress or benefit surviving spouse/partner/family;

   b. whether the disclosure will also disclose information about the family/others;

c. whether the information is already public knowledge or can be anonymised;
d. the purpose of the disclosure.

In comparison, the GMC's guidance to doctors on confidentiality is rather comprehensive; in fact perhaps more comprehensive than that given to nurses by the NMC, or those given to physiotherapists by the IIPC. Nurses and other healthcare professionals with clinical responsibility to deliver patient care can benefit from reading the NMC guidelines at the website given above and comparing these with the GMC guidelines on confidentiality even though the latter were written primarily for doctors. In-depth knowledge hurts no one. The GMC principles are sound and can be applied to nurses, physiotherapists and other clinicians. From the many sources on confidentiality consulted to write this chapter, it can be stated confidently that confidentiality in clinical care is *not* an absolute professional or moral obligation. There are circumstances when nurses, doctors and other health professionals are obliged, ethically, professionally and legally, to preserve patients' confidentiality; but there are also circumstances when they may disclose in the public interest. You are also advised to visit the BMA website at http://www.bma.org.uk/ethics/confidentiality.Confidentiality BiggerPicture.jsp for a more extensive coverage of confidentiality and disclosure. See in particular the BMA's (2010)*'Confidentiality and disclosure of health information tool kit'*.

Hope and colleagues (2003) suggest that doctors, nurses and other health professionals may *not* breach confidentiality, for example at a dinner party for casual amusement; in a simple careless breach to satisfy others' curiosity; to prevent minor crime or help in a prosecution to secure a conviction for a minor crime; to prevent minor harm to others; or where a healthcare professional is working in a genitourinary and sexually transmitted disease unit. A healthcare professional must not write a report or fill in a form that discloses a patient's confidential information, for example to an insurance company, without the patient's consent. If as a private individual you sustain injury in a road traffic accident and are seeking compensation from another driver's insurers, those insurers cannot get information from your medical notes kept by your doctor unless you agree in writing, with a signature, that they can obtain those notes.

Confidentiality and the nursing student

Like qualified nurses, nursing students have a legal, professional and ethical duty of confidentiality to their patients. You should not betray your patients' confidence. The NMC requires you to inform your patient that you are a student. You should also tell the patient you have an obligation to report to the senior staff on aspects of his/her care, so that at all times (s)he can receive the best care. The same conditions that the law places on the registered nurse, to maintain patients' confidence, are also placed on you the student. I have already in Chapter 2 shared with you the occasion of the young female patient bleeding with a threatened abortion who tried to get me to make her a promise that I would not disclose to the rest of the staff a secret she was about to tell me. I politely refused to commit myself in this, and eventually even managed to persuade her to disclose the information to the senior staff. This proved to be to her benefit as she was able to get medical help she needed.

A position of trust

As a student you are in a position of trust and privilege when you gain information to patients' private data for your education or to help you write a good patient care study as part of your degree work. If you breach patients' confidences illegally, that is to third parties without the need to know, a court could hold you liable for breach of confidential information. Your university and the Trust you are working in may also take disciplinary action against you for such disclosures.

Patients' entitlement to high-quality care

A patient is entitled to expect from you high-quality care, as indeed it expects from qualified nurses (*Nettleship v Weston* [1971] 3 All ER 581). Yet, provided you inform the patient you are a student, most of them will on occasions be sympathetic to your need to learn, and will make allowance for your initial nervousness and less than smooth operation in carrying out nursing care and procedures on them. By the same token I would ask you not to panic over your lesser knowledge and skills compared with a fully qualified, experienced, competent registered nurse, because even patients expect that as a student you need to learn and must on occasion consult with and seek the guidance of your mentor where you lack the necessary confidence, knowledge, skills and competencies at given points in your training. It is critical, however, that you operate within the standards the NMC sets for pre-registration students and adhere to the necessary competences domains established. Operate within the limits of your competence. Do not take on without guidance what you are not competent to do. If you feel unsure of what you are doing for the patient, ask your mentor for guidance. It is better to be safe than to be sorry. You should also remember this critical point: if your negligent conduct harms a patient that patient is unlikely to say, *oh well you were only a student, therefore I will not bother to sue the Trust*. Reflect on this.

Student nurses' supernumerary status

In some situations nursing students in placement carry a *supernumerary* status and are not included in the establishment figures. However, it is an established fact that, whilst learning, student nurses contribute to patient care and, given this, are part of the nursing team. Often, the primary reason for having access to patients' confidential information is your need to learn. This, however, could be the basis on which a patient may object to your having access to their confidential notes. It is perhaps also for this reason that the NMC asks you to inform the patient you are student. That patient has the right to ask that you be not involved in his/ her care, although this is unlikely because most patients are aware of your need to learn. Most patients are sensible enough to realise that the nursing student of today will be the qualified nurse of tomorrow. Nevertheless you must not take for granted that you have a right to the patient's confidential notes. Always seek the guidance of your mentor. It seems to me, however, that our patients ought to have a moral (and self-interest) responsibility to help educate tomorrow's health professionals.

Confidentiality regarding nursing care studies and patients' photographs

The GMC advises doctors that patients' consent to disclosure of information for teaching and audit must be obtained unless the data have been effectively anonymised. Relating this to your need as a student nurse, you must be aware that under no circumstances should you carry out *patient care studies* for *publication* or *assessable assignments* without the patient's consent. It is best to get such consent in writing. Even so, the information should be anonymised so that the patient cannot be identified. The same requirement applies to using patients' photographs, e.g. as evidence in patient care studies. You must always seek the consent of your patient to take and use photographs in this way. Even with the patient's consent obtained it is best to limit information that may possibly reveal the patient's identity. Anonymised information can help with this.

Confidentiality in nursing research and other forms of healthcare research

Applications to conduct medical research must properly be passed by appropriate ethics committees. The Nuremberg and Helsinki Codes on healthcare research, and the World Medical Association's Declaration of Helsinki regarding the principles for medical research involving human subjects, apply to nurses too. For further reading on these principles visit http://www.wma.net/en/30publications/10policies/b3/index.html and http://ohsr.od.nih.gov/guidelines/nuremberg.html. Patients must have information about the nature of the research they are being invited to participate in and the researcher cannot proceed with the research if (s)he fails to get the patient's consent. The patient needs to know how data gathered from them will be collected, used and stored; whether the information will be published; and safeguards that will be put in place to prevent his/her identity being revealed. Patients also need to be reassured that research they agree to participate in will not be detrimental to their care.

At a naïve level, the request in Box 6.5 may seem reasonable and harmless. But is it? If adhered to, it means absolute confidentiality by the student nurse. However, the real issue is the possibility that the student would be foolish to agree to this precondition, because the patient may then go on to reveal information that could harm his/her care, or other people, if the secret is not acted on by someone in authority. It will be recalled that, in *Tarasoff v Regents of the University of California* (1976) 551 P(2d) 334, the Supreme Court of California held that a defendant healthcare professional owed a duty of care to a third party against whom a death threat had been made by a patient.

It is dangerous, therefore, to agree to such a request when you do not even know what is behind such a request. Information relevant to the care of the patient must be shared by the team on the basis of a need to know, and to the patient's benefit of course. It is certainly possible that what the patient would have said might have had no serious implications for anyone, but there is every chance that the information may be important to pass up the chain of command. It is reasonably safe to say to such a patient that you cannot give such a promise because the information may be important to his/her care and may therefore need to be passed on to the team. If you felt that telling the patient that you may be forced to pass the information on might make him/her not tell you something that you suspect could be critical to his/her care or that of other patients, then you might wish to exercise a different judgement, perhaps not promising but getting the information anyway. A skilled nurse could achieve this. This way you have not lied to your patients. I have found this tactic has worked well for me, especially when dealing with psychiatric patients who may be potentially dangerous in their interactions with staff, patients and public. In all cases the nurse should remember that ethically (s)he is there to ensure beneficence (the patient benefiting from the nurse–patient interaction), non-maleficence (doing nothing within the

---

BOX 6.5 Student portfolio reflection exercise 6.2

A clinical scenario for critical reflection

A patient says to you: 'Nurse, I want to tell you something, but before I do I want you to promise me you will not tell anyone else.'

How do you think this situation should be best handled and why? Bring your most critical law and ethics focus to bear on this question, and again use your portfolio to help you address the question.

nurse–patient interaction to hurt or harm the patient) and effect justice (ensuring that as far as possible patients are treated fairly). You also have a responsibility to protect third parties.

Summary and conclusion

In this chapter we analysed confidentiality; in particular we covered the following aspects:

*   meanings and definitions – legal, ethical and professional dimensions of confidentiality;
*   whether confidentiality is an absolute or relative moral obligation, and the implications of this for patient care;
*   legal, ethical and professional arguments for exceptions to, and justification for, confidentiality;
*   statutes that regulate confidentiality, including Data Protection Act;
*   whether student nurses' obligation in confidence keeping differs from that of the qualified nurse (the conclusion is drawn that the obligation is no different);
*   comparison and contrast between the GMC and NMC guidelines on confidentiality.

A few key overall conclusions were drawn. Confidentiality is crucial to the therapist–client relationship, which relies on trust. Confidentiality has legal, ethical and professional dimensions, and, although healthcare professionals are professionally obliged to maintain patients'/clients' confidences, confidentiality is not an absolute moral, ethical or professional obligation, because there are critical times when consent may be breached, ethically and legally, to protect third parties. Comparison of the GMC and NMC guidance on confidentiality is interesting, and shows that the GMC guidelines are more comprehensive. Nurses can benefit from reading the GMC's guidelines, selecting those issues that appertain to them.

7 Negligence in healthcare

Objectives of this chapter

After reading this chapter you should be able to:

- demonstrate an understanding of negligence and its implications;
- explain why a study of negligence is crucial for nurses;
- explain what patients must do to successfully win a negligence case;
- explain standards and duty of care – legal, professional, ethical, contractual and voluntary – and how breach of these may be negligent;
- discuss *damage*, including causation issues and nursing implications;
- explain the distinction between tort law negligence and criminal negligence and their significance to healthcare practitioners;
- use your portfolio to address the problems in the student activities.

Introduction

This chapter will help you to understand the concept of negligence, in terms of what it is, the many professional implications of negligent nursing practice, how to avoid giving negligent care, what a patient would need to demonstrate in order to win a negligent case and how by following your professional code of conduct you can reduce the possibility of you and your employer even being cited for negligence.

Negligence and its costs

Negligence costs the NHS a lot of money. The Department of Health (DoH, 2003b) in a consultation paper reported that in 1999–2000 the NHS spent nearly £400 million on negligence claims. Mason, Laurie and Aziz (2006) point out that the NHS annual clinical negligence bill rose from £1 million in 1974/5 to £446 million in 2001/2. The *Daily Telegraph* (2000) reported a doubling in cost of NHS negligence claims over 10 years. The *Daily Telegraph* (2010) also reports that the cost of settling negligence claims in the NHS has increased to £15 billion, diverting much-needed cash from patient care. In its annual report the NHS Litigation Authority (NHSLA, 2010) reported that in 2009/10 there were 6,652 claims, a 10 per cent increase over 2008/9, which in turn recorded an 11 per cent increase over 2007/8. A staggering £769 million was paid out for clinical negligence claims in 2008/9. Cost continues to climb. In individual claims of up to £50,000, legal fees claim the most. This suggests that lawyers are getting richer out of the NHS and tax payers getting poorer because of increasing negligence payouts. Nurses, doctors and other health professionals can do much to stem this astronomical escalation of negligence payout, thus reducing the burden on the tax payers' purse – your purse and mine when we work and pay taxes on our earnings. Not only is the legal costs of reaching settlements greater than the damages (payment awarded to claimants such as patients and their relatives), but it seems too that the perception of huge sums being paid out for clinical negligence is encouraging others to claim, spiralling costs out of control. Moreover the rate at which claims are settled is slow. On average settlements for 1999/2000 took five and a half years (National Audit Office, 2001). Nurses need to do their best to push up nursing care standards. In fact all health professionals need to play their part, doctors particularly since many large payouts are linked to negligence claims against standards of medical practice.

Historical perspectives and implications

Hendrick (2000) points out that liability for clinical negligence has a long history, dating back to the fourteenth century. Most prominent negligence cases seem to concern doctors; for example *Bolam v Friern Barnet Hospital Management Committee* [1957] 2 All ER 118; *Maynard v West Midlands RHA* [1984] 1 WLR 634; *Whitehouse v Jordan* [1981] 1 All ER 267; *Bolitho v City and Hackney Health Authority* [1997] 3 WLR 115. However, members of any of the clinical professions could find themselves being sued for negligence. Many negligence cases have been settled out of courts, so reported cases do not tell the whole story. It is important, therefore, for nurses to be knowledgeable about negligence and to do their best to reduce it. Besides the financial cost there are many benefits to be gained by health professionals and patients from reduced negligence incidents. For example, high standards of care that does not injure patients contributes to their recovery and reduces their misery from pain and suffering, as well as the misery they and their families may experience fighting negligence cases. Health professionals will also benefit from high standards of care that aim to reduce negligence claims because they will not have their names and professional reputation dragged through the courts as respondents in patient negligence suits. High standards of care that reduce risks of negligence claims are likely to remove the public perception of lots of money to be had from making negligence claims. Thus we in England could pull back from the more litigious culture that prevails in America. It is good for no one except lawyers perhaps!

Justifying a study of negligence

Nurses' roles have extended as they have taken on many of the roles only doctors used to perform. Some nurses now diagnose, prescribe, treat minor injuries and undertake minor surgery, suture wounds, order radiography, erect central venous lines and so on. These developments lead to a greater possibility of things going wrong. Alongside this phenomenon, technology such as the internet has increased patients' knowledge of illnesses, diseases and treatment options, thus making patients more likely to challenge medical decision making and pursue negligence claims. Awareness of new 'miracle' drugs, advancing surgical procedures and increasing protective human rights legislation are raising patients' expectations. This new culture, philosophy and attitude may raise patients' expectations and cause them to be more ready to sue when they perceive something has gone wrong.

As Mason, McCall Smith and Laurie (1999, p. 215) note, patients no longer accept that their injury is a simple accident; they believe that 'somebody, somewhere must be made to answer for what happened'.

The media have also had a marked influence on patients' readiness to sue. The tabloid press tends to sensationalise successful negligence cases and vast payouts, thus raising the public's consciousness about their right to compensation for negligent medical and nursing care. Yet only a relatively small number of victims of clinical negligence bring a claim and of these 76 per cent fail (Mason, Laurie and Aziz, 2006). Can you imagine how much worse the financial picture would look if a greater number of victims of clinical negligence were to come forward?

Personal refection: common mishaps in hospital giving rise to negligence claims

My long experience as a nurse working in hospitals alerted me to the many things that have gone, and could go, wrong and spiralling cases of clinical negligence claims: patients falling out of beds or jumping over cot-sides; patients being given the wrong medication, or not having their medication administered at all; the wrong limb being amputated in operating theatres; patients given infected blood products that caused them to develop HIV/AIDS and hepatitis; patients having their sound kidney removed instead of the bad one; injections via the wrong sites; women having their 22-week pregnancy mistaken for 32 weeks' gestation and having their premature fetuses induced with consequential non-survival; patients being given the wrong diagnosis, leading to the wrong treatment or no treatment at all; patients suffering from failed sterilisation; patients having swabs left in their bodies following surgery; and many other mishaps. Careless practices and omissions; clinical practice blunders; I could go on!

It is fitting that patients affected by careless clinical practice should feel that somebody somewhere must account and pay for negligent practice. This chapter continues by looking at the notions of *standards* and *duty of care*, and what constitutes negligence that patients could sue and obtain monetary compensation for.

Definition of negligence and prerequisites for a successful negligence claim

Nursing negligence means carrying out a nursing care act carelessly so that it injures your patient. It could also mean omitting to carry out a nursing act for your patient that you were duty bound to do, such that the omission has harmed your patient.

In a more strict legal sense negligence is failure to act in a way that a reasonable person would act, or to do something or omit to do something that a prudent person would not do or omit to do (*Blyth v Birmingham Waterworks* [1856] 11 Ex Ch 781). In this famous case Baron Alderson in establishing facts and basis of the case defined negligence as follows:

> Negligence is the omission to do something which a reasonable man, guided upon those considerations which ordinarily regulate the conduct of human affairs, would do, or doing something which a prudent and reasonable man would not do. The defendants might have been liable for negligence, if, unintentionally, they omitted to do that which a reasonable person would have done, or did that which a person taking reasonable precautions would not have done.

In order for a nurse, doctor, physiotherapist, a NHS Trust, or any other clinician or healthcare agency to be liable for negligence, the claimant (person bringing the claim) must prove three things:

1. that the clinician/caring agency/NHS Trust or other person or body being sued owed him/her a duty of care.;

2. that duty of care and standard imposed by the law had been breached;
3. that breach had caused harm or injury to the claimant/patient, entitling him/her to compensation/damage.

What do we mean by a duty of care and how does it apply to nurses?

A nurse (doctor or any other health professional) does not owe a duty of care to the world at large, neither are these professionals obliged to act as 'good Samaritans'. The claimant must show that a duty of care was owed to the patient concerned. It is up to the court to decide whether the claimant has proved that a duty of care was owed to the patient, that it had been broken and that breach had caused the patient's injury. The facts of a case will determine these things.

A *duty of care* is an obligation on one party to take reasonable care to prevent harm being done to another party. Applying this to nursing, nurses have a legal, professional and ethical obligation to take reasonable care to prevent harm to their patients. The legal test for duty of care in negligence was laid down by the House of Lords in *Donoghue v Stevenson* [1932] AC 562. In this case the Lords held that the manufacturers of ginger beer owed a duty of care to the ultimate consumer, even if that consumer had not purchased the ginger beer directly and so had no direct contract with the seller/manufacturer. How is this possible?

The *Donoghue v Stevenson* case is summarised here. The friend of the person who purchased the ginger beer (in an opaque bottle) had drunk half of it before discovering it contained a partially decomposed snail. She claimed the drink made her ill. As the drinker was not the purchaser, and therefore had no purchasing contract with the manufacturer or the retailer/seller of the ginger beer, the question was: would a duty of care be owed to the friend who consumed the ginger beer? The House of Lords held that such a duty was owed.

In this famous case Lord Atkins established the *'neighbour'* principle by stating that:

> You must take reasonable care to avoid acts or omissions which you can reasonably foresee would be likely to injure your neighbour. Who then in law is my neighbour? The answer seems to be persons who are so closely and directly affected by my act that I ought reasonably to have them in contemplation as being so affected when I am directing my mind to the acts or omissions which are called in question.

Applying this ruling to nursing, it can be taken as read that as long as the court (in the light of the evidence) takes the view that as a competent healthcare practitioner you should have reasonably foreseen the possibility that your act or omission would have armed your patient, then you will be held liable for your negligent act or omission. The *neighbour* principle suggests that the health professional and the patient have a 'legal' ('neighbourly') relationship. Never hurt your friend or neighbour. As a nurse (the patient's 'legal' neighbour) you must take care not to hurt the patient. As the patient's 'legal' neighbour you owe him/her a duty of care. If your conduct (act or omission) (unintentionally) breaches this duty of care, you will be liable in the tort of negligence, for any injuries caused. This is called the 'neighbour principle' or the 'neighbour test'.

'Neighbour' here is a legal entity, a legal 'closeness' or 'proximate' relationship. The fact that the nurse exists to treat the patient and is actually doing so implies that a nurse–patient relationship exists. This is a 'legal neighbourly' relationship. This means that the nurse must ensure that when (s)he applies his/her mind to plan the patient's care, (s)he must ensure that there is no foreseeable potential harm to the patient from that plan of action. Equally, (s)he must ensure that, in planning that care, giving and evaluating the outcomes, there are no omissions on his/her part that could cause harm to the patient.

Legal concept of reasonable competent nurse within the nursing process

Nurses are expected to apply the *nursing process* to patient care. This means *assessing*, *planning*, *implementing* and *evaluating* care to sound professional standards. In *assessing* patients' problems and needs, nurses need to make sure assessments are thorough, comprehensive and accurate, and take into account the best available research and NICE evidence as well as the patients' input. Their consent is crucial. The assessment must consider the patient's holistic needs – physical, psychological, social, religious, economic and other needs. The assessment must not wittingly (criminally) or unwittingly (tortuously) introduce flaws, including omissions that could *reasonably* be foreseen would harm your patient. The word 'reasonably' is important, as the law expects a *competent* assessment to be carried out by any *reasonably competent* nurse. The law is not assuming some expert, 'super duper' nurse, just a *reasonably competent* nurse, undertaking a reasonably competent assessment, care planning, execution and evaluation of care outcomes. Whether you are a registered nurse or student the law empowers the patient to expect competence. The NMC also expects competent practice that protects the patient and gives him/her the best chances of recovery. The reasonable competent nurse will be judged on the basis of competent performance, not on the basis of an expert nurse or nurse consultant. The patient assessment, care planning, delivery and evaluation of care must accord with the principles laid down in the Bolam test of clinical competence (*Bolam v Friern* HMC [1957] 1 WLR 582).

The *'foreseeability' principle* in negligence is crucial. The court takes the view that a reasonably competent nurse must be able to foresee risks and problems (effects and side effects of treatment) and take evasive action, even advising the patient to expect these. The reasonably competent nurse must also be aware that crucial omissions on his/her part can cause difficulties/harm for his/her patients. Therefore as a nurse try to avoid omissions that could hurt your patient. If you miss or fail to effect reasonably competent nursing steps and care that another reasonably competent nurse would not miss, you will be liable in the law of negligence.

To whom does a nurse owe a duty of care?

A nurse does not owe a legal duty of care to just about anyone. (S)he owes this duty to the patients (s)he is responsible to care for. This is not a duty to the world at large. When you qualify as a nurse, your contract of employment and your job description are a good guide to the patients for whom you owe a legal, ethical and professional duty of care. *Do you owe a legal or even a professional or ethical duty of care to the passenger on the same aeroplane as yourself flying out to Spain for your holiday?* Legally you are not obliged to act as the 'good Samaritan' and volunteer to care for a fellow airline passenger. Professionally you are not obliged to do so either. However, you may feel morally obliged to help such a person, as one kind human being to another. This is on the moral ground that if you were the unfortunate sick person/passenger on such a flight you would want someone to help you. Best of all you would want someone, if you had the choice, with medical training to help. Morally, you may be thinking that if the ill passenger were a relative of yours, you would want someone to help them too. However, legally and professional you strictly do not have an obligation to volunteer your professional service. Professionally the NMC (2008a) Code does not compel you to volunteer your professional service to just about any member of the public. It stipulates that in an emergency you may want to volunteer help, and, if you do, you must care for the person to the best of your ability, in the light of available resources. Legally, however no law in England compels you to volunteer care to an airline passenger you do not know. It may interest you to know, too, that in an emergency situation, such as looking after a collapsed fellow airline passenger, if you volunteer to help, where equipment and clinical resources may not be adequate, the standard you will be judged by may be lesser than that against which you would be judged caring for a patient in a fully equipped hospital (Judge Mustill in *Wilsher v Essex Area Health Authority* [1987]).

Personal reflection on acting as a nurse in an emergency on a train

I recall being a passenger on a train boarded at Euston bound for Birmingham. The public address system had asked if there was a doctor or nurse on board to help in a clinical emergency. Legally, I was not obliged to respond. However, there was a professional and ethical conscience that stirred me into action. It turned out that one of the passengers had collapsed in the toilet. I noticed that he was in a pool of blood. He was obviously in shock; his rapid feeble pulse, pale colour, sweaty skin and staring eyes told me so. He was rather pale and very confused. Does the fact that I initiated clinical assessment of this man and started to render him first aid mean I had taken on the role of his nurse? The answer is yes; I had now come to owe him a duty of care.

I had held out my hand to declare that I was a nurse. The call said 'Is there a nurse or doctor on board . . . ?' I was now obliged to take the best care I could of this man. For me and perhaps for the man too, the situation ended satisfactorily when I persuaded the train personnel to telephone ahead to secure an ambulance to take the man off the train to a hospital, before the next schedule stop. It was my professional judgement that the man might not make it to the next scheduled stop at Coventry, so he was put off to an ambulance crew in an emergency stop at Watford Junction. I was pleased and relieved to hand over the man to the ambulance team, thus ending my legal and professional obligation to the man. Hopefully, my intervention helped the man. I had not just performed an ethical and moral obligation to help a fellow man, but I had taken on and now discharged my legal and professional duty of care to him. Some weeks later a letter arrived at my house from the train company thanking me for my help and informing me the man was fine and well and had left hospital.

Regarding the statement made earlier that, in such clinical emergencies as the train and airline, the standard to which one is held is lower, Judge Mustill (in *Wilsher v Essex Area Health Authority* [1987] QB 730, at p. 749; [1986] 3 All ER 801, at p. 812) stated that, if a person is forced by an emergency to do too many things at once, then the fact that he does one of them incorrectly 'should not lightly be taken as negligence'. Khan and Robson (1997, p. 122) have stated:

> Sensibly, the court will not expect a doctor working in extreme conditions to achieve the same results as his colleagues operating within the confines of a hospital and will not judge the defendant's conduct too harshly simply because, with hindsight, a different course would have been adopted had the situation not been an emergency.

In the normal course of events, however, the standard of care in nursing and medicine is that dictated by the Bolam test.

Acting in emergencies outside work: GPs' situation

The situation with a general practitioner (GP) is a little different from that of a nurse passing the site of an accident in which a person needs emergency medical help. A GP is required to provide medical help to those in his/her practice area needing help following accidents or emergencies. This arises from the GP's contractual obligation to his/her health authority and in accordance with the National Health Service (General Medical Pharmaceutical Services) Regulations 1974, SI 1974/160, Schedule 1, para 4(h) and the National Health Service (General Medical Services) Regulations1992 (SI 1992/635) paras 40–1. Similarly, a hospital's accident and emergency (A&E) department owes a duty of care to any patient who turns up there (*Barnett v Chelsea and Kensington* [1969] 1 QB 428). An ambulance crew called to an accident owes a duty of care to those injured (*Kent v Griffiths (No. 3)* [2001] QB 36). The last two rulings may have implications for any nurse who finds him-/herself part of an ambulance crew or part of the A&E team admitting patients in an emergency.

Duty of care under care contractual relationships

In the NHS caring situation, the duty of care owed to patients comes under *tort* law of negligence, not under contract law. However, duty of care also occurs in contractual relationships where, for example, a patient is privately treated by a doctor, nurse or physiotherapist in a private practice. Clinical injuries in these circumstances reflect a breach of contract, a breach of promise to take reasonable care. NHS patients have no contract with NHS trusts, NHS-employed nurses, doctors, physiotherapists and so on. Hence they cannot sue in contract.

Is it fair, just and reasonable to impose a duty of care?

By way of public policy courts are unwilling to widen duty of care to just about anyone. There have to be limits or negligence costs could overwhelm the state. The legal position in respect to duties of care in tort is to ask the question: it is fair, just and reasonable to impose a duty in the given situation? Furthermore, is the relationship between the claimant (patient claiming damage through alleged negligence) and the defendant (the nurse, doctor etc.) sufficiently *proximate* such that harm that flows from the defendant's actions or omissions was *reasonably foreseeable*? In other words, *how directly might a patient be affected by a nurse's behaviour – action or omission?* The answer is 'very directly', because of the closeness of the professional proximate relationship. The more direct the likelihood of harm the more likely it is that a duty will be imposed upon the clinician. There is no doubt that nurses owe their patients a duty of care. If they breach it and cause harm they are liable in the tort of negligence.

Do nurses owe a duty of care to the patient's relatives?

In imposing a duty on a party the law will ask: how fair and reasonable is it to impose this duty? One might then ask: do nurses owe a duty of care to patients' relatives? In some cases they do. It all depends on the *proximity of relationship* to those relatives and whether it is seen as fair and reasonable to impose such a duty. Given that the duty is owed to anyone who is reasonably likely to be affected by the nurse's act or omission, nurses can find themselves owing a duty of care to the patient's relatives and visitors too. On this note, as a nurse you are reminded to ensure that you should not create predispositions in the clinical settings that could cause visitors accidents and injuries. Making sure your clinical setting is physically not cluttered by objects or people is important to prevent foreseeable situations such as accidents. Do not have too many visitors cluttering up the ward or so many people around the bed that you can hardly move. Look out for loose objects – chairs, cables, rugs, mats, loose carpets – that can trip up people. People will find it difficult to escape in an orderly manner from a crowded ward if a fire breaks out. Nurses must take steps to reduce risks of accidents in the ward, whether to patients, relatives, visitors or other staff. If the *proximity* of relationship is close (as defined by Lord Atkins) then a duty will be owed. There is proximity of relationship between nurse, patients and visiting relatives.

The law believes in that which is fair, reasonable and practicable and sets a limit on potential claimants' capacity to claim. When visitors leave the ward and are out on the public roads, the proximity of relationship between them and the nurse is broken. If the nurse is now on his/her way home and sees one of those visitors in a motor vehicle accident, that nurse does not by English law have to stop, let alone offer medical help, unless the nurse him-/herself was involved in the accident. On the grounds of public policy alone, there must be a limit to which a duty may be imposed on others.

In *Fairlie v Perth and Kinross Healthcare NHS Trust* [2004] SLT 1200 (OH), the view that a father was owed a duty of care by the health board, in respect to alleged distress he suffered from being accused of abusing his daughter, who had undergone allegedly negligent psychiatric care, was not accepted by the court. Why? The court maintained that at no point did the father come into any 'special relationship' with the attending psychiatrist. This leads one to ask: can a duty of care be owed by a healthcare professional to a third party affected by the patient's act or omission?

Khan and Robson (1997, p. 71) state: 'In appropriate circumstances the legal duty of care may be owed by the health carer to a third party affected by the patient's acts or omissions.' However, in respect to the scenario outlined in Student activity 7.1 (Box 7.1), Khan and Robson believe that the English court may take the view that the healthcare professional should have persuaded the patient not to commit the act intended, or should have had him treated in a way that acknowledges his expressed intentions. They doubt that such a duty would be owed under English law because it would be difficult to establish the 'reasonable foresight test'. English law may refuse to accept that it is 'fair and reasonable' to expect a health professional operating within a professional and confidential relationship to breach that confidence and inform a third party of the patient's intention. There are perhaps alternative views on this case. What is yours?

BOX 7.1 Student activity 7.1

Scenario based on a true case

Imagine that you are a qualified nurse counsellor working in psychiatric nursing, but who also provides counselling services to students at a university, to which you are part-time contracted. In the course of his treatment one of your patients (a university student with a paranoid psychiatric illness) tells you that he loves a certain woman (another student), but she does not love him and regards him as only a friend, not a lover. The patient further reveals to you that, if he cannot gain the woman's love as a sexual partner, he is going to kill her. You are very concerned about this express threat, but decide to do nothing about it for fear of breaching the nurse counsellor–patient confidential relationship. You have not informed the female student under threat (a student known to you) of the impending threat to her life. Equally, you decide not to inform the university authority of the threat. Subsequently your patient (the male student) goes out and kills the woman. The victim's relatives bring a case of negligence against you and the university, seeking compensation for the death of their daughter.

Use your portfolio to analyse what you consider to be your situation in law and professionally. Although you are a qualified counsellor you are registered as a nurse with the NMC and use your nursing status as part of your counselling role.

Reflecting on the scenario in Box 7.1, to what extent do you think the claim against you and the university would be likely to succeed? Write your response in your law and ethics portfolio, ensuring you provide legal, professional and ethical rationales for your response. Try to be as analytical as you can. After doing this, read on for some pointers.

Food for thought in relation to Student activity 7.1:

- The patient/client has a paranoid illness. Ponder on the implications of this.
- A third party is at risk. What does the NMC code say in this context?
- What does English law say about duty of care to patients/clients/third parties?
- What happened in the US case of *Tarasoff v Regents of the University of California* (1976) 551 P (2d) 334?
- What about notifying the university authority? Rationale for your answer?
- What about exploring with your client his feelings of hate for the girl, why he would want to do such a thing, the implications for all?
- What about persuading your client to consider discussing his feeling of hate and paranoia with the girl he claims to love, his potential victim?
- Have you considered talking to the potential victim about the situation and her possible predicament? What would you be hoping to achieve here? Explore in your own mind the confidentiality issues involved here.
- What about exploring with the victim the need for her to take precautions, even discussing her situation with her family?
- Have you explored the situation you face with more experienced and knowledgeable counsellor colleagues? To what avail? What does your professional body tell you about working within the limits of your competence? Dangers and implications of working outside your capability and capacity?
- The English court may well take the view that, since both the patient and the potential victim are students at the same university and may be somehow under university influence and 'control', then the female student should have been warned by you and the university authorities to take reasonable care and precaution.
- Khan and Robson (1997) think that sharing client-confidential information with a known third party whose life is under threat may not be tolerated by a British court. What do you think? Exercise some critical reasoning here. What in your nursing Code tells you to be aware of serious risks to third parties and your professional obligations here?
- In America the above scenario was indeed a reality, and, in the roughly similar case [*Tarasoff v Regents of the University of California* (1976) 551 P (2d) 334], the Supreme Court of California held that the defendant healthcare professional (a psychologist) owed a duty of care to the third party: the female student who had been murdered. The male student, who had a psychiatric illness, had said that he would go out and kill his fellow student if she refused to have him as a lover. He did precisely that. He was pathologically obsessed with this woman. The Supreme Court of California said that the known third party was also due a duty of care, and that the psychologist involved should have warned her. What are your thoughts on this?
- The NMC, whilst imploring you to respect the patient's right to consent, privacy and confidentiality, also warns that there may be compelling reasons to breach confidentiality, such as where not doing so would place your patient and other known third party at serious risk of harm. Reflect critically on other likely situations that may force you to breach patient confidentiality.

Duty of care to a third party

In the American case above, the Supreme Court of California took the view that the healthcare professional was not justified to just sit back and argue that as the third party was not his patient he owed no duty of care towards her. The court further held that the healthcare professional had a positive obligation to exercise reasonable care to protect the potential victim from the impending danger which was *reasonably foreseen*. Moreover, the court took the view that the duty of confidentiality was outweighed by the duty to the third party. A number of UK authorities, for example Khan and Robson (1997), are of the opinion that this case would not have succeeded under English law for the reasons given above.

Read the scenario in Box 7.2 and then address the question that follows. I suggest that you use legal reasoning and arguments to analyse the scenario. Use the law and ethics section of your portfolio to record your answer.

Suggestions in response to the student activity question in Box 7.2

Some reasoning

The woman could sue but it is doubtful that under current English law she would win. Under English law, the health professional's duty of care is first and foremost to his/her patient with HIV. It does make good and responsible professional sense, however, to inform your HIV-positive patient of the risks he poses to his sexual partner by having unprotected sex with her. Moreover, try to persuade him to inform his partner of his HIV status. You do not have the right under English law to breach confidentiality by telling the woman of her partner's HIV status, even though morally and ethically you feel you ought to. There may be occasions when a healthcare professional may breach confidentiality and may be protected under English law, such as when a court of law requires you to, or in cases where the

---

BOX 7.2 Student activity 7.2

Scenario based on a true case

You are the nurse treating a male patient who has tested positive for HIV. You know that this patient is in a steady relationship with a woman with whom he has a number of children. You counsel the patient about the danger of unprotected sex and advises him strongly to tell his partner of his HIV status, as his unprotected sex with her imposes a considerable risk of her contracting HIV. You subsequently find that the patient has not told his partner of his HIV status and so you again strongly advise him to do so, threatening that if he refuses you will take it upon yourself as a responsible healthcare professional to tell the partner. The patient insists that you not do so, and moreover states that if anyone tells his partner about his HIV status it will be he and not you the healthcare professional. The patient still has not informed his partner and she later tests positive for HIV.

Student activity question

Can the woman in this scenario sue the healthcare professional as owing her a duty of care to inform her of her lover's HIV status and failing to do so?

public's health would be seriously undermined, or under certain public health regulations and of course under the Road Traffic Act 1988. However, the above scenario situation is not one of these conditions.

The situation in America

In America, although a similar case (*Bradshaw v Daniel* [1994] Med L Rev 237) was one that concerned Rocky Mountain spotted fever, rather than HIV, the Supreme Court of Tennessee held that the physician concerned owed a duty of care to the third party (the man's wife) even though this woman was not the doctor's patient. The court held that the doctor–patient relationship imposed upon the doctor a positive duty to warn the wife of the foreseeable risks of getting Rocky Mountain spotted fever from her husband. It was the view of the Supreme Court that the physician should have reasonably foreseen the injury, in this case the possible contagion, Rocky Mountain spotted fever, and even consequent death, to the third party. The husband had recently died from Rocky Mountain spotted fever. In fact he died only a short time before his wife started to show symptoms of the disease. The son brought the action against the physician on the grounds that he was negligent not to have told his mother of her risk of exposure to the disease.

If we look at Lord Atkin's 'neighbour test' in *Donoghue v Stevenson*, it would be very difficult to establish that in both cases above, if they were tried under English law, the neighbour test applied. Moreover, under English law, it might not have been considered *fair*, *reasonable* and *just* to expect the healthcare professional to owe a duty of care to the two third parties in the two scenarios described.

Some conditions under which public healthcare services owe a duty of care

A public service caring agency, for example the NHS, without doubt owes a duty of care to all patients it accepts for treatment. A GP owes a duty of care to all the patients on his/her lists. Can a doctor or a clinical nurse specialist, or a medical assistant or a triage nurse, for example, refuse to accept an emergency case that turns up in the accident and emergency unit of a hospital for treatment? The answer is no. The reason for this is that the hospital presents itself as offering emergency care, a really public statement that it will provide emergency care in all circumstances. If it finds that it is about to be overwhelmed by a preponderance of emergency cases, probably because of a major disaster down the road, then it is considered expedient and obligatory to inform the ambulance service to try to 'shunt' emergency cases elsewhere. It cannot turn away those who turn up for emergency care. In *Cassidy v Ministry of Health* [1951] 2 KB 343, Lord Denning stated that when a hospital holds itself out as offering hospital care and a patient

> puts himself in the hands of a hospital he expects there to be sufficient qualified people and adequate facilities to look after him properly and hopefully make him better; if that fails to materialise then it is fitting that the health authority should be made liable.

In *Kent v Griffiths* [2000] 2 WLR 1158; [2000] 2 All ER 474, it was established that the ambulance service also has a legal duty to respond to a call for help. The implications of these principles are clear. Under the terms of their contract of employment nurses must make every effort to ensure that the services that their employers publicly claim to offer are in fact in readiness. If you are the doctor or nurse making the everyday clinical and management decision with respect to admitting and treating patients in an emergency situation, and you find that the service is falling short in terms of its ability to respond effectively, it is your duty and obligation to bring this to the attention of your employers.

Student nurses demonstrating duty of care and anticipation of emergencies

As a student nurse you may well ask yourself why the ward manager requires you to check emergency, as well as other, equipment regularly, perhaps daily, to ensure their working order. The answer is self-evident: be prepared at all times to deliver the care you publicly declare is your business or that of your employer. You should do nothing to breach the duty of care you have to your patient. If you do, then you may be liable for negligence, either yourself directly under *primary liability*, or your employer under *vicarious and/or primary liability*. As Mason and colleagues (2006, p. 305) have pointed out, although currently the health service itself bears the entire costs of negligence litigation, 'there is, of course, nothing to stop a patient or claimant suing an individual', meaning a doctor, nurse, physiotherapist or other healthcare professional.

As was alluded to in Chapter 2, it is important for nurses to make sure they have proper insurance indemnity cover against anything going wrong in their care and for which they may be cited as having primary liability for the injured patient. In practice, however, under the NHS indemnity scheme patients are more likely to sue the NHS Trust rather than an individual nurse or other health professional who may not have the means to pay compensation. This does not, however, prevent an NHS Trust from trying to recover its losses by claiming against the nurse's, doctor's or physiotherapist's personal indemnity insurance. So far there is no evidence of this taking place in the UK – yet.

Duty to keep professional knowledge and skills up to date

As a nurse you also have a duty to *keep yourself informed and up to date*. This is both a professional and a legal responsibility and obligation. The NMC (2004) states at paragraph 6.1:

> You must keep your knowledge and skills up-to-date throughout your working life. In particular, you should take part regularly in learning activities that develop your competence and performance.

The NMC's (2008a) revised Code supports the above guiding principle.

The law also expects the healthcare professional to keep up to date with major developments in his/her profession. The law does not expect you to know everything there is to know. It nevertheless expects you to continue your professional development in terms of new knowledge, skills and competencies beyond the point of your graduation from university and registration with the NMC. In the case of *Crawford v Board of Governors of Charing Cross Hospital* [1953], *The Times*, 8 December, CA, the plaintiff had developed brachial palsy from his arm being kept in the same position during an operation. The anaesthetist was alleged to be negligent for allowing this to happen. Six months prior to the operation an article had come out in *The Lancet* pointing out just such an eventuality. Was the anaesthetist negligent? The Court of Appeal thought not. Lord Denning said:

> It . . . would be putting too high a burden on a medical man to say that he has to read every article appearing in the current medical press; it would be quite wrong to suggest that a medical man is negligent because he does not at once put into operation the suggestions which some contributor or other might make in a medical journal. The time

may come in a particular case when a new recommendation may be so well proved and so well known, and so well accepted that it should be adopted, but that was not so in this case.

Is there a legal duty to tell the truth to patients when things go wrong?

Do nurses have a duty to tell the truth? This question of veracity or truth telling is one that is frequently posed within ethics literature (for example, Hawley, 2007; Newham and Hawley, 2007). Hendrick (2000) points to a number of sources that appear to suggest that nurses, like doctors, owe patients a duty of *candour*; that is a duty to inform them when something has gone wrong. Mason and colleagues (2006) point out that the senior judiciary (particularly Lord Wolfe) seems to be in favour of a move towards candour by medical professionals. In *Naylor v Preston AHA* [1987] 1 WLR 958, Lord Donaldson stated that 'in medical negligence cases there is a duty of candour resting upon the professional man'. Healthcare professionals have a duty to inform patients that they have a right to sue.

In *Gerber v Pines* [1935] 79 Sol 13, the court pointed out that when a foreign substance was left in a patient's body the doctor had a duty to inform the patient of that fact, even where there was no negligence. This picture seems to suggest that nurses are in the same position as doctors, and do have a legal duty to inform patients of where their professional care has damaged the patient, or has gone wrong somehow. In reality however, is this likely to happen? Only time will tell.

My feelings from an experiential perspective are that, as clinical negligence claims spiral in the UK and patients become more aggressive about suing for negligence, there might be a greater temptation than hitherto for healthcare professionals not to deliberately reveal mishaps for fear of being sued. Thus this might lead to a growth in defensive clinical practice. Whether or not there is a substantial legal basis for nurses telling their patients when something has gone wrong, there is certainly an ethical duty to do so, especially where the mistake can be put right and other nurses can benefit from knowing how the mistake happened and how it may be prevented and put right. Such candour presents opportunity for effective clinical reflection that can only promote professional growth and development.

Duty to protect patients and clients from themselves

For those of you working within the mental health (MH) and learning disability (LD) specialty the duty to protect patients/clients from themselves can be very real at times. In assessing a patient with a MH/LD problem it is worth asking yourself: is this client a risk to him-/herself? Patients suffering from some forms of depression may be particularly vulnerable to committing suicide and need to be carefully observed. In other cases vulnerability to suicide may result from the drug that the patient is taking, as some drugs, particularly in patients with certain constitutions, may render patients at risk of committing suicide. Some may have hallucinogenic side effects persuading patients to kill themselves. Patients who are admitted to hospital for drugs overdose should, in the first place, be suspected of deliberately attempting to end their life, until further observations and investigations prove otherwise. Until circumstances dictate otherwise, such patients need to be carefully managed and supervised, including, if possible, giving them round-the-clock observation, although in law hourly observation may be enough, even if morally questionable. By this I mean that, as some of the cases below will show, a court may be satisfied that hourly observations of patients with suicidal tendencies may be enough to satisfy the reasonable standard of care expected. Limited resources sometimes preclude more frequent observations.

In the case of *Selfe v Ilford and District Hospital Management Committee* (1970, 114 Sol Jo 935; [1970] 4 *British Medical Journal* 754) a 17-year-old male had been admitted to hospital following a drugs overdose. He had a history of suicidal tendencies, yet the nurses failed to observe him effectively. He was nursed on the ground floor of a ward, which had a total of 27 clients, three of whom were also suicidal risks. The three nurses on the ward knew of the client's suicidal tendencies, yet they made it possible for him to have access to an open window. All three nurses disappeared from the observation scene simultaneously. One nurse was attending to another patient, whilst another went to the loo and the third to the kitchen. None of them informed the others what (s)he was doing. The patient seized his opportunity to escape onto the roof through the open window. He then threw himself from the roof, seriously injuring himself. The court awarded damages amounting to £19,000, on the basis that the degree of nursing care required was proportionate to the risk of suicide involved, and in this case the nurses had failed to exercise proper duty of care in observation and supervision. The court felt that nursing care supervision had broken down, enabling this man to escape through the window

On the other hand, in the case of *Thorne v Northern Group Hospital Management Committee* [1964] 108 Sol Jo 484, a man failed to win damages for the death of his wife. She was a patient in a suicidal mood. She slipped out the hospital when the nurses were not looking, went home and gassed herself. The court took the view that, although the level of supervision that a hospital should exercise over patients with suicidal tendencies is greater than that exercised over other patients, suicidal patients could not be kept under constant supervision by the staff.

In *Dunn v South Tyneside Health Care NHS Trust* [2003] EWCA Civ 878, [2004] PIQR 150, the court arrived at a decision similar to that in *Thorne v Northern Group HMC*. In the *Dunn* case a mental health patient suffering from a bipolar illness and who was on one-hourly observation evaded the nurses' detection, went home and consumed large quantities of anti-asthmatic tablets, which caused severe brain damage. Her legal team tried to establish that a 15-minute frequency of observation was the standard, not hourly. Moreover, they contended that had the police been informed earlier of the absence without leave they would have found the patient and presumably saved her. The case failed because (a) the court accepted that hourly observations were an acceptable standard given the patient's condition, history and the standard laid down in both *Bolam* and *Bolitho* and (b) it was not an established fact that the police would have intervened to prevent the harm even if they had been told earlier that the patient had absconded.

Standard of care

In most clinical negligence cases the most pertinent issue is whether the healthcare professional involved was in breach of the *professional* and *legal standard of care*. Under English law the test question is: did the healthcare professional's standard of care fall below the standard of the ordinary skilled man exercising and professing to have that special skill? In the landmark case of *Bolam v Frien Hospital Management Committee* [1957] 2 All ER 118; 1 WLR 582] McNair J gave the classic answer when he said:

> The test is the standard of the ordinary skilled man [person] exercising and professing to have that special skill. A man [person] need not possess the highest expert skill at the risk of being found negligent. It is a well-established law that it is sufficient if he [the person] exercises the ordinary skill of an ordinary man [person] exercising that particular art.

(p. 121)

It is important to note, however, that McNair J further stated that the test of that skill:

> is not the test of the man on top of the Clapham omnibus because [that man] has not got this special skill.
>
> (p. 586)

This means therefore that the health professional demonstrating the degree of competence expected of the ordinary competent clinician sets the standard. The professional is the one who follows the correct standard of care – the one that is the professionally acceptable standard followed by that profession. These standards are those regarded as respectable by the body of professional opinion and practice.

The 'average' nurse is expected to reach the level of competence laid down by the NMC. (S)he is expected to have a sound grasp of nursing theory and practice, acceptable caring attitudes, appropriate skills and competencies befitting an ordinary competent registered nurse. Such a nurse would be expected to demonstrate that (s)he had kept up with notable professional changes in the practice of nursing, and was up to date on established and acceptable research evidence that informs current practice. This implies that the ordinary competent nurse is expected to continue to develop beyond the point of graduation and professional registration. (S)he should be able to demonstrate the NMC's (2004) *Code of Professional Conduct: Standards for Conduct, Performance and Ethics* (see also NMC, 2008a,b). Thus the ordinary competent registered nurse must be able to satisfy the following:

> You must keep your knowledge and skills up-to-date throughout your working life. In particular, you should take part regularly in learning activities that develop your competence and performance.
>
> To practice competently, you must possess the knowledge, skills and abilities required for lawful, safe and effective practice without direct supervision. You must acknowledge the limits of your professional competence and only undertake practice and accept responsibilities for those activities in which you are competent.
>
> (NMC, 2004, p. 9)

Returning to Judge McNair's classic definition of the *standard of care*, one would point out that if the healthcare professional's practice conforms to a responsible body of professional opinions, existing at that time, then this is good enough. Alleged negligence could fail under such conditions. Why? The healthcare professional can show that what was done conformed to a body of professional opinion regarded as respectable by the profession concerned. As in the cases of *Bolam v Frien Hospital Management Committee* and *Whitehouse v Jordan* [1981] 1 WLR 246; [1981] 1 All ER 267, a healthcare professional is not liable for negligence if (s)he has acted in accordance with a practice acceptable as proper by a responsible body of healthcare professionals skilled in that particular art.

The implications of the *Bolam* ruling for nurses are as follows:

1. Although the ruling was in respect to doctors, it applies to nurses also.
2. The concept of 'the ordinary skilled man' can be safely translated into the 'ordinary skilled or competent nurse exercising and professing to have those special skills, the skills of a nurse'.
3. As a registered nurse you will not be negligent if the standard of your practice accords with that of the ordinary skilled nurse from within the same specialty.
4. A nurse need not possess the highest standard of skill, or have the skills of a 'super-duper' nurse. Nurses will be judged by their peers. This means that the staff nurse will

be judged by standards of the ordinary skilled staff nurse working in the same speciality and not necessarily by the standard of an expert nurse from that speciality. The clinical nurse specialist will be held to the standard of a competent clinical nurse specialist, and the nurse consultant by the standard of other ordinary competent nurse consultants. The fact that the nurse will be judged by a peer or another nurse who does the same job makes the *Bolam* test an objective one.

5. In the case of an action for negligence against a nurse, the court is likely to call what are known as 'expert witnesses' to testify whether the practice of the nurse being tried for negligence is that expected of a ordinary competent nurse in that specialty.

6. Liability for negligence is placed on the nurse whose practice has fallen below the acceptable standard. Liability is not placed on your colleague, even if you had sought his/her opinion of what to do. You are responsible for your own professional judgement. You can not blame your peer for your mistakes.

7. Nurses must remember that the *Bolam* standard applies not only in giving care but in all areas of nursing – assessment, diagnosis, treatment, forecasting outcome/prognosis, disclosing information – and in counselling within all branches of nursing.

8. The *Bolam* standard is about the level or standard from which a professional nurse may not fall. It is the basal safe level and this implies that practitioners should always seek to improve and enhance their standard. Try and operate above the minimum safe bar. If your practice falls below this you will be liable for negligence.

9. Because under *Bolam* the healthcare professional standard has always been judged by a fellow healthcare professional, then it could be said that healthcare professions have always been seen to set, monitor and control their own standards.

10. Since the *Bolitho* case, however, in future judges will be more likely to challenge the judgement of healthcare professionals, acting as expert witnesses, with respect to whether those professionals had put their minds to the issue of risks against benefits and had come up with conclusions that are logically defensible. Even so, however, judges will be unlikely to reject the opinion of experts in the field. In fact judges will be more inclined to accept the opinions of experts as reasonable.

11. If there are differences of opinion from experts as to how a particular nursing procedure can be carried out, the court is not likely to accept one as better than the other (*Maynard v West Midland RHA* [1985] 1 All ER 635). This implies that nurses do not necessarily have to worry that their method (providing it is viewed as acceptable by other respectable professional nurses) is different from that of their colleagues.

    So long as their methods conform to *a reasonable respectable body of nursing opinions, skilled in the art and science of nursing*, this will be acceptable to the court. This, however, is based on the proviso that the experts have put their minds to the issue of considering and balancing risks against benefits and come up with sound defensible judgements. In other words, other reasonably competent nurses do it (the task or procedure) similarly well and to a reasonable acceptable standard. Equally, other nurses who do things differently may also be justified on the same grounds. Nurses need to make sure their practice is grounded in sound research evidence and supported by a respectable body of nursing opinion and practices standards.

12. Given that *Bolam* established a minimum acceptable standard of care, it means that even student nurses must aim to provide that minimum safe and competent standard of care. Patients expect student nurses to owe them a duty of care and to deliver care to the *Bolam* standard. This further implies that if, as a student nurse, you are not certain what to do for your patient, not sure of the acceptable standard, and you do not feel competent

to perform the nursing skill, then you should consult with and ask the qualified nurse for guidance. If the qualified nurse in turn instructs you on a particular procedure and you perform it as directed, and it goes wrong, (s)he has to accept responsibility and liability. However, you are still obliged to query when and where you feel a practice is wrong even if it is performed by a senior colleague. If you consult your superior you are upholding the relevant standard of care (*Wilsher v Essex AHA* [1988] 2 WLR 557; see Box 7.3).

13. If as a nurse you take on a task that has been delegated to you and which you are not competent to perform, then you will be negligent should you cause harm to the patient through your substandard practice.

14. The standard of care must be established in relation to the job description, in other words the post in question, and not to the individual post holder's rank or his/her personal ability, since duty needs to be aligned to acts to be performed, rather than to the person occupying the post. (Inexperience is no defence against a claim of negligence.)

BOX 7.3 The case of Martin Wilsher (*Wilsher v Essex AHA* 1988)

The case of little Martin Wilsher (*Wilsher v Essex AHA* [1988] 2 WLR 557) supports the view expressed at item 12 in the list. In this case Martin Wilsher was born three months premature. He needed oxygen to live and an inexperienced junior doctor, having consulted with a registrar from whom he sought guidance, inserted a catheter into one of Martin's veins rather than into one of his arteries in order to monitor his oxygen levels. Clearly, the senior doctor had failed to spot the mistake. Some time later a senior registrar came along and made the same mistake as the junior doctor. The catheter had therefore failed to monitor Martin's oxygen levels and it was alleged he suffered retinal damage, causing blindness, a condition known as retrolental fibroplasia. Martin's legal team thought that the increased oxygen had caused the condition in question. The trial judge awarded £116,199 to the child for his injury.

The Health Authority appealed, saying that the standard of care delivered was appropriate and that the plaintiff had failed to establish that the excess oxygen was the cause of the damage. One of the most critical points that came out the appeal was the view of the Court of Appeal that there is *no concept of team negligence*. Each team member has responsibility to observe the standards of the unit as a whole. The court also decided that, although inexperience is no defence against a claim of negligence, the junior doctor was not negligent given that he had sought the guidance of his superior, the registrar. The registrar was negligent in failing to note that the junior doctor had placed the catheter into the vein rather than the artery, and for doing the same thing himself. Hence the health authority was vicariously liable for the registrar's negligence.

It is worthwhile noting that, as the child was unable to prove that his retinal damage was as a direct result of the doctor's blunder, the House of Lords ordered a retrial to establish causation of damage. This never took place as the parties settled out of court.

Another critical principle that was established in this case is the view that Health Authorities (now NHS Trusts) can be *directly liable for negligence if they fail to staff their units with adequate numbers of staff and skill mix*.

A word of warning to all nurses

I must warn all nurses reading about the *Bolam* test that the fact that 'Nelly' has done her nursing 'this way' for the last 20 years does not necessarily mean that this 20-year-old method is still the correct one. Registered nurses must continue to question practice in the light of emerging sound research evidence. This is because a procedure or practice that may have been acceptable as respectable 10 years ago may no longer be respectable. Your day-to-day clinical practice must be soundly evidence based, for, as the case of *Bolitho v Hackney Health Authority* [1997] 3 WLR 1151 has shown, the Lord Lords were unanimous that the courts must not just accept the views of doctors (or other healthcare professionals) who testify for doctors (other colleagues) that a particular course of action is respectable and professionally acceptable or competent.

In addition, the court must satisfy itself that the experts giving the evidence in support of the doctor (healthcare professional) have 'weighed up the risks and benefits' and arrived at a 'defensible conclusion'. However, it is widely believed that the courts will in future be unlikely to depart from *Bolam*, because in the vast majority of cases the issue that distinguishes experts in the field are of a particular type most likely to demonstrate the reasonableness of that opinion. (So through *Bolitho* the courts expect to observe logical decision making, in which risks have been weighed against benefits by those giving the 'expert' evidence, and that a defensible conclusion had been reached.)

In the light of the Wilsher case are extended role nurses expected to operate to a higher standard? Just a word of caution for nurses who now take on extended roles previously undertaken by doctors. It must be recalled that, in the Martin Wilsher case, Lord Justice Mustill had said that in the context of health professionals occupying posts in units offering specialised service, the standard is not just that 'of the averagely competent and well-informed junior houseman . . . but of such a person who fills a post in a unit offering a highly specialised service' (1986, 3 All ER 801, p. 813). Does Lord Justice Mustill's statement imply an elevated standard of care, above that of the ordinary competent practitioner founded on *Bolam*? Second, does the Wilsher case mean that nurses who now take on extended roles, previously undertaken by doctors, must demonstrate the same medical standard, including knowledge, skills and competencies? *Logically, this must be the case*. This suggests, amongst other things, that the extended role nurses must possess the same level of knowledge and competencies as the doctors who previously performed those roles. Given this, extended role nurses will be judged by the standard of other competent extended role nurses who are clearly operating to the professional standard of the post in which the post holder is performing. This standard must in logic be that of doctors who previously did the job.

My advice therefore to nurses about to take on extended role functions is to make sure they are properly prepared for the role, to a standard consistent with the skills, knowledge and competencies that define an 'extended role'. Those specific role standards must be clearly defined. From this it may be concluded that, in a negligence case in which a nurse in an extended role is implicated, the standard by which (s)he will be measured is that defined by the role. Extended role nurses will therefore be judged 'by the standard of the reasonable doctor' (McHale and Tingle, 2001, p. 76).

What is the acceptable standard if there is a difference of opinion in terms of a standard clinical procedure? Applying the *Bolam* test to nursing, the courts are not likely to choose between two respectable competing practices or procedures, as to which one is better. The court is likely to determine if both procedures are respectable in the eyes of expert nurses in that field, providing risks have been balanced against benefits and a defensible conclusion has been reached. In essence then, the simple fact that your practice or procedure varies from another nurse's does not necessarily mean you are negligent. If the nurse as the defendant can demonstrate that another respectable body of nursing opinions (nurses) would have conducted themselves in a similar manner, the chances are that the court will find that the defendant nurse is not negligent. However, as indicated above, since *Bolam*, the courts will expect the expert nurses giving evidence in support of their colleagues to demonstrate that they had considered all the risks against benefits in a logical way and had reached a 'defensible conclusion'. In *Bolitho*, Lord Browne-Wilkinson, however, made the point that:

> In the vast majority of cases the fact that distinguish experts in the field are of a particular opinion . . . But if, in the rare case, it can be demonstrated that the professional opinion is not capable of withstanding logical analysis, the judge is entitled to hold that the body of opinion is not reasonable or responsible [however] it will seldom be right for a judge to reach a conclusion that views genuinely held by a competent medical expert are unreasonable.
>
> ([1997] 4 All ER 771 at 779, [1998] 39 BMLR 1 AT 10)

Mason and colleagues (2006) point out that in *De Freitas v O'Brien* ([1995], 25 BMLR 51; [1995] 6 Med LR 108, CA) the court did not go overboard to bolster up the conservative approach to assessing the acceptability of a body of opinion, but instead states that the responsible body of opinion need not be large. In other words as few as a couple of experts (fellow healthcare professionals) may be enough to convince the court that the action taken was the right, reasonable and acceptable one. Thus *De Freitas* is regarded as supporting the notion of the 'super specialist' (Mason *et al.*, 2006, p. 314) whom the court may well accept as being able to perform procedures mere mortal surgeons and run-of-the-mill practitioners may regard as being inappropriate or too risky. The Court of Appeal in *De Freitas* also confirmed that the *Bolam* test does not require the body of professional opinion to be large. These views have led many to criticise *De Freitas* as having given a licence to super specialists within the medical profession to take unacceptable risks. If this is true it is perhaps a good thing for the purposes of pushing the frontiers of clinical sciences even further, because innovative clinical practice does depend to some extent on more than average risks being taken some of the times. If we did not have specialists who are prepared to take risks, this could threaten the advancement of clinical practice. I do not think we need to worry too much about giving an unrestricted licence to innovative super specialists willing to take risks to advance medicine, because the court retains the right to decide when a risk taken is unreasonable and indeed too risky.

How does the above relate to nursing practice, especially to those of our more innovative practitioners? Would their departure from the standard practice be regarded as negligent should anything go wrong? The answer must be that the court would be prepared to look at the logical reasoning behind the departure before making up its mind. The court could be expected, under *De Freitas v O'Brien*, to conceive of the possibility of a limited number of high fliers within the profession being confident, capable, able and willing to depart from the standard mundane practice for the perceived benefit of patients, especially where perhaps standard procedures and practices had failed to work for the patient concerned. Judges are smart, sensible and practical individuals who have the ability to make decisions in relation to risk taking in clinical practice: risk taking that is based on such considerations as what is best for the patient; what could work for the patient when all else appears to have failed; what may be seen as credible practice in the light of new research; justified experimentation to establish new and successful practice procedures, and try out newly found remedies to validate practice and research. I realise that the more faint-hearted among us may gasp at my suggestion, but if risks are not taken, provided those risks can be justified, we do not stand much chance of enhancing the standards of clinical nursing, medical or physiotherapy practice.

The most important final statement under 'duty of care' must be the view that if a nurse or any other healthcare professional breaches a duty of care to their patient (s)he has certainly satisfied one of the three criteria the patient has to prove to win a negligence claim.

Causation of damage

In order for the claimant to win his/her case (s)he must prove that there is a causal link between the breach of duty and the harm suffered. *Factual* causation is perhaps the most difficult one to prove of the three factors necessary for liability in negligence to be found. Although a nurse may have breached his/her duty of care, the claimant still has to prove that the breach caused the injury or at least materially contributed to it, or increased the risk of the injury occurring. The claimant has to prove causation on the *balance of probability*, in which case the court has to be satisfied that the claimant's version of evens is 50 per cent likely. What is also critical is the possibility that the harm alleged to have happened was *reasonably foreseeable*.

The claimant is likely to win the case if (s)he can prove that:

1. 'but for' the defendant's negligence the injury would not have occurred (the so-called *but for* test); or
2. the defendant's negligence materially contributed to the injury, or increased its risk; or
3. where the claim is for negligent non-disclosure of important information relevant to the care, had the claimant been informed, of risks for example, (s)he would never have agreed to the treatment.

The general rule is for the patient/claimant to prove his/her case, namely that the injury has come about owing to the defendant's negligence. It is not for the defendant to prove that his/her negligence did not cause the injury. Hendricks (1997) draws attention to the fact that causation can be difficult to prove because of time lapse between the alleged incident and the trial. Jaded memory and sometimes inadequate documentation may be handicaps. Sometimes there is more than one factor of causation, in which case it may be possible for the defendant to show that, as well as the causation factor (s)he is alleged to be responsible for, there are a number of other factors that may be responsible. In this case the claimant may be unable to prove that the alleged causation is indeed the one, or, if it does contribute to the damage, it may be difficult to state categorically to what degree or extent. In multiple causation factors the evidential burden is on the claimant to prove causation. All three factors of negligence must be present: duty owed, duty breached, and breach leading to the injury.

In the classic *but for* test, the claimant is actually saying: but for the defendant's negligence I would not be in this situation; I would not have suffered this injury. In the case of *Barnett v Chelsea and Kensington Hospital Management Committee* [1969] 1 QB 428, the claimant had drunk some tea, and unknown to him there was arsenic in it. He suffered severe vomiting and turned up in casualty for medical attention. The casualty doctor did not examine him but sent him a message to go away and see his own doctor. Shortly afterwards, the patient died of arsenic poisoning. His widow brought an action in negligence. She lost, because although the doctor did not deny negligence in failing to see the patient, let alone examine him, it was not his lack of care that caused the patient's death. In fact the arsenic poisoning had been too far advanced for any treatment to be successful. So here we find a claimant failing to establish causation of injury. Had the doctor seen the patient it would have made no difference to his death. My advice to the nurse, doctor or other healthcare professional reading this case and its outcome, which was legally in the doctor's favour, is not to be complacent in practice, because any healthcare professional who behaves like this casualty officer could find him-/herself facing severe disciplinary action, professionally and from his/her employer.

Failure of negligence claims where there are two or more causation factors

Returning to the Martin Wilsher case (*Wilsher v Essex Area Health Authority* [1988] WLR 557), it was this multiple causation issue that caused young Wilsher to lose his case. The trial judge had awarded Wilsher £116,199 for his injury; the Health Authority appealed. The Court of Appeal considered that the senior doctor who had guided the junior doctor was negligent. The House of Lords reversed the decision of the Court of Appeal. It held that excess oxygen was only one of the five known causes of retrolental fibroplasia, and all five factors were present in the child. So, on the balance of probabilities, it had not been proven that the excess oxygen was the effective cause of the blindness. The scientific evidence which purported to signal that excess oxygen was the actual cause of the blindness was in doubt, at best inconclusive or ambivalent. The House of Lords did suggest a retrial to establish causation, but the parties settled out of court.

Even where there are only two possible causes of the injury, proving direct causation can be equally problematic for the claimant. In the case of *Kay v Ayrshire and Arran HB* [1987] 2 All ER 417, a two-year-old child was being treated for meningitis. By some error of calculation, he had been given 300,000 units of penicillin instead of 10,000 units. He survived as remedial action had been taken to rectify the problem. The Health Authority admitted liability and offered the parents an amount for the additional pain and suffering the child had experienced. The boy had developed deafness and the parents sought much more compensation from the Health Authority, pointing out that the boy's deafness was due to the penicillin overdose. The case eventually reached the House of Lords, which held that the parents had not proved the causation factor because there were two possible causes of the deafness, (a) meningitis itself and (b) the penicillin overdose. So, although negligence was not denied on the basis of the Health Authority owing a duty of care to the boy and breaching that duty by administering an overdose of penicillin, the case failed on the causation element.

Material contribution and materially increasing the risk tests

In the case of *Bonnington Castings Ltd v Wardlaw* [1956] AC 613, the court held that the claimant need only prove that on the balance of probabilities the defendant's negligence materially contributed to the damage in order to recover the whole of his loss. The material evidence of this case was that the claimant contracted a silica dust-induced disease of the lung – pneumoconiosis – at work. The inhaled dust came from two possible sources: the production source, for which the defendant could not be responsible; and the inhalation of the silica dust due to the defendant's failure in his statutory responsibility to install adequate extractor fans. Medical evidence testified that the claimant's disease arose from both sources of silica dust. As indicated above, the court was satisfied that the claimant needed only to prove that on the balance of probability the defendant's breach materially contributed to the injury. Although in reality it was impossible to say just how much the defendant's breach had contributed to the injury it was sufficient to infer that it had materially contributed to it.

With respect to the claimant's only needing to establish that the breach had *increased the risk of the injury* let us look at the case of *McGhee v National Coal Board* [1973] 1 WLR 1. The claimant alleged that as a result of the defendant's failure to provide washing facilities he contracted dermatitis. The defendant admitted negligence in failing to provide washing facilities. The evidence was not conclusive that the claimant developed dermatitis from the lack of washing facilities. However, if the defendant creates a risk it is justified to make him/ her liable. Yet all that was certain was the fact that there was an increased risk of dermatitis from lack of washing facilities; the percentage of the risk was unknown. A risk may or may not materialise but if the nurse creates it (s)he can expect to be liable for it.

Reasonable foreseeable consequence and the eggshell or thin skull rule

Let us assume that as a nurse a patient sues you for negligence. As the defendant you would be held to have caused the damage only if, all other conditions of negligence being present, the court decides that the damage was a reasonable foreseeable consequence of your breach of duty. However, the extent of the damage and the manner of its occurrence need not be foreseen for the patient (claimant) to win his case (*Crossley v Rawlinson* [1982] 1 WLR 369). What does this mean?

There is an exception to the rule that the damage must be reasonably foreseeable. This exception is known as the *eggshell skull rule* or the *thin skull rule*, otherwise known as, 'take your claimant as you find him'. If the claimant has a 'hidden' weakness that you knew nothing about, and that he himself knew nothing about either, and because of your negligent action the patient's/claimant's vulnerability makes him suffer the damage more readily, you are still responsible for the damage, as though your claimant were a person of normal 'fortitude', constitution or strength. You cannot say: but he already had a weakness. It will not wash with the courts. In the famous case of *Smith v Leech Brain and Co Ltd* [1962] 2 QB 405, an employee was burnt on the lip by a piece of molten metal. He contracted cancer of the lip. This cancer apparently spread throughout the rest of his body and he died as a result. The court held that the amount of damage suffered by the patient as a result of the initial burnt lip 'depends upon the characteristics and constitution of the victim' (p. 415). What does this mean? It simply means that the initial damage (the burnt lip) was reasonably foreseeable as a result of the defendant's negligence and, even though an additional constitutional or personal characteristic weakness of the victim may have encouraged the cancer to spread, the defendant is still responsible for all the damage caused, not just for the foreseeable cancer of the lip occurring from the initial burn. You are also responsible for the consequential secondary cancer spread and the resultant death.

Break in the chain of causation and the concept of *novus actus interveniens*

The claimant's claim will fail if there is a break in causation. Where the action of a third party intervenes to break the chain of causation (i.e. between the original negligent act and the claimant's injury), the court has to decide if liability for negligence is now passed from the initial (allegedly) negligent person to a third party. In other words, does the intervening act constitute what we call in law a *novus actus interveniens*? The *novus actus interveniens* can be the claimant him-/herself or the third party.

Third-party *novus actus interveniens*

In *Prendergast v Sam and Dee* [1989] 1 Med LR 36, a GP's writing on a prescription was so bad and indecipherable that the dispensing chemist misread the prescription and the patient suffered a brain damage as a result. Was the chemist or the GP to blame? The GP claimed that the chemist's failure to query his illegible handwriting had caused a break in chain of causation. The GP failed to impress the court, which held that it was foreseeable that the chemist would dispense the wrong drug because of the GP's illegible handwriting.

The initial negligence must in some way cause the damage; so in *Yepremian v Scarborough General Hospital* [1980] 110 DLR (3D) 513, were not the GP's failure to diagnose appendicitis but instead the carelessness of the operating surgeon was the reason for the claimant's injury, the GP could not be held liable in negligence. For the treatment of the third and intervening party to be seen as a valid *novus actus interveniens* the action of the third party (the intervener) must be seen to be unreasonable and lacking care.

Consider Student activity 7.3 (Box 7.4).

Although we are dealing in this chapter with civil cases for negligence and not with criminal cases, it is important, I feel, to refer to a criminal case (*R v Blaue* [1975] 1 WLR 1411) in which the defendant criminal had claimed that the victim's action had broken the chain of causation in the victim's death. In this case the defendant had stabbed the victim, who refused to have a blood transfusion on religious grounds, as a result of which she died. She (the victim) was a Jehovah's Witness and she claimed that her religion prevented her from having a blood transfusion. Did the defendant's claim that the victim's action (failure to accept the blood transfusion) was a valid *novus actus*? Should her refusal to

---

BOX 7.4 Student activity 7.3

A scenario

You are a nurse and a friend of yours comes all the way from Devon to spend a day with you at your house in Birmingham. He is accompanied by a friend you had never met. Whilst at your house your friend's friend reveals that his varicose veins in his leg have started to bleed again. He had these bleeding varicosities treated surgically a year ago and was not expecting that they would start to bleed again. You recommend that your friend's friend pop into a Birmingham hospital casualty department for first aid before returning to Devon for substantial treatment. It is late in the evening and both decline, saying it is getting late and they must head for Devon. You decide in the circumstances to apply a pressure dressing you had in your medicine chest, but strongly advise your friend's friend to call into his local Devon A&E department that same night for a doctor to examine his leg. He gets back to Devon, goes to bed, sleeps and the following two days goes about his normal business, ignoring your advice to seek further medical help. Two days later he notices considerable haemorrhaging above the dressing and his toes rather blue and cyanosed. By the time he seeks medical help it is too late to save his leg (which had become gangrenous) from amputation. He sues you for negligently applying the pressure dressing, claiming you had become his nurse and owed him a duty of care which you breached by wrongly applying the pressure dressing.

Problem

Analyse the above situation, using all the necessary legal arguments you can muster. Be sure to include a discussion on duty of care, breach of duty, and whether you consider that the patient's failure to heed your advice to seek further medical help had become a valid *novus actus*.

accept the blood transfusion which would have saved her life be seen as the real cause of her death, instead of the defendant's action? No! The court held that there had been no break in the chain of causation. The act of the defendant (the stab wound) had caused the victim's death.

In fact it has been argued by a number of writers (e.g. Khan and Robson, 1997) that the defendant need only take reasonable steps to mitigate his damage. Moreover, religious reasons for refusal of a treatment are most likely to be seen as valid and reasonable. 'It should never be unreasonable to make a decision according to one's religion' (p. 195).

In *Emeh v Kensington and Chelsea Area Health Authority* [1985] QB 1012 the plaintiff (a woman) had sued in respect of her child being born seriously handicapped following a botched or really negligently performed sterilisation to prevent her from conceiving a child. She had learned of her unexpected pregnancy at 20 weeks' gestation, but had declined an abortion. Was her action a *novus actus* as the defendant doctor claimed? The defendant won at the court of first instance. However, on appeal, the Court of Appeal over turned the decision. In fact Lord Justice Slade said that the defendant had by his own negligence put the plaintiff into a situation where she was faced with the very dilemma she had tried to avoid in the first place by having herself sterilised. In reality she under went a sterilisation so as not to get pregnant.

Could the health professional's omission as a breach cause the damage or injury?

The unusual court decision in the case of *Bolitho v City and Hackney Health Authority* [1993] 4 Med LR 381 is worth discussing here. In this case a young child had been admitted to hospital suffering from breathing difficulties. The paediatric registrar, who was summoned by the nursing sister to see the patient, had refused to do so. It was alleged, and the registrar admitted, that he was negligent to refuse to attend the child. However, the court was unable to decide whether the doctor's non-attendance was the cause of the patient's injuries as it was not clear what action the doctor would have taken had he attended. The patient's (claimant's) lawyers contended that had the doctor attended he would have intubated the patient and this would have prevented the patient's ensuing injuries. The defendant registrar contended that if he had responded he would not have intubated. Both lines of medical reasoning were supported by expert medical evidence. This naturally made it impossible for the court to decide whether the doctor's action had caused the child's injuries, or exacerbation of his condition. Why? The court was not certain what action the registrar would have taken, because here we had one body of expert and respectable body of medical opinion saying they would have intubated and another saying they would not have done so. The court held that, where the breach was omission, it was necessary to decide which course of medical action would have been followed had the doctor attended and discharged his duty. To decide on the course of medical action the court had to rely on medical experts. As there was a conflict of medical opinion, in other words there were two equally respected bodies of medical opinion, as required under the *Bolam* test, and the patient could not prove that failure to intubate was contrary to appropriate medical practice, his claim failed. It failed on the grounds of being unable to establish causation of damage.

Where then there are two alternative courses of medical opinions and therefore pragmatic medical actions, the defendant just needs to show that (s)he acted in accordance with one of those opinions and thus his/her action is medically sound. Thus Khan and Robson (1997) conclude that the *Bolam* test is not just applicable to *standard of care*, but also linked to the issue of *causation of damage or injury*.

Lost opportunity or loss of a chance

There are instances when the patient as a claimant might cite loss of opportunity to recover normally or fully as the cause of his/her injury; or (s)he may cite lack of the chance to get appropriate treatment or lack of opportunity to get better from his/her illness. These cases are very difficult to win as they are constructed on the belief that, *but for* the defendant's negligence, one would have stood a chance of being treated, or securing a cure/making a full recovery, or having one's illness correctly diagnosed and so on. Where the patient's claim in negligence is on the basis that the defendant's breach of duty prevented him/her from making a full recovery from his illness, (s)he must establish on the balance of probabilities that, *but for* the defendant's breach (negligence) his/her chances of a full recovery exceeded 50 per cent.

The leading case here is *Hotson v East Berkshire Health* Authority [1987] AC 750. In this case a boy fell from a tree, injuring his hip. He attended the hospital, where he was examined but discharged without radiography being performed. Five days later he returned to the hospital, where his injury was diagnosed using radiographs of the hip. He was treated successfully but suffered avascular necrosis of the head of the femur. This problem gives rise to permanent hip joint deformity. The defendant admitted negligence. However, the real question was: what exactly was the patient's loss? Expert medical evidence had indicated that even with immediate treatment this type of fracture had a 75 per cent chance of developing avascular necrosis. The patient's argument was that the defendant robbed him of 25 per cent of his chances of a cure. Both the court of first instance and the Court of Appeal worked on the basis that the boy was entitled to 25 per cent of any damage that would be allowed for his type of injury. However, the House of Lords overruled the decision, pointing out that the proportionate award was incorrect and the boy should recover all or nothing. As he had had only a 25 per cent chance of not getting avascular necrosis his case failed.

Khan and Robson (1997) have argued that what the plaintiff (the boy) had to argue, properly, on the application of the *Bonnington* case, was that the delay had materially contributed to his injury (avascular necrosis). He needed to establish a 51–49 per cent likelihood that had the defendant not been negligent in delaying his radiography, and therefore his correct diagnosis, he would have stood a chance of making a full recovery. On the basis of the case of *McGhee*, the boy could have argued that the medical delay had materially increased his risk of avascular necrosis; just like how the absence of washing facilities in *McGhee* had increased the risk of the man contracting dermatitis. The *Hotson* case is just another proof of how difficult and burdensome it is for the claimant to prove the causation of damage factor in a negligence claim.

Non-disclosure of vital information as a causation factor

It has been argued that if a healthcare professional fails to provide the patient with vital information about risks, and that patient has treatment which subsequently goes wrong, then that patient can sue in negligence. Khan and Robson (1997) have argued that to frame a claim for damage due to non-disclosure in negligence is not very clever because of the difficulty the patient will have proving causation of damage. It would be better to frame the claim in trespass to the person, because in negligence, once the patient had overcome the *Bolam* test, (s)he must then have to prove that, had (s)he been warned of the risk(s) involved in the medical approach, (s)he would not have accepted the treatment. In the vast majority of cases the patient's claim will fail on the point of proving that had (s)he been told of the risk (s)he would not have accepted the treatment. The difficulty comes from the reality that the court will be most likely to hold that, on balance, the plaintiff would still have undergone the operation. This seems a reasonably sound assertion to make, because in reality, from one's personal experience as a clinician, how many patients, after knowing of the risks involved in their treatment, actually then refuse to go through with the treatment? One would submit that there are very few. Patients are unlikely to miss out on a chance of being treated, whatever the risk, because they are most certainly likely to feel that by not accepting some form of treatment, especially after extensive medical consultation, they leave themselves open to no treatment at all, and consequently no hope of being healed and the possibility of dying.

Importance of explaining risks to patients

Knowing the risk, would the patient have accepted the treatment? In order to demonstrate this, a subjective test may be applied. An important authority here is the case of *Chatterton v Gerson* [1981] QB 432. This was an action brought in trespass. The material evidence in that case was that the patient, Mrs Chatterton, had given her consent to Dr Gerson to accept his treatment for intractable pain. The basis of her case was that, although she had received the treatment that was explained to her, she had not been warned of the side effects: numbness and loss of muscle power. In fact the defendant had explained to the patient that she would suffer some numbness and a possible temporary loss of muscle power in her leg. However, in reality total numbness of the leg was manifested, together with impaired mobility. Mrs Chatterton argued that she had not in reality given her consent to the operation as the doctor had not informed her of the real risks associated with the surgery. The court held that since the patient had been informed in fairly broad terms about the procedure her consent was real. Thus any claim should have been brought in negligence. What is more, the court was not convinced that had the patient learned more about the procedure she would have refused to have the surgery. The court rejected the implication of the lack of informed consent and found for the defendant doctor on the question of trespass and on the related issue of negligence.

In the *Chatterton v Gerson* case Judge Bristow said:

> It is clear law that in any context in which consent of the injured party is a defence to what would otherwise be a crime or a civil wrong, the consent must be real. Where, for example, a woman's consent to sexual intercourse is obtained by fraud, her apparent consent is no defence to a charge of rape . . . When the claim is based on negligence the plaintiff must prove not only the breach of duty to inform, but that had the duty not been broken she would not have chosen to have the operation. Where the claim is based in trespass to the person, once it is shown that the consent is unreal, then what the plaintiff would have decided if she had been given the information which would have prevented vitiation of the reality of her consent is irrelevant.

We will return to the law relating specifically to consent in the chapters covering consent and confidentiality.

Although the plaintiff lost the Chatterton case, by contrast it is important to note that in a claim for 'wrongful birth' from a failed vasectomy, where lack of precise information about the slight risk of reversal of the vasectomy manifested itself, the case was won by the plaintiff. This is the case of *Thake v Maurice* [1986] QB 644. In this case the patient's (the plaintiff's) wife had not contemplated pregnancy as she knew her husband had had a vasectomy, which would have prevented him from ejaculating sperm during sexual intercourse. So, being pregnant and blissfully unaware of this (as her husband was, in theory, sterile) until it was too late to have the pregnancy aborted, Mrs Thake was unable to exercise what would have been her preferred choices, (a) not to become pregnant in the first place or (b) to terminate the pregnancy in good time, certainly well before 20 weeks when it would have been safe to do so.

So in the *Thake* case we see how a failure to inform the patient of specific risks, however small, led to the claimant successfully suing for compensation for 'wrongful birth'. This goes to demonstrate to nurses and all healthcare professionals the importance of warning patients of known risks, irrespective of size. If you fail to do so you run the risk of being liable in negligence. You also leave yourself open to being accused of trespass to the patient's person in the sense that you have carried out some procedure on him/her which (s)he did not consent to. Another important principle that arose from *Thake v Maurice* is the fact that the court made it clear that the standard of care for negligence law is the same as that expected under a private contract for healthcare.

In my view, no comfort should be taken from the *Chatterton v Gerson* case, in which the judge said that once the procedure was explained in general terms informed consent had been gained. In reality, the standard of care does not fall with time. If anything it rises, and therefore today it is reasonable to expect the court to be more satisfied that all the risks (however small) had been carefully explained to the patient [in language (s)he can understand] than to be just told that explanation of procedures had been given in 'general terms'. For a healthcare professional, it is much better to run the risk of being labelled as 'too detailed' and 'pedantic' in one's explanation of risks to patients than to be found wanting from one's failure to explain to the patient the risks involved.

Failed female sterilisation

There is evidence of negligence cases that have been won by female patients for failed sterilisation. In *Emeh v Kensington and Chelsea and Westminster Health Authority* [1985] 2 WLR 233, Mrs Emeh, who already had three children, underwent an operation for sterilisation to stop her from conceiving any more babies. The operation was carried out in May 1976; however, in January 1977, Mrs Emeh found out that she was pregnant again; she was in fact 20 weeks pregnant. She refused to have an abortion and in fact gave birth to a child with major *congenital defects*. The child would require constant medical and parental management. She sued for an unwanted pregnancy, for the birth and the rearing of the 'abnormal' child. Although the trial judge recognised that her sterilisation had been negligently performed, he only awarded her damages for the period before she found out she was pregnant, stating that she was not entitled to damages beyond the point where she discovered she was pregnant, as she had refused to have an abortion.

On appeal to the Court of Appeal Mrs Emeh won her case, on the grounds that, since the objective of the sterilisation was to stop her from becoming pregnant in the first place, it was not reasonable or fair to expect her to have an abortion. She won damages for the negligent performance of the sterilisation, for future earnings, pain and suffering up to the trial, and for amenity, pain and suffering during the life of the child.

It is now good law that a woman's refusal to abort following conception upon a botched sterilisation is perfectly reasonable. Refusal of abortion in the circumstances does not limit damages. Similarly, a duty (legal or moral) to have an abortion or secure adoption for the child born out of an unwanted pregnancy, through a botched sterilisation, or a sterilisation negligently carried out in ignorance on the part of the obstetrician that the woman was pregnant at the time of the sterilisation operation, is not imposed on a woman (*McFarlane and Another v Tayside Health Board* [1999] 4 All ER 961 HL).

By comparison, in the case of *Allen v Bloomsbury Health Authority and Another* [1993] 1 All ER 651, a woman was sterilised four weeks into her pregnancy, unknown to herself and her obstetrician. The Health Authority accepted negligence and awarded her £96,631, which included an amount for future cost of looking after and educating her child.

However, by 1999, in the case of *McFarlane and Another v Tayside Health Board* [1999] 4 All ER 961 HL, [2000] 2 AC 59, the House of Lords addressed itself to the question of whether, in a case where medical negligence led to an unwanted pregnancy, but to the birth of a healthy child, the parents were entitled to damages covering the rearing of the child. The court held that the woman was not entitled to an amount to cover the upbringing of the normal healthy child, but could be awarded compensation for pain and suffering during the pregnancy and during parturition, and for financial loss linked to the pregnancy. This decision was based on what is known as 'public policy decision', that is to say there should be a limit to the imposition of liability for economic loss on a healthcare professional. The imposition of unlimited liability for economic losses in these situations is not fair, just, reasonable or a good public policy decision. To recover economic losses linked to bringing up normal healthy children, regarded as a blessing by society, would not be perceived to be moral or legally fair and just and could affect the principle of 'distributive justice', which focuses on a just allocation of burdens and losses on members of society (Dimond, 2005, p. 389).

If the failed sterilisation was in a woman who was disabled would the situation be different from the one in the McFarlane case?

Unfortunately no. This was the decision in *Rees v Darlington Memorial Hospital NHS Trust*, *The Times Law Report*, 21 October 2003 HL; [2002] 2 All ER 177 CA, in which a blind mother, Mrs Rees, underwent a negligently performed sterilisation; she had felt that her progressive blindness would prevent her from properly discharging her responsibilities as mother. She delivered a normal healthy child and sued for compensation to help bring up her child. The House of Lords rules that Mrs Rees's case was similar to *McFarlane and Another v Tayside Health Board* [1999] 4 All ER 961 HL, [2000] 2 AC 59. However, the Law Lords acknowledged that the lady was a victim of a legal wrong and awarded her a convention sum of £15,000 to be added to her damages for the unplanned pregnancy and the birth.

Res ipsa loquitur

It is possible for the claimant to sue simply on the basis that the negligence *speaks for itself*. In other words, it is self-evident that the defendant damaged the claimant. This is known as the doctrine of *res ipsa loquitur*, the thing speaks for itself. It is then up to the defendant to prove that his/her conduct did not injure the patient. As a number of writers have argued, *res ipsa* does not shift the burden of proof from the claimant; it merely infers negligence, which the defendant must successfully refute, or 'rebut' as we call it in law. Framing a claim on *res ipsa* is not easy to win. However, there may be situations when a patient is simply unable to say exactly in what way the defendant harmed him; for example he may have been unconscious at the time of the injury. To win a negligence claim on the basis of *res ipsa* the claimant must establish two things: (a) that the defendant was in control of the situation and (b) that, but for the course of events over which the defendant had control, the injury would never have occurred, and moreover it would certainly not have occurred in the normal or ordinary course of events (Khan and Robson, 1997).

In *Cassidy v Ministry of Health* [1951] 2 KB 343 the claimant suffered from *Dupuytren's contracture*. He was operated on for the condition and following surgery he discovered that four of his fingers were stiff. Lord Denning found for the claimant in the Court of Appeal where he held that *res ipsa* (the thing speaks for itself) was appropriate as the operation itself was clearly indicative of negligence. As the defendant was in control of the operation he was responsible in law for the problem that resulted from it.

In the case of *Mahon v Osborne* [1939] 2 KB 14, a swab was left in the patient's body during a surgical procedure. The plaintiff won the case for negligence on the basis of *res ipsa* although only on a majority decision. Clearly, the evidence of a swab being left in a patient's body is indisputably a negligent act; the situation speaks for itself. However, a word of warning was given by a dissenting Law Lord, Lord Justice Scott, who said that it would be wrong to apply *res ipsa* as a matter of course, and the plaintiff should be able to prove that the defendant's act lacked the necessary care. The case must be very obvious and clear cut for the court to apply *res ipsa* (Khan and Robson, 1997).

I think most nurses, and certainly those who work in operating theatres, will agree with me that for a swab to have been left in a patient's body reflects obvious negligence on the part of the surgeon. When I worked in operating theatres, it was my experience that swab counting at the end of the operation, before final wound closure, was so critical that one would have to be somewhat negligent and careless to allow a swab to be left in the patient's body. One hopes this case will heighten the awareness of theatre nurses responsible for supporting surgeons, and the surgeons themselves, of the criticality of a careful swab count before the patient's wound is finally closed.

In *Ludlow v Swindon Health Authority* [1989] 1 Med LR 104, the court was unimpressed by the vague account of the patient that she was awake throughout her caesarean operation and experienced pain during the surgery because the defendant was alleged to have failed to administer halothane during the operation. It should be a clear inference that, had the patient been able to establish without doubt that she could feel the pain associated with the surgery as the surgeon operated on her, she would have won her case for negligence on the basis of *res ipsa*.

Criminal negligence

This topic will be touched on very briefly here. Although clinical negligence tends to be a civil matter, dealt with under tort law of negligence or under contract law where patients have private contracts with their private (non-NHS) doctors, nurses, physiotherapists or other healthcare professionals, history has shown that in certain cases the degree of clinical negligence can be so 'gross' as to give rise to a criminal prosecution. Apparently, criminal prosecution for negligence is growing. Ferner (2000) located 17 British cases between 1970 and 1999. Criminal liability for negligence is limited to prosecutions for manslaughter (Ferner, 2000; Mason *et al.*, 2006). The criteria for criminal liability in negligence are that a professional duty of care existed, that the duty has been breached and that the breach has given rise to 'gross' professional negligence. The harm is specifically the death of the patient.

As stated above, the negligence must be gross, severe and extreme, and considerably more than that for negligence in a civil case. Moreover, the court has to be satisfied that the criminal negligence of the defendant went beyond a mere matter of compensation to the victim, and demonstrates disregard for the life and safety of the patient, and satisfies the State's criteria of a crime deserving of punishment.

The case reflecting criminal negligence that always comes to my mind, first of all, is that of *R v Adomako* [1995] 1 AC 171, in which an anaesthetist failed to notice that his patient was distressed because that his endotracheal tube had become dislodged. The patient entered into cardiac arrest and died. Evidence suggests that the patient had become disconnected from his oxygen supply for about 4.5 minutes before the Dinamap machine, which monitored the patient's blood pressure, sounded an alarm. Although the anaesthetist then did a number of checks on the machine and gave atropine to correct the patient's blood pressure and pulse rate, he did not check the endotracheal tube; this demonstrated gross negligence and recklessness. He was convicted for involuntary manslaughter, appealed and lost at both the Court of Appeal and the House of Lords. The House of Lords stated that 'gross negligence' calls for 'an egregious failure' to demonstrate a minimum standard of competence and gross dereliction of professional duty of care.

From this case it is reasonable to infer that any nurse whose carelessness is so gross as to lead to a situation where a patient dies should expect the possibility that (s)he may be prosecuted and tried for manslaughter. It must be noted here that in manslaughter the defendant has not, as in murder, deliberately, wilfully and intentionally committed the act that led to the death. Intentional killing is murder, as in the case of Dr Shipman.

Some key learning points within this chapter

For a patient/client to successfully sue for negligent practice (s)he must show three things: (a) that the nurse owes him/her a duty of care (that nurses owe their patients a duty of care is axiomatic); (b) that the nurse has breached that professional and legal duty of care; and (c) that the breach has caused a damage or injury.

Although most landmark clinical negligent cases concern the practice of doctors, the principles enshrined in them also apply to nurses and other healthcare professionals involved in direct care. The NHS may have to pay out for breaches by its employees, such as nurses, doctors and physiotherapists, under the principle of vicarious liability, but its hospitals may also have to face direct liability for negligence as they have a direct duty to care for patients.

General practitioners, unlike NHS-employed dentists, community physicians, hospital doctors and nurses, have no Crown immunity and so must directly carry liability for their negligence. GPs are also vicariously liable for the negligence of the nurses and other people they employ to provide patient/client care. Negligence cases against NHS employees such as nurses are brought in tort law, rather than contract, as NHS patients have no contractual relationship with NHS employees. However, any nurse, doctor or physiotherapist who proposes to conduct his/her craft in a private context, and who is negligent in so far as (s)he provides substandard care, may be sued in the law of contract. This means then that healthcare professionals who have a private contractual relationship with their patient/client, or those who decide to act as 'good Samaritans', must have suitable indemnity insurance cover.

Even if you are employed as a nurse by an NHS trust there is nothing to stop a patient/client from suing you direct for negligence. However, at the present time negligence litigation involving the NHS is handled by the NHS Litigation Authority (DoH, 1996). The issue of clinical negligence is a growing concern, and can expect to grow exponentially in an era when patients and clients are becoming more litigious. In assessing your chances of being involved in a clinical negligence case, remember this: most clinical negligence cases are settled out of court and so do not reach the law books and journals, so do not weigh up your chances on the basis of the relatively small number of cases made public. Be careful to provide only high-quality care to your patient/client.

The costs of clinical negligence is alarming and the possibility of nurses being sued for negligence is ever growing as the nurse's role extends and as we push the frontiers of nursing and medical practice ever wider and deeper, thus creating more chances of things going wrong. The standards by which a nurse will be judged is still predominantly that established in the *Bolam* case, although since the *Bolitho* case nurses who provide expert evidence to the courts for or against their colleagues must be prepared to justify the standard they deem, and recommend to the courts as, acceptable on the basis that they have seriously considered all the risks against benefits and have come up with a sound and logically defensible conclusion.

Student nurses particularly must be aware that their lack of experience and proper competence and their 'novice' status are no excuse in law when it comes to a court deciding that the care received by the patient/client was of a substandard quality. The *Bolam principles* are strictly applied to qualified nurses as they are to students, and for this reason as a student nurse you must make sure that you give your patient the highest standard of care, and certainly not a standard that falls below that which the ordinary and reasonably competent qualified nurses would have given in the circumstances considered (*Nettleship v Weston* [1971] 2 QB 691, [1971] 3 All ER 581; *Wilsher v Essex Area Health Authority* [1987] QB 730, [1986] 3 All ER 801). Therefore, if you are uncertain of the care to give, make sure you seek the guidance of your qualified mentor.

Summary and conclusion

This chapter:

- Covered negligence and concluded that negligence claims in the NHS are rising, with major financial implications for the NHS. Nurses definitely need to understand the principles of negligence and how negligent practice can impact upon them. Good nursing care can help to reduce the number of patients' negligence suits.
- Examined the factors that need to be present for a patient to succeed in a claim of negligence against a nurse (or other healthcare practitioner) and/or a healthcare provider such as an NHS Trust. The burden of proof that the clinician has been negligent lies with the patient.
- Examined the notion of a *standard of care*, and linked this to the concept of *duty of care* and *negligent clinical practice*. To this end the principles of the *Bolam test* were examined in terms of how they relate to the nurse's *standard of care* and the place of these principles with respect to negligent nursing practice. *Bolam* is under threat and so in future nurses and other professionals need to ensure their care standard is based on the best available research evidence, taking into account risk factors involved.
- Proposed and argued how a *duty of care* may arise under *law*, *professionally*, *ethically*, by virtue of one's *contract as an employee*, and by a nurse's *voluntary actions* in a private or public setting. Within this, the chapter points out how important it is for student nurses to be able to make links with important duty of care principles as found in *Donoghue v Stevenson*, 1932.
- Covered the concept of *damage* and issues around *causation of damage*. The chapter explains the implications of damage for the nurse and other healthcare practitioners. The potential and actual financial and professional costs arte so great that clinicians need vigilance to produce faultless care always.
- Examined the distinction between tort law negligence and 'criminal' law (gross) negligence, and discussed the implications for the healthcare practitioner. Clinicians who commit gross negligence can end up in jail.
- Provided opportunity for the student to analyse a number of patient care scenarios using theory from negligence law, using such an approach, together with critical reflection, to enhance the development of the student's individual professional portfolio.

8   Ethics in nursing
The case for ethics

Objectives of this chapter

After reading this chapter you should be able to:

- discuss why the study of ethics and ethical decision making is important to nurses;
- talk about how we develop and use our moral and ethical values and the implications for healthcare;
- demonstrate relationship between moral values/beliefs, ethics, professional code of conduct and patient care;
- further develop your ethics and law portfolio through reflection on patient scenarios.

Introduction: why is a study of ethics crucial to nurses and other health professionals?

The way we live our lives and care for others – or do not care for them – is not free of ethical and moral considerations. Our actions are governed by our thinking, attitudes, values and beliefs. Even if we would like to feel that our conduct is influenced by other considerations, law, ethics and morality also influence our reasoning and behaviour. For example, the law relating to theft will punish us for the act of stealing from our fellow men/women, but at the root of this is the moral belief that no person should be deprived of property by a thief. Aware of the legal consequences of stealing we may also be discouraged from stealing. Our cultural values may tell us it is wrong to steal; moreover, what we steal someone may have worked very hard to acquire. Even thieves may sometimes have their conscience pricked by what they have done to others, namely depriving them of their earthly possessions. This indicates that even thieves may have a sense of what is right and wrong. We may also refrain from stealing because of possible consequences, such as the risk of being caught and punished.

When we care for our patients in the best way we can we are doing so not just because we have a legal duty so to do, but also because, hopefully, we have come into nursing with certain caring moral and ethical values and beliefs. We may be imbued with notions of caring for the sick, caring for those less fortunate in health than we are at that particular time, caring for those we perceive to need our skills and expertise. In doing so we are seeking to demonstrate values of compassion, kindness, honesty, fairness, justice and other qualities that we feel will enrich the human experience. These are values we may consider to help us contribute to or achieve a *good life* for our patients. So, whether or not we deliberately plan to base our care on moral and ethical values, inevitably our professional judgements and reasoning to some extent are governed by who we are and what values we possess. Having said all of this, therefore, nurses need to ensure that patient care is based on sound ethical and moral values. This chapter therefore has an ethical underpinning, covering how we develop and use ethical and moral values, links between professional code of conduct and ethical and moral values and the very essence of the importance of a study of ethics to nurses.

NMC influences on appropriate ethical decision making in practice

You are not learning about moral and ethical values because it is a fashionable thing to do. You are learning about values because we know there are good and bad values and they can influence our thinking and behaviour towards others. It is imperative to remember that you live in, and are part of, a society where everyone's needs and concerns are probably viewed as equally important as your own. You are also learning about caring values because your professional body, the NMC requires you to. Indeed, in its *Standards for Pre-registration Nursing Education* the NMC (2010a) states that:

> The public needs to be confident that nurses will:
> * Deliver high quality care;
> * Deliver complex care [indeed it is impossible to do this without a sound understanding of values, ethics and ethical decision making];
> * Act professionally, with integrity, and work within agreed professional, ethical and legal frameworks;
> * Practice with *compassion* & *respect*, maintaining *dignity* & *wellbeing* [of your patients].

NMC four domains of professional values

Under *Standards for competence* the NMC requires you to achieve competencies for practice under four *domains*: professional values; communication and interpersonal skills; nursing practice and decision making; and leadership, management and team working. All of these need sound understanding of ethical principles to achieve.

Under the domain *professional values*, the NMC requires you to:

* practise autonomously and provide safe, *compassionate*, *person-centred*, evidence-based nursing that values and accords *dignity* and *human rights*;
* demonstrate *professionalism* and work within recognised professional and *ethical frameworks*;
* promote the *rights*, *choices* and *wishes* of adults and, where appropriate, children and young people, valuing *equality* and *diversity*;
* practise with confidence, according to the Code (NMC, 2008a), recognising and addressing 'ethical challenges relating to people's choices and decision-making about their care', acting within the law to help patients and their families achieve 'acceptable solutions'.
* practise in a *holistic, non-judgemental, caring and sensitive* manner that *avoids assumptions*, *supports social inclusion*, *recognises and respects individual choice*, and *challenges inequality, discrimination* and *exclusion* from access to care.

See Box 8.1 for a student reflection.

Under the domain *communication and interpersonal skills*, we note the NMC requiring you to:

- communicate *safely*, *effectively*, with *compassion* and *respect*;
- demonstrate *listening* and *empathy* skills, responding *warmly* and *positively* towards people of all ages who are anxious, distressed or facing other health problems;
- establish and maintain *partnership* and effective therapeutic relationships with other professionals and the patient and his family through effective, *non-discriminatory communication*, respecting *individual differences*, *diversity*, capabilities and needs;
- be aware of your *own values and beliefs and the impact this may have* on your communication with others;
- respect 'individual rights to confidentiality and keep information secure and confidential in accordance with the law and relevant ethical and regulatory frameworks'.

Box 8.2 contains another student reflection.

Under the competency domain of *nursing practice and decision-making* (NMC, 2010a) we note that the NMC calls on nurses to use professional and ethical values in caring. For example, be compassionate, respect patients' culture and value systems, protect patients' dignity and individuality. Promote self-care, value peoples' choices and give person-centred care whether dealing with children, young adults or older people, irrespective of whether they have physical, mental or learning disabilities. You are further reminded by the NMC that you 'must be able to recognise when the complexity of clinical decisions requires specialist knowledge and expertise'. Even under the competency domain of *leadership, management and team working* we note the NMC's requirement that 'All nurses must be self-aware and recognise how their own values, principles and assumptions may affect their practice'. Reflect on both of these domains in Box 8.3.

Professionally driven ethical and moral values and beliefs

From the NMC's position as outlined above, it is evident that ethical decision making is imperative in nursing care. We recognise too that not only do we use our own moral values systems to influence caring decisions, but our professional body demands that our practice be informed by some specific ethical principles, such as *respect for autonomy*, *confidentiality*, *compassion*, *individual rights* and *freedoms*, *diversity within the patient population*, *cultural* and *individual differences* and *values within ourselves and patients*, and the criticality of constantly being aware of how our own value systems can impact on those of patients. Above all, the NMC reminds us that caring is sometimes a very complex task,

---

BOX 8.1 Student reflection 8.1

Reflect on each point mentioned under the domain of professional values and come up with some ideas of your own on how you would achieve the stated objectives in the patient care setting.

BOX 8.2 Student reflection 8.2

Reflect on each point mentioned under the domain of communication and interpersonal skills come up with some ideas of your own on how you would achieve these things in the practice setting.

BOX 8.3 Student reflection 8.3

How do you think your own value system may impact on the nursing care you provide for your patient? A few thoughts to use in this reflection – consider:

- values as good and bad;
- self-perception a crucial place to start – why?
- importance of working cooperatively/collaboratively, e.g. in our families, with friends/other groups, thereby transferring such values to multiprofessional and interprofessional working, including with clients, patients, relatives and other health professionals;
- truth telling, or lying;
- respect for people's
  - individual autonomy
  - individual rights, values, beliefs
  - individual and cultural health beliefs
  - individual and cultural norms of behaviour
  - views around dietary matters
  - right to justice, equality, beneficence, freedom of thought and religious beliefs etc.

requiring *complex decision making* that calls for constant appraisal of our individual moral and ethical positions. We owe it to our patients/clients to do the 'right thing', including working with them, being guided by sound moral, ethical and professional code of conduct to enable achievement of personal health goals. In the process we must demonstrate respect for patients' own moral values and belief system. If we do not value and respect patients' own value systems we cannot justifiably claim to be respecting their autonomy and rights to their own beliefs and values. Moreover our excessive preoccupation with our own values may set up the potential for conflict with patients, devaluing them as individuals with their own values and belief systems.

Opportunity to explore values, beliefs and nursing ethics using your portfolio

Later in this chapter I have presented you with an opportunity not only to explore the nature of individual moral values, beliefs and professional nursing ethics, but to demonstrate the use of your professional portfolio in exploring ethical issues. You are also given the opportunity to look at ethical catastrophes from history that will hopefully guide your thinking as a nurse, ensuring non-repeat of these catastrophes in your own practice, and also ensuring that your professional behaviour can be justified on caring, humanitarian ethical grounds. Beauchamp and Childress (2001) have identified *four major ethical principles* on which we can base our care of patients and clients. These are respect for *autonomy* (self-directed behaviour and determination), *justice* (fair play and treatment), *beneficence* (thinking and behaviour driven towards helping other to benefit from what we as professionals do for/with them) and *non-maleficence* (doing nothing that will hurt the people we care for). Before we examine what these principles are in more depth, let us look at what we mean by *moral values* and what the term *ethics* really means.

Morals and moral values

The term *morality* comes from the Latin word *moralitas* which defines manner, proper conduct and character. Morality is a state of our being, the way we live our lives, our thinking and conduct that say whether we are good (right) or bad (wrong). Thus we may refer to a person as having (or being of) good *morals* or *bad morals*, meaning the person is viewed as being governed by a particular *teaching* or *sense of value* and *beliefs*, maybe according to a particular religion, culture or philosophy. Thus, we may choose to be *honest*, *caring* and *compassionate* nurses, and be looked upon as possessing a *sound moral code of conduct*, or we may choose to be *dishonest*, *uncaring*, hurt our patients and be described as *immoral* and *uncaring*; characteristics that will surely deny us the right to call ourselves *health professionals*. Wikipedia, the free online encyclopaedia, defines the term 'health professional' as a healthcare practitioner who offers services for the purpose of improving people's health and treating their diseases, mental or physical (at http://en.wikipedia.org/wiki/Mental_health_professional). The fact therefore that as nurses we regard ourselves as professional caring people means that to hold destructive, negative and uncaring, dishonest, immoral and non-compassionate values towards our patients would deprive us of the status of being called healthcare professionals.

Distinction between morality, immorality and amorality

In our communities we may, if we like, choose to be *dishonest*, *disrespecting* of other peoples' views and property (e.g. stealing and plundering), and hence be described as *immoral*. On the other hand, our *individual* and *cultural value system* may make us behave kindly or unkindly towards others within our communities. If we are labelled as *immoral* those doing the labelling are likely to see us as non-conforming, bad and evil, perhaps as unwholesome characters intending to upset the social balance and order within our society. Whereas *immorality* (that which is bad, wrong etc.) is the opposite of *morality* (right and good), there is yet another related concept that we call *amorality*, which is viewed as possessing an indifference towards, disbelief in, or unawareness of, any defined moral code. To be *amoral* is to believe in no standards or principle whatever (Johnson, 2008, pp. 102–103; Superson, 2009).

Reflect on whether you would consider a gay male patient immoral, or a woman having an abortion immoral, or a daughter forging her ill mother's will immoral. In your answers, whatever they are, try to find reasons to justify the position you take.

Ethics

Whereas *morality* simply describes personal cultural, religious and philosophical sense of values of right or wrong and relates to describing codes of conduct that is acceptable or unacceptable (to the society we live in), *ethics* is the *study of morality and morals*. Whereas morality is viewed as having potential to cause benefits or harm, the actual looking at and analysis of morality in this purely descriptive sense puts the concept under the umbrella that is known as *descriptive ethics*. *Ethics* is that branch of *moral philosophy* that *studies* how people behave and conduct themselves. Do they conduct themselves in a *good* or a *bad* way? As a branch of philosophy, *ethics* is the *study of morally acceptable or unacceptable behaviours*. As Beauchamp and Childress (2001, p. 1) put it, ethics presents various ways of understanding and examining 'moral life'; thus there is *normative ethics*, which aims to answer the question of which *moral norms* we should accept and why. See Portfolio-based student activity 8.1 in Box 8.4.

BOX 8.4 Portfolio-based student activity 8.1

'Norm' refers to a standard of behaviour that is representative of a group. Can you think of any particular norm that defines nurses as a professional group? What are these norms? Use your portfolio to write them down. Does any theoretical, research or academic source support your views? Which? Use them to reference or support your own conceptualisations. (Ethical theories attempt to analyse and justify these norms.)

Non-normative ethics is divided into *descriptive ethics* (a factual and methodical way of studying how people behave ethically) and *meta-ethics* (an understanding of how and why people behave and react the way they do, the explanations they give for their behaviours and the study of the ethical language, concepts and methods of reasoning they use). In its normative context, *morality* describes what is right or wrong (according to the society doing the describing and undertaking the evaluation) irrespective of what specific individuals think. For example in one society fighting may be encouraged as a norm, whereas in another it may be frowned upon. *Normative ethics* then is like a truth of morality, the ideal that is acceptable as either the right or wrong thing for that particular society. Hence normative ethics is relative. So, if we take up this relative ideal moral sense, we may say, for example, 'that act is immoral' and hope everyone in that society understands. We are describing a shared 'moral truth' for that society (this moral truth may be unacceptable in another society). This is different from saying that some people believe that the act is immoral. The latter is a not a moral truth or it would be defined in a more independent and objective way, and agreed by all, as in 'that act is immoral'. So morality has two principles – descriptive and normative morality – and ethics is the study of that morality. Hence we have descriptive and normative ethics. Meta-ethics tries to understand why people behave the way they do. Meta-ethics therefore asks: why?

Nursing ethics: what is nursing ethics and how is it derived and used?

Nursing ethics is for me the use of ethical reasoning and awareness of the place and function of moral principles in making nursing decisions. For example, we seek patient's *consent* before we treat them or disclose what they tell us because we respect their right to *confidentiality* and self-*determination*. We respect their right to decide if we can treat them and if we can disclose to others what they tell us about themselves. We seek their consent so as not to hurt their feelings, and to respect and value them as autonomous individuals who are entitled to their privacy and dignity. (This is also a legal and a professional requirement, not just an ethical one.) Here we are subscribing to what Beauchamp and Childress (2001) call the *ethics of autonomy*. In this we are recognising patients' right to self-determination, which includes their right to agree to, or refuse to agree to, our touching them or disclosing information they tell us about themselves, and their right to withdraw their consent to treatment even after they had initially given that consent.

Nurses need to have a clear understanding of the ethical principles and theories and the moral codes and values that they are using to make caring decisions. We as individual nurses (or simply people or members of society, putting the title 'nurse' aside), are not devoid of *personal* and *idiosyncratic values*. We are not *value-free*. So there is a sense in which we need to realise that when we make nursing decisions (in fact decisions in any part of our lives) we bring our state of *morality* and *ethical values* to bear on those decisions. Hence why the NMC (2010a) tells us to be aware of 'own values and beliefs and the impact [they] may have on' patients and clients. Hence the reason the NMC further reminds you to respect 'individual rights to confidentiality and keep information secure and confidential in accordance with the law and relevant ethical and regulatory frameworks'.

Need for sensitivity in ethical decision making

In our professional decision making we are also drawing on *established ethical principles*, *cultural* and *religious* norms, *professional values*, *codes* and other *guidelines of professional practice*. The sooner we become aware that our individual and personal value systems influence our attitude, thinking, feeling and conduct, the sooner we will become aware of the need to ensure that the resultant behaviour (which is after all, what the patient senses, feels and can describes) is also *not value free* and therefore we must ensure such behaviour is guided by attitudes and values we can defend on the grounds of being *just*, *fair*, *respectful*, *honest*, *sincere*, *warm*, *helpful*, *caring*, *people/patient-centred*, rather than self-centred values. Indeed Dogan and colleagues (2009, p. 687) support the reality of 'culturally determined value systems' that are crucial in understanding health and illness and in determining health interventions and care objectives. Moreover, Banja (1996) proposed that *culturally determined different value systems between health professionals and patients* were correlated with the complexity of medical ethical conflicts. Furthermore, different values between patients of a defined religious group and health professionals of a different religious persuasion can lead to prejudice and discrimination (on both sides) that can cause major problems and ethical dilemmas in the caring context (Dogan *et al.*, 2009). Indeed the NMC (2010a) reminds you that as a nurse you 'must not discriminate in any way against those in your care'. *Self-awareness* is one of the most essential and fundamental qualities and prerequisite to effective caring. We need to strive to give patient-centred, rather than self-centred, care, putting the patient and his/her health beliefs at the centre of care as far as it is possible and professional to do so. Clearly, where a patient's self and health belief makes him/her request from the health professional a remedy or care measure that is illegal or which would confound sound professional judgement, values and standards, then the health professional cannot comply and the patient needs to be told this, but with sensitivity. If we are not self-aware of the influence of our thinking and personal value system in our nursing decision making and behaviour, we will not realise that we are being unfair, untruthful and prejudicial towards our patients. If it is at all possible do not separate the patient from his/her inherent value system and health beliefs. Do so only where you are unreservedly convinced that the patient's health beliefs and values are detrimental to his/her health and well being. If in the Rastafarian culture the smoking of 'weed' is a valued attribute, but as a nurse you are aware of the links between smoking 'weed' and psychotic episodes or between the mere factor of smoking and lung cancer, then you owe it to the patient to point this out. Here you are not necessarily seeking to separate the Rastafarian patient from his/her cultural practices and beliefs but you are pointing out the health risks inherent in the cultural practice.

Indeed, we noticed above that the NMC (2010a) in its publication *Standards for Pre-registration Nursing Education* states that nurses must establish and maintain *partnership* and effective therapeutic *communication* and relationships with other professionals and the patient and his/her family through effective, *non-discriminatory communication*, respecting *individual differences* and *diversity*. In the philosophy of caring the NMC also requires you to use the best available research evidence to inform your practice. This includes being aware of the various ethical positions you and your patients may take, but trying always to find acceptable, ethical and moral solutions that as a nurse you can defend, using sound professional standards, values and ethical principles.

Do not fall on your sword of 'I know best'

We will fail as nurses if we are providing care purely on the basis of what we idiosyncrati-cally think is suitable for the patient, rather than on the grounds of what the best research evidence tells us, and also on the basis of sound ethical, moral and legal frameworks. We should also as far as it is professionally possible take into account *the patient's own value system and health beliefs*. This is not to say we must give in to what the patient wants, no matter what. Indeed, as pointed out above, what the patient wants may not be perceived professionally safe, legally or ethically correct. What the patient asks for may not be in keeping with professional guidance or in the patient's best interest. For example, however much the patient asks us to end his/her life, we cannot do so because, although we may share the patient's ethical view that it is better to die rather than to ensure the intractable pain of bone cancer, to help him/her end his/her life with a lethal cocktail of drugs would be illegal, even if ethically we felt comfortable about it. This is a point where ethical reasoning and expectations may conflict with legal principles. We cannot give the patient a treatment option that we know to be against nursing protocols or our professional code of conduct, or simply give a treatment we know is unethical.

Ethical strength to challenge the law

However, ethical reasoning allows us to challenge the law, so that, should the majority of society be in favour of euthanasia is cases of severe intractable bone pain, then through the democratic process we may wish to persuade our government to change the law. We could do so through well-organised pressure groups, maybe through a referendum on the issue and so on.

How do we acquire our moral values, whether or not we bring them to bear in nursing decision making?

Before we focus further on ethical principles used in nursing let us learn about *how we form moral values and attitudes and whether we bring them/any into nursing*. We may have taken for granted that our moral values of right and wrong are essentially part of us. As adults, our values are part of us, formed and used because we exists as part of society and can, and do need to think, not only of ourselves and our own individual needs, but of the wider society's as well. But how did we acquire personal moral and ethical values?

Influence of socialisation on moral and ethical value formation

In the same way that nursing and medical ethics have received contributions from a number of sources and disciplines, for example social anthropologists, sociologists, philosophers, theologians, lawyers, judges, economists, doctors, nurses and other health professionals (Herring, 2008), so we have acquired our earliest moral values that we bring with us into nursing from a variety of social interactions: self with family; emulating influential role models; interaction between self and school, church and social clubs' influences; work and friendship groups' persuasions; and so on. Research has shown that *social interactions* influence children's development of moral values. Whereas Piaget's early twentieth-century work ascribes the development of moral reasoning to the process of growth and *maturation*, Kohlberg (1980) sees the development of moral values, particularly in boys, in terms of levels of thinking based on chronological ages and on the mental challenges that society puts to the individual. However, Haidt (2001) proposes a social intuitionist theory in which it is argued that moral evaluations come from immediate intuitions and emotions, with ethical reasoning being described as part of moral philosophy which deals with important questions about how and why human subjects conduct themselves. The certain fact you will have learned from the immediate preceding account is that moral values and its acquisition can be explained by a number of different theories.

In the early 1960s Albert Bandura's research demonstrated that when children observed adults being aggressive towards inflatable toy dolls they themselves became aggressive; an indication of how our social environment can influence our values of right and wrong (Bandura *et al.*, 1961). Miller and Bersoff (1992) conducted cross-cultural research to see if socio-cultural factors influence moral behaviours, especially when faced with moral dilemmas. Using US and Indian research subjects (children and adults) the researchers posed to the research participants a dilemma faced by a man travelling to his best friend's wedding, where he would be the best man. At the train station his wallet and ticket were stolen, threatening his ability to get to the wedding. However, the opportunity to steal a train ticket presented itself. The research subjects were asked: what should the man do? The results of the study showed that on average 84 per cent of the Indians would meet their social obligation (to arrive at the wedding on time and carry out the best man's tasks) by stealing the ticket, whereas only 39 per cent of the Americans would. This result suggests that children's views of morality are *at least shaped by their social and cultural value systems*. But what did Jean Piaget find?

Piaget's work on moral reasoning and development

Jean Piaget's work in the first half of the twentieth-century suggests, on the other hand, that children's moral development has much to do with systematic changes in children's thinking due to *maturation*. He used various approaches to work out how children think about rules and in making moral judgements in two different ways, his so-called *two stage theory*. For Piaget, children younger than 10 or 11 think about moral dilemmas by regarding *rules* as *fixed*, *rigid*, *unalterable* and set by adults or divine authority. Thus children of this age are more likely to view the morality of a situation in more *objective outcomes* rather than *subjective motives or intentions*. Rules are not to be changed. Furthermore, breaking rules carries consequences, for example punishment, which must be avoided. Thus a young child who hears of a child breaking 15 cups in order to help his parents would regard that child as naughtier (breaking more cups) than a child who broke just one cup in the process of stealing some cookies. Older children at a less concrete, greater formal operational stage are, however, more likely to view the one-cup breaker as naughtier, because of his unacceptable or bad motive. Older children base their moral judgements on *intentions*; that is, the motive underlying the act being judged. The older child's view is more relativistic. (S)he understands that rules are relative and is it possible to change them, given the situation, for instance if everyone agrees. It is my view, however, that in spite of any strength in Piaget 'maturation' theory there is a sense also in which the child's development and formation of morals, attitudes and beliefs are governed and influenced by socialisation to a certain degree.

A multiplicity of influences in development of moral reasoning

You are now an adult student nurse who may have changed your moral values many times before this point in your life. Patients also change their moral values over time, altering their expectations of health services, which can bring complications and challenges for nurses

(Rest and Narvaez, 2009). With respect to change of moral outlook, please try to look back on, say, when you were aged five to seven (if it's possible to remember that far back). You may find that at that stage of your development you regarded rules as handed down by God, your parents and teachers and so on. Rules then may have appeared fixed and unchanging, compared with how you now think as an adult. Hopefully you now think of rules in more *relativistic* ways. If you can find the necessary reflective, research and well reasoned evidence to convince the ward sister about the need to change a certain style of care giving, you may well be successful. When I came into nursing the status quo around wound treatment was to put egg white on wounds. I could not find any evidence to support this practice. I soon began to question the practice in the wards I worked on. Even if there were then no concrete evidence of an alternative approach I used the sceptical literature that also questioned the approach of using egg white to treat patients' sores. Today the practice is not in evidence as far as I know. New research evidence brought forward new approaches to treat wounds. Our attitude towards egg white as good wound treatment has changed. When I did my adult nursing placement in the general hospital I noticed how aggressive and uncaring the health professionals were towards patients who had been admitted to A&E with deliberate drug overdoses. Emergent values, beliefs and attitudes that signal the criticality of healthcare professionals being empathetic and sympathetic towards patients who attempt suicide by drug overdose, the reasoning that such patients were crying out for help, have, I believe, led to a more humane caring approach today. Crain (1985) argues that adults tend to view rules as not being sacred or absolute, but as means to getting along cooperatively, and as means to an end. This tells us that we do not have to accept unpleasant, unhelpful and unkind status quos. We can change them.

Kohlberg's work on moral reasoning and development

Progressing from Piaget, Lawrence Kohlberg demonstrated that moral development does not stop at the age of 10 or 12, but continues into much later teenage life. This suggest that as individuals, with new knowledge, skills and experience, we may be persuaded to change our attitudes, opinions and values towards certain things and situations. Working with 10-, 13- and 16-year-old middle- and working-class boys (initially) in Chicago, Lawrence Kohlberg's research demonstrated that intellectual development and moral reasoning continue beyond Piaget's commencement of the formal operational stages of 11 or 12 years of age.

Kohlberg put scenarios containing moral dilemmas to his research subjects. One scenario told the story of a husband named Heinz who had a wife dying from cancer. He knew that a local druggist had developed the only cure (radium) but he was selling it for 10 times what it costs him to develop. Heinz tried every legal and fair means to borrow the $2,000 needed to buy the cure, but could only raise $1,000. The druggist insisted on the full amount, even when Heinz pleaded with him to let him pay the balance later or sell it to him at $1,000. His wife's life depended on it! Heinz stole the drug. Kohlberg asked his subjects whether they thought Heinz should have stolen the drug. From the various answers from different age groups, Kohlberg concluded that moral reasoning develops through six stages:

Level I

Stage 1: preconventional morality level. Similar to Piaget's first stage of moral thought, children believe what is right to be what authority figures say is right. Being morally good is to do what powerful authority figures such as parents, teachers and God say is right, thus escaping punishment. It is about obeying rules and the law and avoiding punishment. At this stage young children do not yet speak as belonging to the wider society (preconventional morality). They view morality as external to themselves; what their parents and other authority figures command them to do. Do or be punished! Rules are fixed and must be obeyed unquestionably.

Stage 2: individualism and exchange: Children see that there is more than one right view handed down by authority. Different individuals hold different points of view, one person being free to pursue his/her own interest, and another person an entirely different personal interest. Even children who think like this should appreciate that, whereas one patient may not wish to have his/her gangrenous foot amputated, another mentally competent patient may wish so to do. As an adult student nurse you should be able to take the debate much further, advancing cultural, philosophical, ethical, legal, moral and professional standards of care reasoning to justify patients' possible stances. Here you are recognising that different patients have different viewpoints.

Level II

Stage 3: conventional morality level. Kohlberg argues that at this stage children (teenagers of 13 or so) value good interpersonal relationships. Morality is not about a simple deal that Heinz could strike with the druggist. At this stage the expectations of the family and the wider society are paramount. Thus good morality is to behave in good, acceptable ways, possess good motives, caring interpersonal feelings, love, empathy, trust and concern for others. It is about being people-centred, problem-centred, rather than self-centred. Thus at this stage children in the research would argue that Heinz could justify stealing the drugs to cure his wife, because life is precious, more important than property – his love for his wife being viewed as more acceptable than the druggist's greed to sell the over-priced cure for $2,000, ten times the cost of making the drug. (Reflect on current situations in the NHS where Trusts are saying that, because of the high cost of some drugs, they are unable or unwilling to have them prescribed for certain cancer patients. See also Box 8.5.)

Stage 4: maintaining social order. Young people think in terms of being good people, having good caring motives towards others, even those outside the family. Their concerns shift towards maintaining the integrity and order of society; thus they view good behaviour as crucially obeying the law. Thus Heinz will realise that if he steals the drug he can save his wife's life; however, the consequences are that he faces the court for theft. Even if he hopes to be able to persuade the judge to let him off lightly, he expects the judge to uphold the law and punish him appropriately. Although, as a nurse, you may think in terms of consequences, for example not breaking the law for fear of going to jail, hopefully you are beginning to think in terms of people-centred, problem-centred care, doing what is best for the patient, whilst keeping within legal frameworks. Our practice should be positive, consciously doing what is best for the patient, not negative or defensive practice, just doing what is required to avoid being sued.

Level III

Stage 5: post-conventional morality level. This is viewing morality in terms of social contract and individual rights. People want to preserve their society as a functional, non-chaotic whole, even if that society is not seen as a good one. Hitler's well-ordered German society was totalitarian, well organised but not a moral ideal. It preached hatred of one section of the society, whilst loving and respecting the other section. Thus stage 5 people, argues Kohlberg, are able to judge society in a

BOX 8.5 Reflective exercise

What are your thoughts on the next situation described? The ward you work on has just paid £3,000 to purchase a brand new plasma TV set, having the latest technology. One of your patients with mental problems is in a very aggressive mood, with truculent behaviour and threatening to break up the TV. He and others are also slightly at risk. What action should be taken?

I guess that even 13- or 14-year-olds would be able to see that, should an aggressive psychiatric patient begin to break up the ward furniture, trying to prevent him from hurting himself, other patients and staff themselves would be a most important priority. Trying to save the ward's very expensive television set at the expense of people being hurt cannot be justified morally or professionally. People are more important than property. A TV set can be replaced; a person cannot. Professional standards and your code of conduct ask you to put patients at the centre of care, always addressing the need for patient safety and the safety of others in your care, other members of staff included. You also have a moral, ethical and legal duty of care to put patient interest over that of property and inanimate possessions. The ethic of beneficence requires you to ensure that patients benefit from your action, not harmed by them (the ethical principle of non-maleficence). Even at stage 3 of Kohlberg's moral reasoning model, young people think in terms of being good individuals, having helpful and caring motives towards people, even if it is only towards those close to them, for example family members. Kohlberg says that this arises not from pure imitation but through mental reasoning. This point suggests that as a health professional you should be concerned to develop your reasoning power and be prepared to accept that you may be challenged on your moral values, which you may have to change in order to be an effective caring nurse possessing the moral values and ethical principles that your profession demands of you.

more abstract way, a theoretical assessment that involves stepping back and asking critical questions such as: what values, rights and beliefs should this society value? People should feel free to put forward their ideas on what makes a good society on the basis that all will benefit from implementing such ideas, not just Aryan people, but Jews too, black and white, brown and yellow, all people irrespective of their ethnicity. There are certain basic rights and liberties such as the right to life, the right not to be punished without a trial, and the right to autonomy in decision making related to one's and other people's healthcare. Individual rights and liberty must be protected. Unfair laws can be changed but by democratic order whereby everyone has the same opportunity to be involved in the change process. Relating this to nursing, one nurse may believe in euthanasia, another does not; one patient may support euthanasia whereas another disagrees with it; but through the democratic process, should the government of the day within the UK put the idea forward that the nation should vote on whether or not we legalise euthanasia, then every qualified voter would have the opportunity to vote in a general election or a special referendum to decide for or against euthanasia. At stages 5 and 6 we should be advocating against any nursing measures we believe to be wrong or inappropriate, even if such measures appear to be the norm at the time. If Adolf Hitler's generals had done this, in the seemingly ordered and organised German society, they would have been unlikely to face the death penalty in the Nuremberg trials.

Stage 6: universal principles. Crain (1985, p. 123) sums up this stage by saying:

> Stage 5 respondents are working toward a conception of the good society . . . (a) pro-
> tect individual rights, . . . (b) settle disputes through democratic processes. However,
> democratic processes alone do not always result in outcomes that we intuitively sense
> are just. A majority may vote for a law that hinders a minority. Thus Kohlberg believes
> that there must be a higher stage – stage 6 – which defines the principles by which we
> achieve justice.

Kohlberg argues that, unlike Piaget's findings ascribed to a process of growth and maturation, his levels of moral reasoning are not attributed to genetic determinants as blueprints for moral development and reasoning. He argues that his stages emerge from the individual's freedom to think about moral issues. Social influences are only important in that they create opportunity to stimulate and challenge our mental processes, our mental reasoning. Thus, as we are motivated and challenged about our moral position, we are being aided to come up with new and more comprehensive positions. Social interactions challenging our thinking must be open and democratic. We must respect, however, that environmental influence are at play in the development of moral reasoning. We must give ourselves and our patient space and time to think; give patients the opportunity to think and make up their minds about whether they want to follow a proposed course of treatment or not. Patients have a right to reject a treatment even if they cannot demand one of their own choice. Similarly, we need to give young people a chance to develop their own reasoning, not pressurise them. The English court in *Gillick v Norfolk and W. AHA* already acknowledges that children of 16 are in some cases fully able to think logically in determining whether they should have certain treatments even if their parents object. Kohlberg argues that the approach of mentally challenging people's ethical positions is best for encouraging their further moral development, taking their level of thinking and moral reasoning to higher stages. For you, the nurse, the implication is that some of your patients whom by virtue of chronological years you may call children (under 18) are able to demonstrate very serious and clear ethical and moral reasoning necessary to inform their decisions about accepting medical care even when their parents are refusing. So 16-year-olds may be deemed to be competent to make healthcare decisions, and if they are Gillick competent they can certainly consent to treatment. The message here is that we should obey the law, appreciating that each individual is unique and must be assessed with this in mind.

Banerjee (2005) argues that where parents encourage reasoning, rather than physically punish a child to conform, such a child is more likely to develop positive moral values. Banerjee argues that:

> In fact, research evidence shows that parents' use of physical punishment may be related
> to greater levels of aggression by young children towards their peers. Children are more
> likely to learn positive moral values from their parents if they are helped to understand
> those values through explanations.

Criticism of Kohlberg's theory of moral reasoning

Kohlberg is not without his critics. His theory is culturally biased, being based purely on Western philosophical values and tradition, ignoring Eastern philosophies (Simpson, 1974; Crain, 1985). It is also criticised as being sex or gender biased, being based on research on US male subjects only. Carol Gilligan (1982) another eminent Harvard University professor, criticised Kohlberg's research for its male orientation. She argues that, whereas moral reasoning in males revolves around rules, legalistic arguments, rights, formal justice and abstract principles, in female morality principles are focused on interpersonal relationships, compassion and caring ethics. Women are likely to want to maintain good relationships, even after an argument in which participants took differential positions.

Consequence of our socialisation and morals learned

One of the consequences of our socialisation is the moral values learned; a further inevitable consequence of our learned morality is the resultant behaviours that arise from these states of thinking, attitudes and moral positions. As the ethics of consequentialism shows us, every behaviour has both a motive and a consequence, which we need to be aware of in order to be good, caring nurses. If we are taught to study consequences as a way of determining that morality of our actions, we will always seek to justify conduct on the basis of how we perceive and value consequences – the ethical principle of utilitarianism. If we believe the rightness or morality lies in the nature of the act itself (deontological ethics) we will always be inclined to look for moral justification in the nature of the act itself. If we are brought up to value the rational approach termed cost–benefit analysis we will always be seeking to assess cost against benefits; for example, we may seek to do something based on the utilitarian principle that we will pursue this approach because it will benefit the majority – the principle of regard for the greatest good or happiness of the greatest number as a morality rule. But this may not be entirely appropriate in nursing and medicine, where patients in the minority may get overlooked. So in nursing and medicine, therefore, we may have to use a combination of utilitarian and other principles, for example operating to our belief in God, divine healing and other faith principles that we cannot logically explain. We may, correctly, value happiness over misery, life over death, that truth telling is good and worthwhile because this is seen as contributing to the good life. Having values has implications for our professional thinking and behaviour and is also a basis for realising ethical dilemmas, or being faced with two equally valid approaches to solving a problem and not being sure which to pursue. Our patients are uniquely different people, with different moral positions, values and health belief systems. Taking one medical or nursing approach could help some but not others. So what should we do? These are some of the moral dilemmas and contradictions our own moral beliefs let us face each day. So how do nursing students think we acquire these values that make up our sense of morality and therefore our ethical reasoning and how can we use them in healthcare practice? The work of Piaget and Kohlberg has already provided some answers.

How does a small group of student nurses believe we develop moral values?

When I put the above question to a group of 32 first-year undergraduate nursing students recently. Their answers, provided in a 500-word essay, revealed wide-ranging ideas on how we come to develop our moral values. The students' short essays revealed the following perceptions, views and understandings of how we develop our moral standpoints. In our earliest years, the students argued, we start to form associations or links with others. We call this *socialisation* or *social interaction*. We are being *socialised* into the world. Our earliest associations are with parents, our mother, father, brothers and sisters, cousins, grandparents if we are lucky enough to have them, our parents' friends and associates, and so on. We learn a lot in these early years even if we are not consciously aware we are doing so. As we are so dependent on others we learn a lot from them. We learn that our mother (perhaps our father too) cares for us. They feed us, wash and change us, keep us warm, play with us, talk to us, perhaps even coo at us, even though sometimes we do not understand what they are saying. However, we know when people are kind, warm and loving to us and when they are not. Hopefully, our parents make us happy.

On the other hand they may make us sad, depending on how they treat us. If they are unkind to us they may treat us in a rough manner, hurt us, pinch us or even squeeze us to a point where we feel pain, and so on. If they are kind to us they do not do any of these horrible things. Instead they care for us with gentleness. As young as we are we can sense when people are warm and friendly to us and when they are unkind and horrible. From these early interactions we begin to form attitudes towards others; for example we feel warm and close to those who are warm and kind to us. Those who are rough and unkind to us we do not feel so warm to. From these interactions we begin to form our own *value systems* – recognising kindness from unkindness, love from hate, honesty from dishonesty, caring from uncaring and so on.

As we grow older we become more aware of our parents through contact, their own conduct and behaviour, attitudes, verbal exposition and reasoning with us. They teach us certain values: kindness, respect for others, warmth, gentleness, honesty, loyalty, how to act lovingly, calmly and so on. We continue to learn values throughout our lives, learning many of these from relationships outside our families. For example, although in our earliest years we may not learn how to value and handle money, as we grow older we may learn this value, perhaps by first going to the shops with our parents. As we grow older we continue to learn new values from our family but also from other wider social interactions, for example with friends and associates, nurses, health visitors, doctors, nursery nurses and teachers, playgroups leaders and other children. We learn from school, church, social clubs and other social interactions. We are now becoming more *independent* but we are still learning our values from others through our social interactions. When we learn to read we learn even faster about other people's values and beliefs. If we are Christians we may learn to read the Bible; if we are Muslims we may read the Koran; and so on. We may begin to learn many 'divine' values; for example, if Christians, the Ten Commandments that tell us not to steal, lie or kill, to honour our parents, love our neighbours and so on. We may not have such experiences if, for example, our parents are atheists, who do not believe in God. There are of course many, many interdependent ways of learning values but we do not have time to cover them here. Try to make a start using Box 8.6.

Bringing our personal values into nursing

We can learn good values and we can learn bad ones. We can learn caring values or uncaring ones. By the time we get to university we have a well-formed value system that is ready to be built upon or even changed, especially if we perceive that some of the personal moral values learned earlier are now in conflict with professional codes of ethics and conduct. If we hold values such as prejudice and racism, dislike of people with disability, hate for people who are gay or lesbians, we will experience cognitive dissonance or mental discomfort, because we cannot hold on to these values and comfortably give care that values the opposite of these views. We may have come to nursing with the view that no woman should

---

BOX 8.6 Student reflective question 8.4

Use a page in your ethics portfolio to jot down your reflection on ways in which we learn other than those outlined above.

abort a fetus. However, we will soon learn that women have a legal right to determine what happens to their own bodies. If we must function effectively as a health professional, we are going to have to abide by the professional code of conduct, ethics and performance.

Clash of values

I suggest to you that if your personal moral values seriously clash with your professional ones you are going to find it almost impossible to sustain the journey to becoming a registered nurse, unless you can alter your individualistic position. If you fail to it could mean you dropping out of the nurse training programme. There needs to be a certain consistency between our personal and professional value systems and beliefs. If there is not the state of tension between the two (cognitive dissonance) will be too great to bear, and will not sustain competent professional practice.

Impact of values on behaviour and attitudes

The point I want to impress upon you here is that our personal moral values and beliefs influence our thinking, attitudes to people and situations, and also influence our behaviours. In respect to personal behaviour, our values and our attitudes can make us behave kindly or unkindly, cold or warm, friendly or unfriendly, sincere or disloyal, courageous or frightened and scared, honest or dishonest, and so on. Our value system is adding to who we are, what we are becoming, how we will interact with others and react to situations. Our values can change in the light of new evidence, new learning, new experiences and so on. Someone may set out deliberately to change our moral values. What should be clear here is that if we learn bad values they, like the good ones, become part of us, entrenched. As I said earlier, by the time we come to train as a nurse we have quite a substantial moral value system built up. It is in place, ready to influence our approaches to ethical decision making.

Our values and attitudes can influence our professional interactions with our patients. This is crucial. The fact that as human beings, first and foremost, and second as professional nurses, you have personal and nursing values and a philosophy of life that you use to lead your personal life and organise and deliver patient care, logically implies that those patients/clients for whom you care also have their own individual moral cultural and ethical values and beliefs. These were formed and influenced by those patients'/clients' individual social interactions, in the same way that healthcare professionals' moral and ethical values were formed and influenced by our socialisation.

Patients and clients use their philosophy of life, and moral values and beliefs not only to lead their personal lives, but also to influence their health beliefs, and to respond to illnesses and cope in their interactions with us as healthcare professionals. Most important of all patients' health beliefs influence their progress through an illness, the strength and resolve they develop to cope, including their approach to dying and death.

The aim of good nursing care ethics is to enhance the nurse–patient caring relationship, respecting patients' ethical values and beliefs, as well as meeting national and international ethical standards that define sound nursing care. Nursing values need to be grounded in respect for patients' own cultural and ethical health beliefs, because the people we care for come to us with their own health beliefs that help to make them an integral whole, who and what they are. If health professionals' values do not at least respect patients'/clients' own cultural and ethical values and health beliefs they are unlikely to promote patient recovery. This is not to say that, as nurses, where the evidence points to the patient's own health beliefs as being destructive and handicapping to their recovery we should not point this out. Indeed we should. For example a pregnant woman may tell the nurse, midwife, doctor and others that it is part of her cultural health beliefs to have as many children as possible, never practising any form of birth contraception. However, she has already had five caesarean sections due to inability to have a normal delivery. The staff feels that she faces a real possibility of a ruptured uterus from yet more caesarean births. Irrespective of how the patient feels about having more children on the grounds of cultural and individual beliefs about children, it would be irresponsible of the health professional not to point out to the woman the high risk she faces of sustaining a ruptured uterus that could kill her. Indeed the NMC expects you to be open and honest, protect the health and wellbeing of patients, make the care of people your first concern, treating them as individuals, share with people, in a way they can understand, the information they want or need to know about their health, and deliver care based on the best evidence. Sound ethical practice values people's right to their own value systems, autonomy and self-determination but not if this would make you do something that was unethical, against the patient's best interest or against your best professional judgement. A patient can refuse care but cannot demand it.

Of adult years and possessing mental capacity, patients/clients possess autonomy to do what they think is best for themselves, including refusing treatment if they feel the need to, even without an obligation to explain why. When and where nurses fail to recognise such fundamental human rights they are likely to fail in the provision of sound ethical care or conduct of patient-focused research. Failure to respect correct ethical standards can make a nurse end up treating patients/clients with disrespect and, at times, illegally. The case of the nurses Kevin Cobb and Beverley Allitt are examples of this.

Summary and conclusion

This chapter has focused on:

- Why a study of ethics is crucial to nurses. It concludes that it is essential for nurses and other health professionals to understand and apply sound ethical values to clinical practice.
- The nature of individual moral values and beliefs in the caring relationship. The conclusion is drawn that therapists and patients have their own moral and ethical value systems which interact. Therefore compatibility is necessary for individual, culturally sensitive patient care. Nurses should not impose personal value systems on patients, but value patients' own value system and health beliefs.
- The place of family and the wider community socialisation in morality and value building, and their subsequent possible impact on professionalism. The conclusion is drawn that personal morality, professional ethics, and patients' personal and cultural values are in dynamic interactions within the therapeutic relationship.
- The implication of student nurses bringing their personal value systems (good or bad, caring or uncaring, desirable or undesirable) into nursing. Where individual moral and ethical value systems clash or conflict with professional code of conduct, ethics and expectations, they cause major cognitive dissonance that need to be modified for professional survival and sensitive patient care. If health professionals hold values of prejudice, racism and homophobia they will have to change them or leave the profession, or they will be ineffective carers.
- A study of ethics and an examination of personal value systems, the nurse's and the patient's. This is essential to all student and qualified nurses.

9 The importance of ethical practice

Objectives of this chapter

After reading this chapter you should be able to:

- discuss how absence of ethical principles can lead to human catastrophes and what can be learned from such catastrophes;
- identify and discuss how aspects of professional code of conduct, law and ethics can prevent human catastrophes in healthcare;
- use your understanding of the ethical issues within the Tuskegee and Nazi German experiments mentioned in this chapter to critically examine how health professionals could seriously undermine patients' own value systems and erode their personal, cultural and religious rights to proper ethical standards in healthcare;
- discuss the nurse's moral, ethical and legal obligation to ensure that the historical catastrophes referred to in this chapter are never repeated.

Introduction

We have already noted in an earlier chapter how a number of UK nurses (e.g. the infamous Colin Norris, Benjamin Green and Beverley Allitt) exercised callous lack of respect for moral values, for example one should not kill others. Therefore as a nurse you should remember the ethical principle of non-maleficence that says you should not hurt your patient. Respect your patient's *human* and *legal right to life*. As a nurse you need to value the sanctity of human life. The lack of such value perhaps drove Norris, Green and Allitt to callously murder their patients (in Allitt's case innocent children). Similarly, Dr Harold Shipman disrespected the ethical value of *life preservation* over destruction of human life so badly that on 31 January 2000 he was found guilty of murdering 15 of his patients and suspected of killing many more. Shipman disregarded his profession's specific ethical and professional value to 'maintain utmost respect for human life' (Physician's Oath: Declaration of Geneva, 1948. Adopted by the General Assembly of World Medical Association at Geneva Switzerland, September 1948. Online source: http://www.necef.in/node/6). For a fuller account of the Shipman case read the Shipman Inquiry Reports at http://www.the-shipman-inquiry.org.uk/reports.asp.

The Independent (11 April 2000, 8 July 2000) reported that a male nurse, Kevin Cobb, was found guilty of the manslaughter of a nursing colleague. He was also convicted of drugging three female patients and raping two of them. Such crimes not only are plainly illegal but raise the question as to the moral, professional integrity and ethical values on which these people have conducted their professional interactions with patients. It is important to learn from history.

The catastrophic Tuskegee experiment

We will focus on the Tuskegee experiment, describe it and analyse it, essentially looking for unethical and illegal moves. We will then address the lessons nurses can learn from this experiment.

The Tuskegee experiment (otherwise known as the Tuskegee syphilis study, or the Public Health Service syphilis study) was conducted in Tuskegee, Alabama, USA, between 1932 and 1972. Its purpose was to study the natural progression of untreated syphilis in African-American men, who were in fact poor tenant farmers (sharecroppers) who paid part of their rent by giving up some of their crops to the land owner. To participate in the study the men were given free medical examinations (not treatment), free meals and free burial insurance. They were not informed that they had syphilis, nor were they treated for it. The point I would like you as a nurse to focus on is the fact that, pivotal to the success of this experiment, a nurse by the name of Eunice Rivers (against what should have been sensitive nursing care values, sound ethical human values and morality of fair play, racial justice, right to informed consent before participation in experiments, the best treatment for all patients irrespective of race, and a nurse's obligation to prevent human suffering, especially that of one's own patients irrespective of their race, colour, gender and cultural background) helped to persuade some 399 African-American men with syphilis to be part of this observational study. You must remember that the object of the study was to observe the natural progression of syphilis in these untreated men – not to treat them. The men were observed, examined and tested at strategic points to see how the disease was progressing. Although penicillin was tested and proven to be the drug of choice against syphilis, having been discovered between 1940 and 1943, and widely used by the mid 1940s, for 32 years the Tuskegee experimental subjects were not treated for syphilis. In fact they were actively encouraged not to have the treatment. The US public health authorities even persuaded the US Army drafters not to recruit eligible men from the Tuskegee syphilis research sample, further removing the men's chance of being treated for syphilis. Thus the men's lack of opportunity to have their disease treated was compounded by this additional and deliberate sabotage. This further frustrated the men's chances of treatment and a possible cure. In reality if the men had joined the US Army there was a real chance they would have been treated for the disease.

In reflecting on this case (Box 9.1) one would expect you to include some of the following at least. On ethical grounds, although the men might have reasonably expected their doctors and nurse to tell them the truth (the ethic of *veracity*) and to care for them, they were lied to at each strategic examination when they were simply examined and samples of their cerebrospinal fluid taken, simply to check on the progression of their disease, not to treat them. They did not benefit from the approaches taken; in fact they were denied treatment, which seriously hurt them and their families. This was a disregard of the ethical principle of *non-maleficence*: do nothing to hurt your patient. They were led to believe they were being treated, and there again not for syphilis but for 'bad blood' (Jones, 1981), yet another deception, clearly no benefit to them. They were bribed to cooperate with the experiment,

---

BOX 9.1 Student portfolio activity 9.1

After reading the brief version of the Tuskegee case above, write down in your ethics portfolio your thoughts and feelings about the experiment. Reflect on the *ethical* issues of the case as you see them. I suggest you use Gibbs's (1988) reflective model. Then identify appropriate *ethical theories* that you feel can be used to support your views on why the study was ethically wrong.

promised free transportation to the test centre, free lunches, free treatment (although not for syphilis, as they were not told they had syphilis) – free burials too! This last inducement was wrapped up in more deception since the real motive of free burials was for the medical authority to get their hands on the men's cadavers for further investigative study of the progression of syphilis in their bodies.

One of the biggest ethical problems was that the men *never consented* to participate in the experiment, which went on till 1972, when journalists exposed the horror. By then the horrendous consequences of this experiment (progression of acute to tertiary syphilis, characterised by brain and other internal organ destruction, distortion of body postures, further contagion of other people, including congenital syphilis in babies born to men and women with the disease, excruciating pains, madness and agonising deaths) were irreversible. For 40 long years the 399 men were kept in the dark about their disease when they could have been successfully treated. Gross negligence in my book. This amounts to at least gross negligence punishable in the criminal law under a charge of manslaughter, but more accurately the entire medical team could be viewed as having slowly and painfully murdered the men and their families. Compare the ethical approach in Tuskegee with the ethical approaches health professionals are now expected to respect, by following the Nuremberg Code on medical research ethics.

Another huge unethical dimension to the experiment was *racism*. All 399 men were black and recruited in Macon County, Alabama, where 82 per cent of the population were black, with some 36 per cent of the overall population suffering from syphilis. Of course syphilis had no respect for class or race. Selvin (1984) reports that many rich, titled and famous people had it: people such as King Henry VIII, Christopher Columbus, Queen Cleopatra, King Herod of Judea, General Napoleon Bonaparte, Frederick the Great, Pope Sixtus IV, Pope Alexander VI, Pope Julius II, Catherine the Great, the famous artist Paul Gauguin, Franz Schubert and James Joyce. Here is another racist element: the US Public Health Service, a predominantly white middle-class doctor establishment, decided that only black men would be recruited to the sample. Given that the American Civil Rights movement had not been really active in America at that time and given that racism was still rampant, it is easy to see why this sort of unethical decision making involving negro subjects came about. Pence (2004, p. 278) captured the racial scene in America at the time:

> In the 1930s, American medicine was, and had long been, widely racist – certainly by our present standards and to some extent even by the standards of the time. For at least a century before the Tuskegee study began, most physicians condescended to African-American patients, held stereotypes about them, and sometimes used them as subjects of non-therapeutic experiments.

Another principal ethical weakness in this study was lack of proper documentation and haphazardness.

> The Tuskegee study was hardly a model of scientific research; . . . as a study in nature, it was carried out haphazardly. Except for an African-American Nurse, Eunice Rivers, who was permanently assigned to the study, there was no continuity of medical personnel.

(p. 281)

Spence notes that once the journalist Jean Heller, of the Associated Press, broke the story across America on 26 July 1972, revealing how the US federal government had used poor African-Americans as guinea pigs in this horrible experiment, the world took notice. As would be expected in the very litigious US, a legal action was brought successfully by the men, to seek redress and monetary compensation for the victims and their families. The case was settled out of court.

Ethical lessons from Tuskegee

Try to summarise for yourself the ethical lessons of Tuskegee. Important historical cases such as this should convince us of the need to study ethics and practise medicine and nursing ethically, so that such catastrophes can be prevented. Present and future healthcare decisions need to be grounded on sound ethical principles and practice. One of things I would like to point out to the modern nurse is this: you need not be like Nurse Eunice Rivers, and put up with observed unethical practice or be part of it. You are entitled and expected to stand up and be a powerful advocate for your patient. Your training, now a university education, and your status as a registered nurse empower you to advocate on behalf of your patient.

Tuskegee and up-to-date Department of Health ethical research guidelines

The UK Department of Health (DoH, 2005c, 2008) research protocols for human experiments give much protection to patients participating in research. The UK government set up research committees under the Central Office of Research Ethics Committee (COREC) to vet research applications and protect research participants. Research not approved by an ethics committee cannot go ahead. These tight controls should hopefully prevent a repeat of Tuskegee. Currently, nursing is being practised in a more collegiate, multiprofessional and multidisciplinary healthcare environment where each professional, regardless of his/her named profession, has equal opportunity to speak out (*whistle blow* even) to protect patients' right in nursing care and research. Nurses are now more empowered to protect patients' rights than hitherto. One presumes that in Nurse Rivers's time she may have been just a 'token' in the medical hierarchy dominated by white gentlemen physicians with paternalistic attitudes. They ruled the roost. Things have changed. We are now closer than ever before to a more balanced structured multidisciplinary care team in which nurses need to seize their moment and advocate effectively for their patients.

The potential for a clash of values between patient and nurse

The fact that the nurse has a set of moral and ethical values and beliefs and the patient his/hers means that somewhere in this nurse–patient/client interaction both sets of values, beliefs and philosophies must meet. The potential for a clash of values is therefore very real. It is important for both nurses and patients that there be no serious clash of philosophical values and beliefs that would result in the patient suffering as a consequence, for example in retardation of the patient's progress towards recovery or a peaceful death if this is the inevitable outcome of the patient's/client's illness. It is important that nurses' personal moral value systems do not undermine the patients' (positive) attitudes and response to their illness, and to their progress and positive health beliefs.

Ignorance of patients' cultural ethical values and health beliefs can lead to patients being treated disrespectfully, unethically, and culturally insensitively. A nurse–patient relationship that is fractured by a clash of ethical values, cultural insensitivity, disrespect and insults will not benefit the therapeutic relationship that every healthcare professional needs to foster. Consider how upsetting, demoralising, degrading and potentially destructive of a good nurse–patient relationship either of the following would be: offering a plate of pork to a patient from the Jewish, Muslim or Rastafarian faith; administering blood to a patient of the Jehovah's Witness religion. Cultural awareness is fundamental to sensitive and effective nursing care.

There are other potentially insensitive situations that may upset patients of certain cultures. An Islamic woman may not be comfortable with male midwives and obstetricians in attendance at her labour. A Hindu may have difficulty complying with medication given in capsule form for fear of consuming capsules made from cows and pigs. It may be considered offensive to Jews for a nurse of the Christian faith to handle their dead in certain ways. A Muslim must be buried within 24 hours of death. There are of course very strong underlying values that have given rise to such practices and if they are not observed and respected great offence may be caused to the patient/client and his/her relatives. It can be seen, therefore, how important it is for healthcare practitioners to understand the diversity of cultural values and beliefs that their patients and clients bring to the therapeutic relationship.

Value of learning about some ethical catastrophes in Britain

Analysis of the Tuskegee experimental has demonstrated that misguided ethical conduct by nurses and physicians can cause serious ethical problems. Historically, we note in the UK how a lack of proper ethical safeguards led to other ethical problems. For example, Professor van Velzen (of the Alder Hey Hospital scandal) had, over a period of time, unilaterally decided to remove organs and tissues from children's cadavers during post-mortem examinations, without parental consent (Report of the Royal Liverpool Children's Inquiry, 2001). Moreover, his action was illegal as it contravened the Human Tissue Act 1961. Historical examination of the negative influences of poor ethical decision making by healthcare professionals shows how such dilemmas can be prevented in future. The UK cases of Dr Shipman and nurses Kevin Cox and Beverley Allitt demonstrate that health professionals can lose their sense of rationality and sound ethical reasoning to patients' detriment. Safe and sound ethical guidelines must be kept in place.

How helpful are ethical guidelines from the NMC?

Please refer to Boxes 9.2, 9.3 and 9.4 for Student portfolio activities 9.2, 9.3 and 9.4 and do the exercises. Use your law and ethics portfolio to record your effort.

The exercises in the three boxes are designed to help you to reflect on and consolidate your learning in respect to the ethics material covered in this chapter. Moreover the excises will help you to cement your understanding of relationships between ethics, your NMC PCC, your nursing practice and your use of portfolio to enhance your learning and professional development.

It is self-evident for discussions about nursing ethics and sound ethical practice to focus on the nurse's code. The code is the nurse's professional guiding light. It is important for the nursing student to examine his/her own moral beliefs and values brought to the profession in the light of the nurse's code of conduct and ethics. It is important to look at the code and match it up with your personal moral values and beliefs and see if there are conflicts in the relationship, because, if there are, they need resolution to free up your thinking so that you can act with sensitivity, caring and sound moral judgement in your nursing activities. Constant re-evaluation of your value systems alongside analysis of the NMC Code, together with the necessary adjustments, is required throughout your professional life.

A useful question for continuous self-examination is: is my own value system still compatible with my professional obligations and aspirations as a nurse, and does my personal value system continue to benefit the nurse–patient therapeutic relationship? If you do not continually balance the two value systems, your *cognitive dissonance* will

---

BOX 9.2 Student portfolio activity 9.2

Get hold of a copy of the NMC 2008 Code, Study it and write down in the space below, or in an appropriate section of your developing law and ethics portfolio, those code guidelines that you consider to be essential for sound *ethical* practice. Give reasons for your choice.

BOX 9.3 Student portfolio activity 9.3

Reflect on those guidelines you identified in Student portfolio activity 9.2 and for each one jot down your thoughts on why you feel it is an *ethical* guideline.

BOX 9.4 Student portfolio activity 9.4

Reflect on the ethical guiding principles from your NMC Code, personal reasoning, ethics portfolio work to date, your nursing practice and on what you read about Tuskegee and write down in the space below critical reasons why healthcare professionals must study ethics as a prerequisite to sound and competent practice.

---

overwhelm you, to a point where you become frustrated, disillusioned, harassed and battle fatigued. Soon the resultant stress and burnout will reduce the effectiveness of your practice and you may even give up nursing prematurely. Renewal of professional spirit is critical for continued successful nursing practice that benefits the patient/client. This renewal comes from constant reappraisal of personal values against expected professional values and standards.

Hitler's doctors and the Nuremberg code of ethics

It is well documented that Hitler's genocide practice killed many millions, Jews particularly. It is questionable whether the doctors and others in Hitler's army who committed such atrocities in their unethical experiments on people, especially those they considered to be 'imperfect', shared any decent personal and professional moral and ethical human values. To establish a pure Aryan race Jews and people with disabilities were put to death. Although this may have been seen as legal under Nazi German law and morally acceptable by Nazi German moral codes, it was certainly inhuman, cruel, illegal, immoral and unethical by Western democratic values. As a nurse you should note that those who later in the Nuremberg trials claimed to have acted under 'superior orders' were still found guilty of human cruelty, murder and genocide, and many were consequently put to death. Such extreme unethical practice in Hitler's world led to much human suffering, which must not be repeated. Hence today if as nurses we wish to conduct experiments involving human subjects we must ensure that consent is obtained, human subjects receive clear information on the nature of the experiments and their rights to refuse are respected, even after initial consent. Nazi experiments caused much human pain and suffering. Experiments like Tuskegee or the Hitler concentration camps must not be repeated. By reading of these historical happenings, hopefully, you are thinking that never would I allow myself as a nurse to become involved in such activities. The cruel ethical practices of the Second World War subsequently led to intense universal ethical scrutiny on human experiments at the Nuremberg trials, resulting in the *Nuremberg code* of ethics. Although experiments on humans can produce great good for humanity as a whole, researchers must make sure participants in research are properly informed of what will happen, the nature of their involvement and participation, effects of the studies, implications for any treatment they are having, and the fact that experiments will not interfere with patients' treatment or their position as patients; most important of all, patients must have properly consented to participate in research before it can go ahead. A number of valuable medical *ethical codes and declarations* since the Nuremberg code, such as the Declaration of Geneva, have contributed to sounder ethical practice in healthcare research today.

Please complete the questionnaire in Box 9.5.

Summary and conclusion

This chapter has focused on examples of how healthcare professionals have subjugated moral, ethical and legal principles to hurt, even kill, their patients. Using known historical incidents such as the Tuskegee and Nazi-German experiments we have noted how disregard of sound moral, ethical and legal values and principles relating to human interactions can lead to human catastrophes that have destroyed not only individuals but have also attempted to wipe out large sections of ethnic and cultural groups. The world would not wish to see a repeat of these catastrophes and nurses and other health professionals can do much to prevent their reoccurrence. The chapter also gave you an opportunity to use your law and ethics portfolio to identify key ethical guidance principles within the NMC Code, analysing their relationship to your own moral value judgements and their application in the achievement of sound ethical practice standards within healthcare. It is hoped that by completing the questionnaire in Box 9.5 you have reinforced your learning in relation to this chapter.

BOX 9.5 Questionnaire

Which of the following murdered innocent children?

a. Dr Harold Shipman
b. Nurse Beverley Allitt
c. Nurse Colin Norris
d. Nurse Eunice Rivers

The ethical principle of non-maleficence says that:

a. You must act to benefit your patient
b. You should promote patient autonomy
c. You should not hurt your patient
d. You should promote justice for patients

Nurse Eunice Rivers actively encouraging the Tuskegee patients with syphilis not to have available penicillin treatment amounts to:

a. Professional cruelty, murder and non-malificence
b. Professional suicide, beneficence and non-malificence
c. Racial justice, cruelty, and lack of autonomy
d. Racial injustice, cruelty and failure to observe non-malificence

Professor van Velzen's decision (in the Alder Hey Hospital scandal) to remove children's organs without reference to the parents breached the ethical principle of:

a. Consent
b. Confidentiality
c. Beneficence
d. Non-maleficence

10 Ethical theories part I

Principlism

Objectives of this chapter

After reading this chapter you should be able to:

- describe major ethical theories and how we may relate them to nursing decision making;
- define and distinguish between *normative* and *non-normative* ethics;
- explain principlism, distinguishing between *autonomy*, *beneficence*, *non-maleficence* and *justice*; explain how these principles can be applied in nursing;
- examine how your Code of conduct and nursing practice relate to ethical theories;
- briefly define *teleological/consequentialist* and *deontological* ethics;
- examine how ethical thinking and beliefs can influence attitudes in patient care, patients' health beliefs, illness and recovery;
- work with others, in identifying self and patient values of importance in nursing and make links between these and the NMC code.

Introduction

We have established in the previous chapter that as nurses we need caring values and beliefs to guide our healthcare practice decision making. It may be useful for you to find out from your next clinical placement what ethical and philosophical values the care team uses to provide care. You may hear the ward manager and members of the team talking about the ward philosophy. What is it? What ethical values drive it? These values represent the normative ethics or ethical theories that guide healthcare decision making. The ward staff may subscribe to the view that all patients must be treated *respectfully* and helped to gain early *independence* and avoid *learned helplessness*. We must tell patients the *truth* and deal fairly with them irrespective of their health status, socio-economic background, race, colour, creed, gender or sexual orientation. We may be told by the ward staff that they value patients' right to decide, consent, refuse consent and so on. We may be told that the ward believes that what it does should benefit the patients and that we should do nothing to harm our patients. We may even be told that on this ward we aim to be fair to staff and patients, and so on. Most of these philosophical or caring principles can be summed up at fitting the ethical principle known as *principlism*. The four major *ethical principles* described under the concept of principlism by Beauchamp and Childress (2001), and which most clinicians and ethical theorists agree guide healthcare practice, are *autonomy*, *beneficence*, *non-maleficence* and *justice*.

Autonomy

Autonomy means respecting mentally competent persons' right to make personal healthcare decisions: consent to/refusal of treatment and which treatment options to accept. People have a right to make decisions relating to how they run their lives, provided the way they do so does not hurt or offend others. We need to remember that we live in a society that is governed by laws and an eclectic mix of ethical and cultural values. Therefore autonomy gives freedom to decide personal behaviour and decision making, providing our autonomous decisions do not offend others. Autonomy demands that we respect patients' right to self-determination even if self determination means choosing to die rather than accepting the treatment offered. Gaining patients' consent to investigations and treatment is to respect their autonomous right to give or refuse consent. Autonomy means asking the competent patient's permission to take his/her blood pressure, record his/her temperature, dress his/her wound, clean out his/her locker, make his/her bed, take him/her for a walk, exercise his/her limbs passively, even to enter his/her house if you are the district nurse.

Behaviours that reflect a position opposite to accepting the patient's right to autonomy are those decisions of a *paternalistic* nature; those that use autocratic conduct to erode patients' autonomy. Patients need to know they have the right to choose and question health professionals, who must be prepared to be questioned by the patient. The patient benefits by feeling confident that (s)he is not being taken for granted, but is respected and valued within the caring relationship. Law and ethics are so closely intertwined that nurses who accept patients' ethical right to autonomy are unlikely to encounter legal and ethical problems such as touching patients without their consent, falsely imprisoning patients, betraying patients' confidence or committing a negligence and criminal act against the patient. The days of paternalistic behaviour by nurses and doctors have long since past.

What happens when patients are not competent to make autonomous decisions? Sometimes patients are not mentally competent to take autonomous healthcare decisions. All adult patients and children who are Gillick competent have the autonomous right to make decisions regarding their care. However, mentally incompetent patients such as the unconscious patient, or some suffering from dementia, severe mental impairment and learning disability, severe Alzheimer's disease and so on, may lack the competence required to make decisions relating to their care. Such patients may not be able to act autonomously and therefore health professionals may have to take decisions in their best interest (Mental Capacity Act 2005). A word of warning. One is not saying here that in the situations cited above the loss of mental competence is always the case or even that it is permanent. In some cases of unconsciousness, for example, the loss of mental competence may be temporary. This means that as soon as the patient regains consciousness and competence (s)he resumes the right of self-determination.

Beneficence

This ethical principle is about ensuring that patients benefit from the caring relationship. This ethical principle involves the healthcare professional balancing benefits against risks and costs, and ensuring that, all things considered, the patient receives the best care. I choose to mention the phrase 'all things considered' because sometimes scarce resources make it impossible to give certain treatments. For example the NHS Trust may not be able to afford the most expensive and arguably the most effective drug. *Deontological* ethical values may determine that the action involved in choosing a particular cheaper drug is the best one for a number of reasons. Under the principle of beneficence, however, even though the drug of choice by the trust is not the most expensive and arguably the best one, on account of scarce resources, the drug chosen must be seen to be according benefit to the patient. For the patient to benefit from the chosen drug, the ethical principle of beneficence demands that (s)he be told of the effects as well as the side effects of the treatment. However scarce resources are, we should not choose treatment options unlikely to benefit the patient. However, even the courts take the view that healthcare managers and clinicians must balance outcomes against cost; a more *consequentialist ethical perspective*, whereby the choice of beneficial treatment option is based on ensuring that the majority is served, although sadly this may be at the expense of the minority.

Sometimes it is possible to question whether in the NHS managerial care decision benefit patients. Sometimes healthcare providers are faced with ethical dilemmas that they make decisions on. Needless to say it may be possible to demonstrate that some patients do not benefit from the decision. For example, one recalls the case *R v Cambridge Health Authority ex parte B (A Minor)* (1995) 23 BMLR 1 CA, [1995] 2 All 129. In this case a 10-year-old girl suffering from leukaemia and needing further chemotherapy, and a second bone marrow transplant, had to forgo the transplant for lack of funding. Her health authority (Cambridge HA) decided at the time not to spend further resources in treating the girl as it believed she would not benefit from yet another bone marrow transplant or chemotherapy. Moreover they thought that they had other more deserving priorities to spend the cash on. Morally and ethically, the decision seemed unjustified. Why should a little girl whose parents had worked, paid tax and contributed to NHS resources be denied further treatment? The reality, though, is that sometimes health authorities have to take very hard decisions. The court agreed in this case that health authorities, now NHS Trusts, do not have unlimited resources. They must simply manage within the limitations of their resources. If we look closer at the decision made, the teleological ethicists may justifiably support the decision on the basis of the possible consequences or outcomes of the decision. For example, the consequentialist may argue that the end result of yet another treatment was certain failure; furthermore, more patients were likely to benefit from the money being spent on this one girl, who the scientist thought would not benefit from the treatment and in fact had only a 20 per cent chance of so benefiting from the treatment. So here we see that sometimes we have to face moral dilemmas and take decisions which we feel we can best justify from our own moral and ethical standpoints. Hence, perhaps, the reason why the NMC states that nurses must be prepared to make difficult decisions and complex decisions. At a logical theoretical level, therefore, it is possible to state that, although nursing ethics aims at giving patients the 'best' care, 'best' may be relative to the overall situation faced. Nursing and medical decisions can be tough at times, yet we must ethically and professionally be committed to prioritising care on the basis of our best assessment of the situation and the contexts. We have to accept also that patients cannot always get the treatment they want. Furthermore if ethically and professionally, using our best professional judgement, supported by the research, we think that the treatment asked for is not appropriate then we are within our professional right not to give it. It is always possible that we may be challenged in law, as Cambridge HA was in the case outlined above. But health professionals must be prepared to defend and justify their positions. Utilitarian teleologists would certainly praise the decision that lead to the majority benefiting from the action.

Non-maleficence

This is the ethical norm that advocates no harm to patients. Florence Nightingale argued that hospitals should do patients no harm. By today's standard, this is quite a paradox because many patients go into hospital and leave with problems they did not take there: deformities from surgery, wrong operation and loss of healthy functional body parts, MRSA and

Clostridium difficile infections contracted in hospital, other forms of wound infections, to mention a few. Such iatrogenesis runs counter to the ethical doctrine of non-maleficence. In trying to prevent harm from coming to our patients we must continue to assess their risks of acquiring harm, educate them and the staff about prevention and do all in our power to stop patients being harmed by medical and nursing interventions.

Ethically, we owe patients a duty of care to protect them from harm. Newham and Hawley (2007) take the view that non-maleficence is a process of actively preventing harm; thus they draw a distinction between positively doing good, as in the case of *beneficence*, and actively preventing harm, as in the case of *non-maleficence*.

Justice

Justice is not the law in its narrow sense. It is a principle of distributing access, benefits, risks and costs fairly and equitably. How do we achieve fairness in healthcare? The case of Child B above questions whether this is possible. To apply justice and equity we need to accept and value differences and diversity. Our patients come from different cultural and religious backgrounds, bringing different ethical values with them. Fairness means recognising their difference and not acting prejudicially towards them. We must not behave unfairly to one group of patient at the expense of another. Traditionally, I believe that in the NHS we have tended to view patients who come with Eastern philosophical values with Western philosophical eyes. This is wrong. We need to be aware of our own and other people's cultural differences and take these into account in nursing them. Justice is about advocating on behalf of all patients, whether they come with a Western philosophical perspective or an Eastern one. We must endeavour to ensure fairness in access, diagnostic and treatment interventions. This is not the same as 'sameness' because we cannot justifiably treat all patients the same. Some come with diabetes, some have hernias, others have heart failures and so on – all different problems. They may share some common symptomatology, requiring similar interventions, but specifically they are different problems requiring different approaches. We can, however, be fair, applying equity with regard to according equality in terms of respect, ensuring equal access, ensuring right to life, consent, confidentiality, and giving the highest standard of care. Justice is not about treating all patients the 'same', as some student nurses sometimes make the mistake of saying in my ethics classes. In the NHS there must be a sense of equal opportunity, meaning all patients' right to fairness, justice, free speech, diagnostic, treatment and rehabilitation services. However, the services will perhaps differ depending on individual needs. Self- and culturally aware nurses will always be in a position to give care in a fair and just way.

Being free to choose does not mean that we should begrudge those who have the means within our society to seek, choose and obtain private treatment. But it does mean that within the NHS we should not put the rich above the poor, whites before blacks, the working class behind the middle class, the educated before the uneducated, the linguistically skilled before the patient with language deficit, Christians before Muslims, Protestants before Catholics, men before women and so on. Fairness does not mean allowing NHS-contracted doctors to use NHS resources to treat patients privately. Fairness is about equality, equity and justice and is much broader than the narrow concept of law. Indeed the law may not be perceived as fair to all. However, justice may motivate us to change the law through democratic means.

Justice is about equal access to healthcare based on individual needs, equal access to privacy, dignity and the highest standard of evidence-based care. The care must be the one considered potentially most beneficial to the individual patient. Incompetent patients must have decisions taken on their behalf in their best interest. This is justice.

Ethical values and beliefs linked to the nurses' code of conduct

Ethical studies and analysis are about critical examination of assumptions, arguments, values, norms and behaviours that people use to guide their lives. As pointed out in an earlier chapter, ethics is the study of moral philosophy, or enquiry into norms, values, right and wrong, good and bad, and what ought not to be done (Gillon, 2003). If we accept these views, we need to have an understanding about nurses' ethical values, beliefs and philosophical thoughts that influence their practice. As we have noted, individual nurses do not always possess the same values and beliefs, as nurses themselves are individuals, with their own individual personality, make-up and life experiences. A mix of values on the side of the nurses and their patients is inevitable and invaluable, as it is likely to foster intercultural understanding. However, Banja (1996) and Dogan and colleagues (2009) have proposed that culturally determined different value systems on the part of patients and health professionals can result in ethical conflicts and may even be a basis for prejudice and discrimination in the understanding of health, illness, caring interventions and therapeutic objectives.

Where one nurse lacks knowledge of the values and belief systems of those cared for, another nurse may possess the requisite knowledge, and therefore be able to share values and knowledge with those who are unaware. So similar and different values and beliefs on the side of the client/patient and the nursing staff can be a good thing, either promoting greater intercultural understanding or stimulating the uninitiated to learn about others' individual cultural and ethical value systems and beliefs. Indeed, in relation to value systems in nursing, the International Council of Nursing Code requires nurses to promote 'an environment in which the human rights, values, customs and spiritual beliefs of the individual, family and community are respected' (International Council of Nurses, 2006, p. 2). Dogan and colleagues (2009, p. 693) suggest that in such an environment the principles of *respect*, *beneficence* and *justice* are 'basic elements'.

Nurses need certain ethical and morally acceptable guiding principles that they can safely use to underpin their nursing practice. Some of these ethical principles are to be found within the NMC Code; therefore it is essential that you study it carefully. Reading the code alone in isolation from ethical theories and principles will not give us enough depth. Therefore we need to study ethical theories and principles on which many healthcare decisions are made. To just accept the principles outlines within code at face value is not good enough as we would be lacking their ethical conceptual underpinning. There must be a sense in which nursing ethics as outlined in the NMC's Code is bound to, and justified by, some profound and fundamental moral and ethical theory. Three of these moral theories – *teleological* or *consequentialist* moral ethics, *deontological* moral ethics and post-modern *care ethics and feminism* – are explained and explored in some detail in the next chapter.

But for now I am asking you to work on the student activities in Boxes 10.1–10.4 to identify: (1) personal values you brought to nursing; (2) ethnic and cultural groups you have

---

BOX 10.1 Student activity 10.1

Self-identification of personal values brought to nursing

Reflect and identify personal values you (personally) brought to nursing. (You may wish to use your portfolio to record your thoughts.)

Example: A sense of wanting to care for my patients, whoever they are, with *kindness*.

BOX 10.2 Student activity 10.2

Identify named ethnic groups from which patients/clients come and list a few personal and cultural values you feel they bring to the therapeutic relationship.

BOX 10.3 Student activity 10.3

Organise a small group of fellow students. Together share your views about those personal values you brought to nursing, their importance to you and to the people you care for. (Use your portfolio to summarise points expressed.)

---

encountered in nursing, together with moral and ethical values you discern they bring into the caring relationships that you need to address and why. Then (3) share your ideas in the first two student activities with a group of your peers and (4) compare your answers with the NMC (2008a) Code.

Now use some of your portfolio pages to work on the case study in Box 10.5, and then compare your answer with the one that follows.

Regarding Mrs Montgomery, I would expect you to have identified the following:

- The fact that the consultant physician took a unilateral and paternalistic decision regarding her resuscitation. She had not been consulted about this important decision, yet nothing in the scenario suggests she is not mentally competent. Her right to self-determination and autonomy have been taken from her.
- Mrs Montgomery's right to information about her condition and to be part of any decision making. She is being treated disrespectfully by nurses, physician and her son.
- Her right to confidentiality has been ignored. Nothing in the scenario suggests she has lost her mental competency to take personal decisions, yet her son has been consulted to help make decisions on her behalf. Furthermore, although he is her son he has no legal right to be informed of her medical condition, let alone assist in decision making regarding whether she lives or dies. It has to be assumed that her mental confusion is transient and stress-related and should not permanently block her ability to self-determine.

    Some legal issues: the Human Rights Act (HRA) 1998 confers the right to respect for privacy and private family life. This is not happening to Mrs Montgomery as her son seems to know more than he should about her condition without her knowledge. The Data Protection Act is being compromised too as confidential data are being shared with her son without her knowledge. She has a right to life under Article 2(1) of the HRA, which states that everyone's right to life shall be protected by law. One may think that this lady's described physical condition and her medical condition remove her right to life, but it may be contested that her stress-related confusion is not permanent, and in all probability would not seriously reduce the quality of her life by enough to deny her the right to active resuscitation. People are living longer these days. Mrs Montgomery may, with care, still live a good quality of life for many years to come, if she receives the right treatment and nursing care. This lady, it could be said, is subject to inhuman, degrading and humiliating treatment that Article 3 of the Human Rights Act makes illegal.

BOX 10.4 Student activity 10.4

Do any of the values you came up with in Student activities 10.1, 10.2 and 10.3 correspond with key nursing and midwifery standards outlined below? (Abridged and paraphrased from NMC 2008a Code.)

Example: Nurses and midwives need to be able to:

- Behave in a way that those they care for will be able to *trust* them with their health and well-being.
- Make those whom we care for our first concern, treating them as individuals and respecting their privacy and dignity.
- Work with and share with others, in order to promote and protect the health and well-being of the patient/client.
- Demonstrate openness, honesty and integrity when caring for people.
- Treat those we care for kindly and considerately.
- Treat those we care for responsibly and objectively on the basis of research evidence.
- Support patients/clients and their families, advocate for them where necessary and help them access relevant health and social care.
- Respect people's confidentiality, yet explain the need to share information with colleagues for the benefit of the patient/client.
- Know when to engage in appropriate disclosure to protect those at risk.
- Value others' contribution to care, whether those others are the patients/clients or other healthcare professionals.
- Act in a way that is non-prejudicial, fair and objective in dealing with people.
- Demonstrate patients' right to self-determination, to refuse or consent to treatment and to contribute to decision making in relation to their care.
- Respect multiculturalism, multi-ethnicity, diversity of language, health and illness beliefs, values, political affiliation, culture and religious beliefs.
- Demonstrate that they have the patient's/client's best interest in mind at all times.
- Recognise the need for clear professional boundaries, including sexual boundaries; not accepting gifts from patient/clients or those close to them if these are likely to ruin the nurse–patient/client relationship and/or lead patients to seek preferential treatment.
- Demonstrate a helping relationship not only to patients and their relatives, but to colleagues, including juniors who need to learn the art and science of nursing; in this, being ready to share knowledge, skills and experience, and work in a collegiate relationship with peers.
- Ask questions and consult where they need to for the benefit of patients.
- Carry out instructions to a very high standard, seek clarification of instructions as required and work only within the limits of one's competence, knowledge, ability and experience.
- Inform authority if others are being put at risk, including blowing the whistle if you think someone is treating patients in a disrespectful and harmful way.
- Demonstrate a willingness to learn, keep up to date and demonstrate the highest standard of care possible.

BOX 10.5 Student activity 10.5

Patient case study

Mrs Montgomery, a 70-year-old diabetic patient, is admitted to the hospital in a state of mental confusion. She looks like a lady who does not care much for herself as, apart from the mental confusion, she appears very dirty and unkempt. It is established that she has one son, who lives many miles away and does not visit her often. In any case they do not get on well and he does not appear to care much about her needs. Apart from her diabetes she also has a heart disease. Further investigations show that her confusion is due not to her diabetes but to severe stress as her husband died very recently. The consultant physician, after consulting with her son, decided that if she arrested she should not be resuscitated. She had not been consulted in the decision. Without her knowledge her son decided to put up her house for sale and in fact sold it within four weeks of her admission to hospital. He had asked the nurses not to tell her and they decided to go along with his request, saying it was not their business to intervene, even though Mrs Montgomery had asked them about her house and how it was being looked after.

Question

What do you consider to be the ethical and legal issues in the above case?

The Freedom of Information Act 2000 gives Mrs Montgomery privacy, which the situation has removed from her. (Read up on the Human Rights Act 1998, the Data Protection Act 1998 and the Freedom of Information Act 2000).

When the NHS was set up it was done on the basis of the person's right to free treatment based on their health needs, not on a factor of age. Ageism is being practised on Mrs Montgomery. Seventy is still a 'young' age by today's demographics.

If her son sells her house without her permission, this is a form of theft. He can be reported to the police by his mother and be prosecuted for theft and deception and for fraudulently depriving the lady of her house. No doubt this is a point Mrs Montgomery social worker and her lawyer will discuss with her.

• Regarding the ethical concept of beneficence, Mrs Montgomery should be seen to benefit from her hospitalisation, not to be harmed by it. Clearly a decision not to resuscitate is one that will inevitably bring her harm. Her son, with whom she does not see eye to eye, has taken this drastic decision to self her house without her knowledge and the nurses have fallen accessory to the decision. It is difficult to see what benefit this decision brings the lady, because, with appropriate care, she may well recover sufficiently to return home to lead a relatively independent and self-fulfilling life. Her house will be gone and in all probability the money raised on the sale; a son who does not visit his mother often, does not get on well with her and decides under these conditions that she should not be resuscitated could easily cheat her out of the money raised from selling the house.

It cannot be seen where positive steps are being taken to help the lady out of her, hopefully, transient confusion state. Stress-induced confusion is treatable, yet we see no measures being directed in the pursuit of this objective, to help return the lady to a lucid thinking state, in which she can once again derive the benefit of autonomous decision making and beneficence.

- As per the Nursing and Midwifery Code, nurses are expected to advocate on behalf of their patients who are in a vulnerable state, yet none of them challenges the physician's unilateral decision not to resuscitate. Neither has any of them advocated for the lady when her son hinted to them he was selling her house without her knowledge. A nurse who is a powerful advocate for her patient should have the knowledge to inform the hospital social worker of the lady's impending predicament, or at least mention to the son the importance of discussing his plan to sell the house with his mother, as she may well recover and be discharged and would probably need her house to return to upon discharge. The nurses are doing nothing that appears to be benefiting this lady.

- Regarding the ethical principle of non-maleficence, by not challenging the physician or the son, the nurses are conspiring, even if on a passive level, to harm the patient. Florence Nightingale once said that the hospital should do the patient no harm. This is not in evidence in the present scenario. The physician's decision is clearly one designed to harm her.

- The ethical principle of justice: justice is about that which is fair, correct and right as per the norms of the society we live in. In the situations regarding 'do not resuscitate', in the way Mrs Montgomery's son decides to dispose of her property, and in the manner in which the nurses failed to advocate on her behalf, in respect to the house and her treatment and 'do not resuscitate' decision, there is no evidence of fair play and justice here.

- The NMC Code advocates that nurses should:
  - Support patients/clients and their families, advocate for them where necessary and help them access relevant health and social care.
  - Respect people's confidentiality, yet explain the need to share information with colleagues for the benefit of the patient/client.
  - Know when to engage in appropriate disclosure to protect those at risk (and Mrs Montgomery is certainly at risk – of death, financial loss and lack of appropriate caring measures).
  - Value others' contribution to care, whether those others are the patients/clients or other healthcare professionals. The social worker could have been called into the situation.
  - Act in a way that is non-prejudicial, fair and objective in dealing with people.
  - Demonstrate patients' right to self-determination, to refuse or consent to treatment and to contribute to decision making in relation to their care.

  None of the above was instituted in respect to Mrs Montgomery.

- Medical ethics, like nursing ethics, requires doctors to take decisions in the best interest of their patients, where patients have lost the mental capacity to decide for themselves. Mrs Montgomery's condition and age do not appear to necessitate a decision of 'do not resuscitate'; moreover if such a decision is to be taken justifiably it needs the input of the team, not just the physician in consultation with Mrs Montgomery's son, whose interest seems to lie elsewhere in any case. The doctor has clearly not taken on board the ethical principles of beneficence, non-maleficence, justice and autonomy.

Summary and conclusion

In this chapter we covered:

- principlism – the ethical principles of autonomy, beneficence, non-maleficence and justice, and how they can be applied to nursing;
- the nurses' code and its relationship to ethical theories, personal values and nursing practice;

- how ethical thinking and beliefs influence attitudes in patient care, patients' health beliefs, illness and recovery;
- the influence of locus of control on patients' personal behaviours;
- the use of ethical knowledge to analyse patient case study/scenarios and develop one's professional ethics portfolio, learning and team working.

The conclusion can be drawn that essentially nurses and other health clinicians use four key ethical principles – *autonomy*, *beneficence*, *non-maleficence* and *justice* – to shape their thinking, ethical decision making and actual care provided to their patients. Ethical principles can be used to analyse issues, dilemmas and problems within healthcare, and thus can be applied to professional nursing care and portfolio building.

11 Ethical theories part II

Deontology, teleology and caring ethics

Objectives of this chapter

After reading this chapter you should be able to:

- explain *teleological*, *deontological* and *feminine care* ethics, distinguishing differences, similarities, strengths and weaknesses;
- explain how these ethical theories may assist health professionals;
- discuss relationships between morality and professional ethics, putting a case together to establish relationships between ethics, law and the nurses' Code;
- demonstrate understanding of *virtue ethics*, and the roles virtues play in ethical reasoning and decision making in healthcare;
- explain the *natural law* theory of ethics, the *doctrine of double effect* and the *principle of totality* in ethical decision making;
- apply Immanuel Kant's formulation, 'treat people not as means but as ends in themselves', to nursing care.

Introduction

In the preceding chapter we looked at the ethics of principlism, discussing *autonomy*, *beneficence*, *non-maleficence* and *justice* in some detail, applying them to healthcare. We also touched upon the wider ethical theories of *teleological* and *deontological* ethical principles. The present chapter focuses more deeply on the wider conceptual ethical theories of *normative* ethics, concentrating on the main subdivisions of *teleological*, *deontological* and *feminine moral theories* and the *caring* ethic. The chapter asks if these theories can help ethical decision making in nursing and the wider healthcare.

Teleological or consequence-based ethical theories

What are *teleological ethical theories*? This group of theories postulates that *what we achieve* by our action (the *consequence*) determines the moral status of that action. If the *end outcome* or *consequence* of our thinking and *action* is judged to be good, then the *causative action* is judged to be *morally right*. Teleologists attach importance to end results; hence we call this group of theories *consequentialist theories*, *end-based theories* or *consequentialism*; all three terms are interchangeable.

Types of teleology

There are three types of teleology.

1. *Ethical egoism*: this type of teleology says that an action is morally correct if its *outcomes* are more favourable than unfavourable only to the moral agent performing the action. Egoism is about self-interest and self-love. Thus an egoist nurse would be more motivated by personal benefits. For her, it is not about what the patient or a fellow nurse stands to derive from the action, but what she stands to gain from it. The philosopher whose name is most commonly associated with this theory is Thomas Hobbes, who argued that the greatest motivator of human beings is *self-preservation*. For the *ethical egoist*, an act is morally right if it serves his/her purposes – self-interest. The ethical egoist chooses action(s) with the best foreseeable consequences for him-/herself. The nurse as an ethical egoist would be keen to see the nurses' duty shift times change, not for patients' and other nurses' benefit, but just for him-/herself.

2. *Ethical altruism* says an action is morally correct if its consequences are more favourable than unfavourable to everyone *except* the moral agent. The altruistic nurse is more driven by the fact that his/her action will benefit others. (S)he is *people centred*, *problem centred*, unimpressed by self-interest and driven by an urge to serve and help others. Thus (s)he would be willing to cooperate with measures aimed at changing the duty rota to benefit patients and other colleagues, not necessarily herself.

3. *Ethical utilitarianism*: this theory says the action is morally right if its consequences are more favourable than unfavourable to *everyone*. Thus in the case of *Child B v Cambridge Health Authority* where the HA decided not to give a further (pointless) bone marrow transplant to a minor, who on scientific evidence would inevitably die (operation or no operation), those HA officers who made the decision not to give a further transplant, but instead to spend the money meaningfully on patients who stood a change of recovering or benefitting from the treatment, could be said to be engaged in ethical utilitarianism. Why? They foresaw the problems and benefits as follows. (a) The child's misery and painful life would persist as she would not benefit in the long run from yet another bone marrow transplant. (b) The money could be used to treat others capable of benefitting from it. Spending it on this group, the HA thought it would not have wasted its budget. There are of course other (opposing) considerations, such as the morality of allowing a youngster to die owing to financial constraint. However, the *ethical utilitarian* is concerned not about the quality of the decision making in itself, but with the consequential benefit by other patients. They may also have thought of the benefit to the youngster; that is, not to extend her suffering by giving her an additional futile bone marrow transplant.

The origins of classical utilitarianism (consequentialism) can be found in the writings of Jeremy Bentham (1748–1832) and John Stuart Mill (1806–1873), although other philosophers espoused the virtues of utilitarianism, among them David Hume (1711–1776), G. E. Moore (1873–1958) and R. M. Hare (1919–2002). The theory is 'utilitarian' because it views actions as worthy if they produce a worthwhile 'utility', a useable and valuable end, a consequential advantage, referred to as 'value over disvalue'. In this sense even death may be seen as worthwhile in removing someone's intractable and untreatable pain. Death is therefore seen as a relief from the intolerable painful situation. Hence utilitarianism advocates the 'greatest good for the greatest number'.

Beauchamp and Childress (2001, p. 341) argue that utility seeks to 'produce the maximal balance of positive value over disvalue (or the least possible disvalue, if only undesirable results can be achieved)'. Let us look further at this theory in the light of a theoretical scenario. Suppose you are a nurse in a ward with 30 very mentally disturbed patients, all of whom are capable of erupting into uncontrollable violence (disvalue). On this particular day, one of the most provocative patients seems determined to stimulate violence in the remaining 29 patients. You know from previous experience that this is a potentially real and explosive, destructive situation. You use all sensible means to calm down the disruptive patient but he does not respond. The utilitarian ethicist would advocate that something be done to stop this patient from causing further violence. To the utilitarian ethicist the means is not critical, just the end: prevent the violent consequence and secure a peaceful ward. For the utilitarian any action chosen is morally correct if it brings about the desirable calm, the value over disvalue. In this scenario the utilitarian is attempting to minimise evil consequence at any cost.

Use of utilitarianism in resource allocation

In resource allocation within healthcare, the principle of utilitarianism is sometimes employed. When resources are scarce, we may seek to ensure money is spent to benefit the majority rather than a few. For example, an expensive anti-cancer drug for one patient may be rejected for one that is cheaper in order to resource treatment for many patients. The case of 'Child B' v Cambridge Health Authority is mentioned above. The material evidence of that case was that the child had had previous bone marrow transplantation for leukaemia; it had failed. Future transplants were clinically, scientifically and statistically predicted to fail. Given this scenario, the HA refused to spend more money on future expensive futile bone marrow transplant. When the HA was brought before the High Court by the child's father for a judicial review, the child lost the case. Why? It could be said that the court operated, inter alia, a *utilitarian* judgement which supported the HA's attempt to use limited resources to maximise the value or care outcomes for the majority of the patients in its area of responsibility. With the limited budget, a larger number of patients could be treated less expensively than a single bone marrow transplant that would fail anyway. The line of ethical reasoning accords with the ethical doctrine of the *greatest good for the greatest number*.

Classical utilitarianism in healthcare

Classical utilitarian principles believe that people are driven by two primary forces/needs: the desires to avoid pain and to seek pleasure ('pleasure principle' or *hedonism*). Jeremy Bentham and John Stuart Mill were *hedonistic* utilitarians, because they conceived utility as *happiness* and *pleasure*. For them, health professionals should always aim to produce the greatest good, the *greatest happiness* and *pleasure* for everyone. It is about happiness at the expense of pain.

Returning to the allocation of scarce resources mentioned above, modern health economists might argue that with scarce resources we should try to maximise healthcare outcomes (benefits) whilst reducing costs to tax payers. Utilitarian philosophy might favour clinicians trying to maximise pleasure over pain. We need to balance cost with benefits. These two views are somewhat extreme and so perhaps other approaches are sometimes required, because sometimes it may be necessary to spend a lot of money to save the life of one individual, particularly where doing so might not necessarily deprive a greater number of their cheaper care option. The reality, though, is that in healthcare management of resources money is never unlimited. We have to manage with what we have, even though we owe it to our patients to keep advocating on their behalf for greater services of better quality.

Limitation of utilitarian principles in nursing

There are problems with utility seeking the greatest pleasure for the majority. First, nursing philosophy is based, inter alia, on equality, attending to the needs of all the patients, not just some. It is good if the majority of the patients are happy and progressing in their recovery, but what about the few who are not? Although, with respect to the violence-seeking client referred to in the scenario above, the *ethical utilitarian* might argue that even he benefited from the state of calm that subsequently prevailed after he had been given a tranquilising, even if painful, injection to calm him down. Second, people do not always seek pleasure and avoid pain. Consider pain-seeking masochists. Furthermore, as Beauchamp and Childress (2001, p. 341) have pointed out 'many human actions do not appear to be performed for happiness'. Highly motivated scientists often work themselves to exhaustion in search of new knowledge or new healthcare treatments; they do not appear to be seeking pleasure and personal happiness. In wars, for example, nurses and doctors who work tirelessly to the point of nervous exhaustion, well beyond the call of duty, to secure further benefits for patients may not be seeking pleasure and personal happiness.

Recent utilitarian philosophers have argued that there are values other than happiness that give intrinsic benefits, for example knowledge, friendship, good health, beauty, personal freedom, autonomy, achievement, deep personal relationships, understanding and enjoyment (Beauchamp and Childress, 2001; Griffin, 1986, p. 67). A third problem is that utilitarians are not agreed on what values should be maximised. For some it is happiness and pleasure; for others it is other *agent-neutral* or *intrinsic goods*; *freedom* and *health* are two of these 'agent-neutral' benefits. John Stuart Mill has added other values, such as *duty, love* and *respect*, to Bentham's *utility, pleasure seeking* and *pain avoidance*.

On the positive side, utilitarianism could encourage nurses to consider the patient's emotion: his/her feeling, such as pain and sorrow. The theory implies that, just as a coin has two faces, a patient's emotion can be sad or happy, or up and down. Under utilitarian philosophy, nurses would be expected to seek and promote *positive value*. Pain and suffering are negatives – the *disvalue* on the reverse of the coin. In essence, this theory suggests a rationale that we can use in healthcare to inform our ethical decision making. Traditional nursing has been criticised for not having a strong theoretical scientific or philosophical base that supports nursing actions and ethical decision-making. Perhaps, then, utilitarianism offers a theoretical rationale for ethical decision making in nursing.

A problem for the utilitarian nurse

A problem a utilitarian nurse might have is that, faced with many alternative actions, a utilitarian philosophy does not tell him/her which action to select. An incomplete theory! Other rationales need to be exercised to guide with respect to which alternative action to pursue. Perhaps, then, in ethical decision making in healthcare we could use, for example, empirical data and experimentally determined evidence to firm up our decision making. Rely on the best available research evidence – a recurrent theme in modern nursing. Even so, the 'best available evidence' could be questionable. Do we mean, for example, scientific and empirical evidence in terms of rate of progress of wound healing? Or do we mean best evidence based on human beings' emotional strength to cope with identified or unidentified personal emotional problems? Or do we mean best evidence based on the (questionable and illegal) belief that, if we allow the patient in severe pain who is grunting heavily in the ward and keeping others awake to die by giving them a large dose of morphine, we are appealing to our idea of a quiet ward as the best reason? The utilitarian might argue that it all depends on the nature of the outcome we are looking for. Hope and colleagues (2003, p. 4) have argued that consequentialism is incomplete as a moral theory because it does not tell us what aspects of the consequences are morally important. Furthermore, if, as Mill says, utilitarianism is valuing pleasure over pain and 'happiness is intended pleasure, and the absence of pain' (Ryan, 1987, p. 278), then there is a problem here for health professionals, in the sense that we cannot always make pain go away and, in any case, pain can be helpful in spotting a major pathology which can be treated. Pain for a patient may be intense psychological agony, despair, gloom, depression, heartache and sorrow that drugs may not simply remove.

Strengths and usefulness of utilitarianism

The strengths of utilitarianism, as a basis for moral philosophical and ethical decision making, lie in the fact that the theory tells us that the consequences of our actions *matter*. We must therefore ensure that, where possible, consequences are good: *value*, not *disvalue*. Consequences should benefit patients. The theory also says that moral actions must follow certain rules, for example the pursuit of pleasure, happiness and freedom from pain. Ethical decision making, therefore, must not be done without rationale and purpose. We need bases and justification for ethical decision making in healthcare. The theory gives some certainty to decision making in stating that *outcomes* and *consequences* are *critical*. It reduces the possibility of conflict, since clear directions as the need for outcomes, based on the nature of action, brings some certainty, thus removing the possibility of confusion and conflict. However, every one may not agree on the consequences aimed for.

In evaluating happiness and unhappiness everyone counts equally. A rich patient's happiness is worth no more than a poor patient's happiness. Thus, as health professionals, we may be encouraged by this theory to treat every patient equally, for example in terms of care principles such as enabling access, valuing consent and confidentiality, respecting patients autonomy, reducing/preventing pain and respecting personal choices in order to promote happiness and pleasure. We also come to realise from this theory that health, happiness and pleasure are essential features of everyone's existence. We *all* have the human needs for freedom from pain, and for love and affection. (The sadomasochist stands outside this formula; so is this everyone? A theory limitation. What about the masochist who seeks pain?)

Weaknesses of the utilitarian philosophy are as follows:

*   Difficulty measuring key components of utilitarianism such as happiness, pleasure, unhappiness.
*   Some actions are wrong even if their consequences are good; for example, it would be difficult to justify killing a patient simply because he has an unknown disease that threatens the entire population. It would be out of the question to kill a mentally incapacitated seriously mentally and physically handicapped person to give each of his useable organs to a number of altruistic scientists who would seem certain to function more effectively in their quest to advance the benefits of the world.
*   It is somehow difficult to justify the value of the majority over the minority because all humans have equal value and should be treated equally.

For some further powerful arguments on the strengths and weakness of utilitarianism, see Smart and Williams (1998).

Deontologically based ethical theories

According to the *Stanford Encyclopaedia of Philosophy* online (http://plato.stanford.edu/entries/ethics-deontological/#PatCenDeo) the word *deontology* comes from the Greek words for duty, *deon*, and science (or study), *logos*. In moral philosophy deontology is about normative ethical choices of what is morally required, forbidden or permitted. Deontology assesses choices about what we ought to do, which action is morally correct, which is wrong. Unlike consequentialism, which focuses on end results to justify the morality of the decision, deontology examines the nature of the decision itself, and thus stands in opposition to consequentialism. In other words deontology says: what we do in our action, the nature of the action itself, determines its moral status. Deontologists have a duty to do that which they consider to be right regardless of the consequences.

If an action is judged the right one to take in the circumstances, even if the consequences turn out to be not so good, ethically the action taken is deemed the right and ethically correct one. Deontologists favour processes over utility outcomes. So for the deontologist, the action to give Child B yet another bone marrow operation is seen as the best course of action because of valuing people over money, the morality of caring for all the patients, not just those more likely to live, and the morality of giving a final bone marrow transplant to please the child and the parents even if in the end the child succumbs and dies.

Divine command deontology and natural law theory

The *divine command* element of deontology says we should take action, live our lives and make moral decisions based on rules and duties from a deity (God). Following on from this, Christians are expected to follow the Ten Commandments, for example do not steal, commit adultery or bear false witness against your neighbour. 'Thou shalt not kill.' The three Abrahamic religions, Christianity, Islam and Judaism, follow some kind of divine command even if there is some slight variation on the theme. Some patients have great beliefs in divine command; hence they pray to get well. Some Muslims pray five times a day. Some patients use their religious values to give them strength to recover from illnesses. It is crucial therefore to respect patients' health beliefs based on their divine beliefs and philosophy. I recall reading about a UK nurse who was sacked from her job as a nurse because she prayed with a patient. If that patient had asked her to pray with him/her then one cannot see much harm in that. However, if the nurse was forcing her own strongly held religious beliefs on the patient, undervaluing the patient's own belief (or lack of belief) in a divine being, then one could see justification in perhaps reprimanding the nurse. Whether sacking her would be necessary is a matter for debate. However, the message to you as nurses is that you should not force your own moral values on patients. Self-awareness is necessary to prevent you from doing this. Cultural competence and sensitivity about others' personal and cultural values are essential prerequisites to effective holistic and culture-sensitive nursing.

Divine command and natural law theory

In a way the *divine command* theory is tied into *natural law* ethical theory. Natural law is not about man-made laws, case law and statute. It is related to the view that everything and everyone comes from nature, which in itself is believed to come from God, a divine being. The theory takes the view that, as humans in God's image, we are capable of rational thinking and behaviour. We are moulded and modified on the Godly image and the behaviour of the great prophets such as Jesus and Muhammad. In this sense God is viewed as a natural law giver, who created man in his own image. That man/woman is empowered to think rationally and to discover natural laws is essentially a feature of natural law theory. Thus it is considered that to act rationally is to act morally, based on rules laid down by God, the clergy and the church. Thomas Aquinas established links between God and the natural law. He pointed out that a rational God made the world and enables it to function rationally. Thus man is able to think rationally and discover his rational, natural laws. Thus many patients come into hospital with a very strong belief in God. It probably helps them through their illnesses because they passionately and fundamentally believe in divine preaching. Hence a hospital may be justified in seeing the need to pay for a chaplaincy service that can provide spiritual support for patients of different faiths. What would be prejudicial would be to allow the Rabbi into the ward to see a Jewish patient whilst keeping out the Catholic priest or the religious representation of the Jehovah's witnesses, the Islamic faith or any other denominational faiths.

In the fourth century ce St Augustine taught that human nature had become corrupt with sinful behaviours, full of lust and greed. Thus, for St Augustine, to be moral was to go against one's natural inclination towards earthly contamination. Moral behaviour was not about self-indulgence but about following rules laid down by God. An example of natural law concerns heterosexuality, man and woman sharing intimate relationships. Natural law theory takes the view that God made man and woman to copulate and bear children, not to form homosexual relationships. Aquinas believed that same-sex copulation is against natural law. Therefore for him homosexuality is immoral and sinful. For Aquinas heterosexuality is the only natural rational sexual relationship. For nurses, what are the implications of such a view for the sort of patients you are going to have to care for, especially in genitourinary units? You are not there to condemn people's sexuality and sexual preferences. Use a section of your portfolio to write down your views on the professional implications of following rigidly Aquinas' view. Can you see some obvious problems? What are they? Reflect on them.

A reality of natural law theory, however, is a tendency for moral values, thinking and behaviour to shift or move on. Moral values do change over time. For example, today many more people than hitherto consider homosexuality to be moral, rational and natural. So, moral views about natural law theory have shifted over time. The Catholic church does not regard abortion as moral; neither does it regard conception in test tubes as natural and moral, since it considers the married couple's sexual copulation as the natural process towards conception. Yet recently Pope Benedict XVI announced that the use of condoms is acceptable in exceptional circumstances (BBC News, 20 November 2010). For more reading on the divine command theory of ethics see http://www.philosophyofreligion.info/christian-ethics/divine-command-theory/. Also for a good foundation in and defence of the theory of divine command read Wierenga (1983). You may also want to access Murphy (2008) for a further clear exposition of the natural law theory of ethics.

Doctrine of double effect and principle of totality

Natural law theory from mediaeval Catholic theology has given the *doctrine of double effect* to healthcare. The doctrine holds that if an action has two effects, one good, the other bad, the action is still morally permissible (a) if the action was good in itself, (b) if the good flows from the action as the evil or bad effect does, (c) if only the good effect was intended, and (d) if there was an important reason for carrying out the action as for allowing the bad effect.

Applying this principle to an example, let us consider a case where a woman is pregnant. She also has a cancer of the uterus which could cost her life if she does not have the uterus removed surgically. The surgery will of course cause her fetus's death even though removing the fetus is an unintended consequence of the surgery, but a side effect of it. The moral question is: can it be morally right to perform surgery that will inevitably kill the fetus? If we return to the theory of utilitarianism above, we will find utilitarians arguing for an evaluation of the best/better outcome. Saving the mother's life is seen as value over the disvalue: her death. She can have a child by adoption. But her life is seen as valued over perhaps the idea of both mother and fetus dying from no surgery at all.

Utilitarians might argue that they want this operation to go ahead because they foresee the possibility that, by allowing the pregnancy to continue, the mother might die from the disease even before the child is born. Thus her death from the cancer might also take the fetus's life, thus leading to two bad consequences instead of one. This would be morally indefensible. But then if we turn to the *deontologists* we will see them saying: in order to determine if an action is morally right the action itself should be evaluated independently of the consequence.

Moreover, *deontologists* hold that some actions are bad or immoral in themselves. Killing is one such action. Deontologists believe that killing is wrong, whatever the planned purpose of the killing. The view is that it cannot be good or moral to use a bad action (killing a fetus) to bring about a good effect (saving the mother). Or can it? In effect, in the above scenario it is not the killing of the fetus (bad) that is the first consideration. We are not intentionally killing the fetus, even to save the mother on this occasion. We are removing the cancerous uterus that, left alone, will kill the mother, but in doing so we face the inevitable unpleasant consequence of taking the life of the fetus as well. A fundamental question is: can a moral theory that considers killing a fetus wrong also justify surgical removal of the fetus in the scenario given? The *doctrine of double effect* is supposed to have the answer to this question. The key point from all this is that the *doctrine* allows for abortions, if the direct intention is to save the life of the mother. The good action, to remove a cancerous uterus, makes this a good or moral action in itself (deontology), and consciously saving the mother's life (the intended objective) also good (teleology). Deontology is a process and teleology a result or consequence of that process/action.

We might want to bring in some legal arguments to show why the inevitable death of the fetus in the scenario given is not a murder, for example that (a) the law permits terminations in some circumstances or (b) a fetus has no legal existence unless it is born alive. The final point l want to make about the doctrine of double effect is this: the doctrine does not support an intended good action if the unintended foreseeable result is worse than the good achieved. Critically, the doctrine holds that there is a distinction between a foreseeable undesirable result and intending that result.

The principle of totality and the need not to judge or condemn your patient

This principle is also derived from *natural law ethical theory* and holds that our body is not something that we own, but something we hold in trust for God. Second, changes are permitted to the body only if those changes seek to ensure its proper functioning. The Bible says the body is the 'temple of God' (1 Corinthians 6: 19). This principle holds that we are given our body by God for a purpose and should not change it for frivolous reasons, for example have plastic surgery to make ourselves 'look beautiful'. The principle of totality would perhaps hold that breast enlargement, sex change, clitoral rings, penis rings, lip spouting, jaw modification for cosmetic purposes and liposuction for better body alignment are frivolous. Yet other deontological moralists might say: if they are done to make the person feel good and less depressed and uncomfortable with self image, fine. As nurses we should not be quick – or slow for that matter – to condemn people on their personal reasons for having cosmetic surgery. What for the external observer is frivolity may be serious therapeutic intervention for the patient. The principle rules out sterilisation as contraception because natural pregnancy opportunity is lost. It rules out vasectomy too for the same reason. It militates against other forms of cosmetic surgery for personal appearance and the social attention it may bring us. The principle also rules out cosmetic breast implants, breast reduction, breast augmentation and so on. These are seen under natural law as vanity. But how will the ethical principle of *totality* work for those who do not believe in God? In fact there are patients, doctors, nurses and other health professionals who, because of their disbelief in God, would not be touched by the ethical morality of body totality. Consider this further in Box 11.1.

BOX 11.1 Student activity 11.1

Use this box to put some arguments forward in favour and against the ethics of *divine command* and *body totality* as far as healthcare decision making is concerned.

Libertarian deontology

Libertarianism as a philosophy holds that people should be free to do as they please provided their actions do not impinge upon the rights of others. *Libertarianism* is further discussed under *contractarianism* to show that there is an extreme view of contractarianism as espoused by philosophers such as the Harvard professor Robert Nozick. We will also look at the Rawlsian justice under the notion of contractarianism as this offers a tension with Professor Nozick's brand of contractarianism. It should be apparent that there is some interlinking between the various philosophical views of morality and ethical thinking.

Contractarianism and social contract theory of morality

Contractarianism says that an action is morally correct if it accords with the rules that rational moral agents would agree to uphold once they had entered into a social 'contractual' relationship for mutual benefit. Hence this theory belongs to the group of theories called *social contract theories* or *contractarianism*. Contractarianism exists independently of belief in God (divine command). Hence contractarianism is a secular theory of morality. It assumes that people are motivated by self-interest and each person in society might want to take all for him-/herself. The theory argues that moral rules evolved to enable humans to get along with one another, in other words peacefully coexist. It is rational and moral for humans to agree to the rules of peaceful coexistence, otherwise there would be a settling of scores with the sword and all would be worse off. So contractarianism is about the politics of peaceful coexistence based on *social contracts* between people.

The English philosopher Thomas Hobbes (1588–1679) held that one of the most detestable conditions of nature was a pre-moral existence, in which people were driven by self-interest. For self-interested individuals life was solitary, poor, nasty, brutish and short. Using reason, therefore, people came to accept that they would be better off if they changed their free-for-all sword-carrying society into one governed by moral rules backed by the force of law. Social contract theory links politics to ethics and asserts that *hypothetical political bargaining* goes on. By 'hypothetical', contractarians mean they do not believe people ever really came together to form the basic social contract. How do these views fit into our present society?

Pence (2004) argues that contractarianism presents *two opposing views*, one which supports 'minimal' government (low government/little official intervention) – the *libertarian view of justice* – and the other which supports 'maximal' government, characterised by more official/government interventions. The *Rawlsian philosophy of justice* supports the latter form of government.

Libertarianism is championed by modern philosophers such as Robert Nozick, who sees forced taxation by government as equivalent to forced labour or slavery. Whereas libertarians might favour minimal government intervention such as only a national army for defence, they are not in favour of big governments, a taxation-financed NHS, disability and unemployment benefits, and, in America, government health programmes such as Medicare, Medicaid, food stamps, hospital insurance trust fund and welfare. Libertarians view these big government interventions as socialism, robbing the rich to pay the poor. With a libertarian philosophical view, there would be fewer hospitals built, and a reduced health service for the poor, the elderly and other vulnerable groups. Libertarians favour the present status quo of the rich owning most property rights, and private health insurance whereby the healthy do not subsidise the unhealthy (Pence, 2004). This libertarian view of contractarianism does not fit comfortably alongside socialism that advocates wealth redistribution. Professor Nozick's view on libertarianism might well balance out with the opposing Rawlsian justice discussed below.

Rawlsian justice

Rawlsians, named after Professor John Rawls (Harvard University) believe that the *social contract* under which people live (*contractarianism*) needs *moral restraints*. Rawls rejected the free-for-all libertarian justice whereby everyone owns whatever goods they can secure for themselves. He also rejected the utilitarianism of maximising total benefit. Instead Rawls developed a theory of social and economic *distributive justice*, relating to how money and goods would be distributed in society. Rawls considered that the most important moral restraint on the social contract is what he called the 'veil of ignorance' (Rawls, 1972, p. 975). This is a thought experiment in which one imagines the type of society one would choose behind this 'veil of ignorance'. It would involve one sitting in some heavenly or ethereal place looking down on a variety of societies. Each society distributes wealth differently. Some societies are rich, some poor; some distributes wealth equally, others unequally. The thought experiment requires the observer to choose to join one of these societies without knowing who you will be within that society. In this hypothetical social contract, no one

---

BOX 11.2 Student activity 11.2

Reflection

Please see if you can identify any patients' rights from the NMC Code; if you can, compare/contrast them with patients' legal rights from the Human Rights Act 1998.

Look at your code of conduct and see if it identifies any rights the patient has and any duty which nurses must carry out.

Then look at the Human Rights Act and see what rights your patients come with to the nurse–patient/client therapeutic relationship.

---

would know any personal information related to self: level of intelligence, age, gender, race, number of children, health, income, wealth or any other arbitrary personal information. The critical question is: which society would you choose to join?

Rawls argues that the only *rational* way to choose under the 'veil of ignorance' is as though you are the *least well-off person in society*. Choosers should opt for institutions that seek to create equality, *unless* some *difference* favours the least well-off institution. Rawls's idea that justice is best secured by the worst-off groups being maximally well-off is known as the *difference principle*. Rawls expressed this principle thus:

> The intuitive idea is that the social order is not to establish and secure the more attractive prospects of those better off unless doing so is to the advantage of those less fortunate.
> (Rawls, 1972, p. 975)

Pence (2004) argues that, under Rawlsian justice, every citizen would have equal access to healthcare unless unequal access favoured the poor. (This would be unlikely!) With respect to reasonably upright professions, such as nursing, law, medicine and physiotherapy, Rawlsian justice would argue that everyone should be trained in one or either of these respectable professions unless training just a few people would favour the less well-off. Rawlsian justice seeks to reduce society's natural inequalities of fate, such as genetic diseases. Therefore it advocates that such health inequalities need good medical care if morality and justice must be seen to be operational. The theory is a form of contractarianism because it assumes that self-interested people use social contracts to define their society. Under the *difference principle* people would permit inequality only if it were advantageous to all.

Monistic deontology

This advocates that an action is morally acceptable if it agrees with some single deontological principle which guides all other subsidiary principles. This theory is linked up with the discussion on Kantian philosophy below.

Rights theories

These say an action is morally right if it respects the rights which all humans have: for example the right to life, freedom of expression, liberty; right to protect our property; right to fight against oppression, unequal treatment, prejudice, discrimination and arbitrary invasion of privacy; right to express our own moral viewpoint. The rights of all parties in a contractual or professional relationship come under this theory's emphasis on rights of individuals (libertarianism).

Rights theory is a moral political philosophy that advocates freedom of thought and action so long as others are not hurt. From this position you may want to consider the rights that your patients have, even those we detain under the Mental Health Act.

Applied to the wider society, however, libertarianism favours a society in which individuals are free to live their lives as they choose provided they do not offend others. In such a society homosexuality would be accepted as there would be a prevailing view that people are free to practise whatever version of sexuality they favour. It follows from this that health libertarian professionals would resist paternalism in favour of the right to personal choices and self-determination.

There are many important libertarian principles and rights in nursing care: patients' right to self-determination, autonomy, consent, confidentiality, privacy, dignity, information for decision making related to care and right to life. Beauchamp and Childress (2001, p. 357) argue that rights are justified claims that individuals and groups can make upon others. Personal choices; the right to decide who touches one's body; the right to agree to or refuse to agree to certain treatments, even if not consenting means certain death.

Duty theories

This deontological moral theory says: *an action is morally right if it accords with some list of duties and obligations*. Duty-based theories take the view that factors other than consequences are important to ethics. For example, it could be argued that we have *a duty not to lie* to each other. Duty theories suggest that it is wrong to lie even if the consequences of telling a lie would be better than telling the truth. Applying this to nursing, one implication is that, even though lying to a patient who has been diagnosed with cancer, by telling him he has not got the disease, might make him feel better, it would be still wrong and unethical to do so.

Telling patients a lie is wrong. Why? Lies conflict with the ethics of *veracity* (truth telling), *justice* and *non-maleficence*. Health professionals are expected to tell the truth. If truth telling is abandoned there is no basis for a trusting therapeutic relationship. If a patient cannot rely on therapists to tell the truth, then that patient would never be sure about the status of his/her diagnosis, recovery rate and prognosis. (S)he would not know whether, for example, to make a will in the belief that death was imminent. The integrity of informed consent is built upon the premise that health professionals tell truths to patients. A patient's consent not based on truth is a fraud, for which the health professional must carry the moral, professional, employment and legal responsibility and consequences. However, unpleasant and distressing truths must be told *sensitively*. This is still different from telling lies. Bluntness can hurt at times.

Some patients in any case might prefer not to know about the very worst inevitable consequence of their illness. However, they have a right to know, but a deadly prognosis can be told with sensitivity. It is not ethical or good psychology to deliver bad news insensitively. Worst of all is to deliver it with an intentional and malicious 'knock out' blow! Not even the most cantankerous patient deserves that! Never hit a man when he is down! In nursing this is cruelty, not in the spirit of non-maleficence. Assess when to give bad news. Often the patients ask for bad news about prognosis when they are ready. Some do not ask for fear of what they may be told. Newham and Hawley (2007) give a good example of insensitive communication, by saying that, having just explained the patient's malignancy diagnosis to him/her, one does not then have to crush the patient by adding a really crushing element, for example that the last ten patients nursed with that diagnosis all died a horrible painful death. Nurses are expected to be sensitive, caring, compassionate professionals.

It must have become clear that *divine command* is also linked to *duties*; divine duties tend to be coached in prohibitive language such as the Ten Commandments, 'thou shall not . . .' Davis (1991) and Hope and colleagues (2003) have pointed out that some of these 'morally relevant' duties include promise keeping, truth telling, not lying and not betraying various rights. One key feature about duty-based theories is that they are built either on the notion of *rationality* or alternatively on *divine command*. As some health professionals do not believe in God, divine command's influence on healthcare ethical decision making is questionable. It might be difficult to reassure a patient on the 'God line' in the absence of certainty. Yet, strangely, I recall a female patient asking me, 'Please would you pray with me?' I found the request rare, but with my Christian background, my faith and belief in God, I was able to pray with her. What was also interesting was the end result of the prayer when the patient remarked, 'I feel so much better, thank you.' She clearly had strong faith in God and must have been examining her faith within the context of divine healing. If divine healing can help, then nursing should do nothing to prevent that. It requires nurses to be accepting of patients and their faith and beliefs in divine healing, as an alternative form of therapy.

I recall a group of nursing undergraduates who went on an overseas elective placement to Jamaica, returning to the university to report that, in the particular hospital they had spent their time, prayer was a common start to the nursing day, and was also used as patient therapy. The local nurses told them how important the daily prayers were to them and their patients.

Kantian deontology

The debate about deontological ethics would be incomplete without reference to the work of the great Prussian philosopher Immanuel Kant (1724–1804). He was a Christian, yet he thought that a sound theory of morality had to be justifiable on grounds other than man's subjection to divine commands from God. He believed that a sound theory of morality should be independent of man's 'inclinations, purposes, or happiness' (Gillon, 2003, p. 16). Kant's moral theory has grounding in *rationality* – the rational nature of human beings to think objectively and logically. Kant (1998) believed that all rational humans would recognise themselves as belonging to the *supreme moral law*: the belief that rational agents (people, unlike animals and inanimate objects) possess an *absolute moral value* that renders them as belonging to what he called the kingdom of *ends in themselves*. Not only do rational beings recognise themselves as belonging to the kingdom of ends in themselves but they also recognise that all other rational agents are similarly ends in themselves.

The above Kantian formulation suggests that we should not take people for granted. We must not 'use' people (patients) but respect them as possessing autonomy, a right to respect

---

BOX 11.3 Student activity 11.3

Recognising Kant's morality in care

Reflective question: Do you recognise any of Kant's moral principles in your own profession? If you do, what are they? What further principles or rules do you think are derived (could be derived) from such a principle? In your reflection please relate to your patient.

and self determination. We could also stretch the point to the patients we treat and the research we invite them to participate in. Patients should not be used as guinea pigs. They must be valued as rational human beings with the right to refuse to participate in research. If we value patients as *ends in themselves*, there is a good chance we will acknowledge their contribution to their care. We will provide them all necessary information for their informed choice to participate/refuse to participate.

Kant also formulated the maxim that a *moral principle* has to be a principle *for all* people. All other principles would be derived from this key principle, which he labelled the *categorical imperative*.

Kant distinguished two kinds of imperatives: *hypothetical imperative* and *categorical imperative*. The *categorical imperative* is the one that issues a command that is not conditional on further objectives. On the other hand, the *hypothetical imperative* is conditional on other purposes; for example, it says 'do this if you want to achieve that'. Kant believed that the *categorical imperative* that says 'do this' without being conditional on any further purpose is the one that would be agreed by all rational persons as providing the foundation for a morality based on *pure reason*. Kant formulated his *categorical imperative* in a number of ways:

1. As a moral agent you should act only on the maxim through which you can at the same time will that it should become a universal law. (A maxim being a principle that directs people's behaviour.)
2. As a moral agent you should act as to treat humanity, whether in your own person or in that of any other, never solely as a means but always as an end.
3. The agent should also act like a king who is creating a universal law for his subjects as ends in themselves.

Going back to the first formulation, has it got any implications for the way nurses and doctors do their job? By implication this formulation is: follow care principles that are so perfect, so objective, so research-based and empirically supported, so removed from misleading emotions, so soundly and rationally conceptualised, that other nurses/health professionals can follow such principles without having to offer justification. For me, the first of these imperatives is the need to treat people with respect: the right not to be lied to, not to be harmed. These care principles are so sound that they need no qualification, clarification or explanation. If we turn to law we note that both the *Bolam test* (give care as per the acceptable body of healthcare opinions in operation at the time) and the principles that arose from the case of *Bolitho* (base acceptable principles of care logically on the best available research evidence, having considered all the risks) are pretty close to Kant's idea of objective *universal law* and *pure reason*. The research evidence supporting care must be able to stand on its own without doubt.

'Do to others as you would have them do to you' is also a powerful moral theme that runs through many different moral theories. Gillon (2003) points out that this theme is embedded in both Islam and Christianity. So whether we are treating a patient of the Islamic or Christian faith we are implored to ask ourselves: if we were in this patient's position, how would we like to be treated? The sorts of rational answers that I think would come back are points such as treat with kindness, respect, honesty, truthfulness and sensitivity. Hardly debatable!

The second Kantian formulation, *treat people not as means but as ends in themselves,* asserts that we should work to the libertarian philosophy that says we should not compromise people's right to freedom, free choice and autonomy for any reason. Gillon (2003) claims that the Kantian principle that people have intrinsic moral value or worth that prevents them from being used as means to ends is also found in utilitarian philosophy. He argues, however, that what is missing from utilitarianism is the Kantian view that people have *intrinsic moral worth* that prevents them being treated as means to an end, no matter how important and valuable that end/consequence is. Hawley (2007, p. 88) argues that Kantian deontology 'is an ethic of respect for clients and patients'; for nurses to respect people's 'rational nature and their inherent dignity'.

Deriving from Kant's moral principles is the idea of his *'perfect'* and *'imperfect'* duties. Perfect duties are rights and obligations which we must observe; there can be no exceptions to such perfect duties as respect all persons, tell the truth to all persons, do not kill people. These fundamental ethical principles underpin most healthcare professionals' code of conduct. The NMC PCC, the GMC's guidelines for doctors and the CSP and HPC rules for physiotherapists state that members of these professions should respect patients' rights to confidentiality and autonomy and their right to give/withhold consent to treatment. The problem is: these principles are not absolute because we note that confidentiality, for example, may be breached under certain conditions even without patients' consent. Therefore, as critical as these professional guiding principles are, they are not absolute as Kant's moral theory demands.

Kant's moral philosophy has been rejected on the grounds of austerity, as an austere, arid, and rigid version of morality (Gillon, 2003). Anyway, as a theory of morality it does remind us that as professionals we have fundamental rational duties to patients. Some are absolute, others are relative, but nevertheless Kant's theory offers some basis for ethical reasoning and decision making.

If I accept the absolute moral principle that I should never harm someone, self-defence is impossible. I could also not tell a lie even if telling one would save a person from dying. There is the question then of what one does when one is faced with a moral systems in which there are *absolute* and *pluralist* moral theories. In *absolutism* we apply the moral principle without exception. In *pluralist moral theory* we have a mixture of fundamental moral principles. There is room here for clash/conflict. This is where we will look briefly at W. D. Ross's *prima facie duties*.

W. D. Ross's prima facie and absolute duties

Ross (1930) believes that the primary purpose of moral philosophy is to list *moral obligations* based on mature personal reflections. He says, however, that some of these obligations may clash. He distinguishes between what he calls *prima facie duties* and *absolute duties*. *Prima facie duties* are moral obligations that should guide our moral reasoning *if there are no conflicting moral thoughts or obligations*. He identifies various moral principles which he feels any mature reflective and intuitive person would accept, for example duties of *fidelity* (keeping promises), *beneficence* (imperative to help others), *not to hurt others* (non-maleficence), *justice* (being fair and equitable in dealing with others), *reparation* (compensating others for the wrong we do them), *gratitude* to those who help us, and *to foster one's own needs and talents*.

Ross says if there is a clash between different prima facie moral duties we have to decide in the light of the circumstances whether it is morally more important to follow one duty or the other. Deciding on the balance is a matter of judgement. This theory is actually implying that there will be occasions when the health professional is going to have to take decisions based on his/her own reasoning, experiences and perhaps even personal preferences. In deciding which action is the right one to take, the healthcare professional needs to weigh up the options and decide on the best course. Hope and colleagues (2003) believe that Ross's duty-based approach to ethics has influenced the four ethical principles of autonomy, beneficence, non-maleficence and justice. For Ross, although the consequences of utilitarianism are important there are other morally important things, such as keeping promises, showing gratitude, helping others when able, and treating others fairly.

Virtue ethics

Virtue ethics is centred around virtues: qualities and characteristics of persons. For example, what are the characteristics of a 'good nurse' or 'a good doctor'? I remember as a student being asked to write a paper on what makes a good nurse. My initial thoughts were on the values, qualities and characteristics I felt I had learned as a child: kindness, caring, honesty and truth telling, hard-working, being ambitious and wanting to achieve in life but not doing so whilst trampling on other people. My late father used to say to me: be kind and fair to others, seeking always to help others rather them expecting them to help you; be nice to people otherwise, 'when you are going down, you will meet them coming up'. Later in my development and study of psychology I came across the work of Piaget and Lawrence Kohlberg and learned that we learn moral virtues not only from our parental, school, church and social clubs' influences but also by virtue of being constantly challenged to critically reflect on our value status, constantly studying whether we need to shift our moral position in the light of new arguments and knowledge. I often ask new first-year student nurses, just coming into nurse training, what sorts of qualities and virtues they think nurses should have. Amongst their answers come values and virtues such as *caring, compassion, warmth, kindness, consideration*. Consider this in Box 11.4.

Origins of virtue ethics

The origins of virtue ethics lie in the work of the Greek philosopher Aristotle in the fourth century BCE. Other Greek philosophers such as Socrates and Plato had also advocated virtue ethics as defining those characteristics that make a person a good person. In moral terms, the right act would be that which is performed by a virtuous person. The virtuous person is blessed with virtues; (s)he exhibits virtues. According to Aristotle (1976) those who are endowed with good virtues (good traits of character) enjoy the best life, *eudaemonia*, which means *flourishing*. This notion is also linked to the sense of deep happiness which the virtuous person experiences. If this were the only definition of virtuous – self-centred, egocentric and self-rewarding – then one might question: how could such a state (or morality) be helpful to other people?

However, when further analysed, virtues have utilitarian purposes. For Socrates, Aristotle and Plato the distinctive virtues necessary to function in society are the cardinal (primary)

BOX 11.4 Reflective questions

Look at the virtues in the text that are often identified by undergraduate freshmen and women and see whether you agree with them. What virtues do you consider nurses should have? Having done this, turn to your NMC Code and see if any of the virtues identified by you are actually identified by the Code. Do you think any of the virtues identified and defined by you could prove handicapping to a nurse? If so, which and why?

virtues of wisdom, the ability to administer justice or fairness when relating to people, courage and temperance (capacity for calmness in times of stress, challenges and adversities). These virtues are seen as desirable since they are likely to lead to good outcomes; for example, the compassionate nurse or doctor may be seen to be exhibiting compassion and caring towards his/her patient who specially needs this type of understanding. Pence (2004) has pointed out that in Greek medicine, if one wants to know what makes a good doctor, the purpose of medicine needs to be known. The same question could be asked of a nurse: what makes a good nurse? The answer may come back as: the purpose of good nursing is to heal the sick, promote health and even help patients to achieve a peaceful death (in the UK, not euthanasia of course). I recall Virginia Henderson's (1966, p. 15) famous definition of a nurse, which says, inter alia, one of the imperatives is to assist the individual sick or well, including where appropriate helping him to *achieve a peaceful death*. This might include keeping the patient pain free. The question is then asked: what virtues are necessary for this? Possible answers may be kindness and compassion. However, virtues alone are not enough, and have the weakness that they do not positively preach technical knowledge; they only define *role-based ethics*.

Limitations of ancient virtue ethics in modern nursing and medicine

Although the virtues cited above are still relevant in today's nursing and medical practice, alone they are not enough to make a healthcare professional a comprehensive and effective moral carer. Aristotle's virtues did not stop doctors acting patronisingly and paternalistically, limiting patients' own intervention and activeness, rather than passivity, in their care. It does not canvass their opinion; it is more inclined to teach patients *learned helplessness* that causes patients' overreliance on carers and overuse of the external locus of control. If virtue ethics condone this paternalistic view, they are not sound ethics. It would not be a complete helpful ethical theory, although no one would deny its partial ability to help with ethical decision making. A complementary approach, using scientific knowledge, research-derived findings about effectiveness of care strategies, communication and interpersonal communication skills, awareness and self-awareness, social, psychological, spiritual and other technological abilities, together with the virtues would make a good combination.

Virtues based on religion are suspect. There are arguments to suggest that people in the West are becoming less religious and less spiritual. The Church of England has sold off many properties because fewer people now go to church. Conversely in some parts of the world religion seems to mean a model of radicalism, hate, irrationality, wickedness and cruelty that may well account for disasters such as 9/11 or the deliberate Bali, Mumbai, London and Madrid explosions that made a carnage of fellow brothers and sisters. Religion-derived virtue ethics need re-evaluation. If virtue ethics are linked to religion and spirituality, they need redefining in the light of observed current changes in people's attitudes and virtuous behaviour.

In Aristotle's time the religious virtues of hope, charity, faith, and compassion rated highly for physicians. Some religious virtues are tied to the idea of 'suffering' – Jesus of Nazareth suffering on the cross. Does this mean the virtuous nurse must suffer with or for her patients? Not a rational perspective. If you suffer too much it depletes your ability to use yourself therapeutically for the good of your patient. Nowadays people even talk about religious virtues that make them fight 'holy wars', in the process killing indiscriminately. Virtue ethics linked to religion need re-evaluation.

The natural law virtue of heterosexual-only relationships is under pressure. We now need to look at virtues that value diversity and deviations; we need virtues that value homosexuality as a person's right to decide his/her sexuality. So we need not only to broaden and bring up to date the traditional list of virtues and what they stand for, but we also need to analyse them in terms of meanings, applications and relevance to today's society.

The ancient virtue ethics of Hippocrates and his brethren held that doctors should not only 'adopt patient-centred ethics but also sanctity-of-life world view' (Pence, 2004, p. 11); for example, do not participate in abortion or assist with euthanasia. These views are becoming dated, as they clash with the modern philosophical view that the patient is the one who decides his/her own fate: self-determination. Patients are perhaps driven by autonomy, natural God-given rights and legislative (human rights) too: the rights to life, privacy, not to be abused, fair trial and so on. Virtue ethics should consider and reflect patients' needs more holistically, sensitively, widely and deeply than hitherto was the case. If the patient considers a pregnancy to be detrimental to her health she should be understood in term of her own personal perspective, and be able to gain the compassion, thoughtfulness and understanding of the physician, nurse and significant others, who may help her to safely abort her pregnancy. She has choices. She has rights; let her be free to exercise them.

Please carry out Student activity 11.4 in Box 11.5.

Feminist moral theories and care-based reasoning

So far we have looked at *teleological* and *deontological* ethical theories. Some have offered useful insight into how modern ethical decision making could be achieved and justified. However, there are shortcomings in those theories, particularly regarding the fact that most were conceptualised through masculine perspectives, too driven by unemotional rationality, and gave too much power to physicians to make ethical decisions concerning patients. Moral reasoning and values development, as the work of Piaget and Kohlberg (in Chapter 8) has shown us, comes in chronological stages for Piaget, and through chronological and environmental stimulation influences according to Kohlberg. However, the latter's research was biased in favour of male reasoning. Criticising the research approaches to the study of moral development taken by Kohlberg, a famous female Harvard professor, Carol Gilligan

---

BOX 11.5 Student activity 11.4

Reflective group work on virtue ethics

Get together with a few of your fellow students and draw up a list of what you consider to be worthwhile virtues of any nurse.

From your list identify those virtues that you consider to be most important/most valuable/most crucial in:

- psychiatric nursing;
- paediatric nursing;
- adult nursing;
- learning disability nursing.

For your list of overall virtues *and* for your sublist based on the nursing branches designated, write a sound justification for the virtues identified.

Ensure that this work is written up in the appropriate section of your ethics portfolio, identifying what you think you have learned from this exercise and how you feel it has contributed to your academic and professional development.

(1982) challenged Kohlberg's work and came up with her own theory of moral development, using female research subjects. She argued that traditional ethical theories largely ignore considerations around family values and relationships. Female values must be brought into the equation. Ethical theories also need to value individuality and individual differences more.

In the 1970s too, *feminism* and a modern movement for patients' rights decided that physicians, particularly men, had too much power in making decisions concerning patients. Women in America begun to question why they were unable to gain health-related information in down-to-earth, patient-friendly language, rather than in the technical, unintelligible, esoteric language of particularly male doctors. Early published ethical theories were largely silent on the contribution of female ethicists. Yet Hawley (1997) argues that female philosophers have made considerable contribution to philosophical reasoning but have not been recognised.

The critical question, whether there is a difference between male and female ethical values, was answered by Gilligan's (1982) study, in which she demonstrated that boys and girls acquire and use moral reasoning abilities differently. Boys tend to solve moral dilemmas by applying principles, rules and precedents and addressing the question: what is the right thing to do? Boys were more likely to be impartial in decision making. Girls tend to resolve dilemmas by suggesting that the right way forward is to discuss the problem with the key stakeholders. Girls were more concerned to preserve relationships. They were more oriented to peaceful, friendly and cordial relationships at the end of a dispute.

Following Gilligan's work, feminist theorists have articulated the view that female ethical decision making values tenets not much valued by men, for example cooperation between members of decision-making groups, trust, friendly relationships and caring. Males on the other hand tend to focus on legal relationships, rational arguments, abstraction, rationality and oversimplification of the problem. Applying these views to medical and nursing decision making, one might expect to note that the male thinking will be along the lines of analysing problems simplistically, looking more superficially at the issues and the people involved, making decisions without necessarily engaging in in-depth discussions. On the other hand, one may expect female nurses and doctors, faced with a clinical dilemma, to call a meeting with the parties, discuss in detail all the issues, listen to all the arguments before arriving at a resolution. From the observations of how women solve ethical problems has come the notion of an *ethics of care*, one that values friendships, trusting friendly relationships, nurturing and love.

A weakness in the ethics of care theory is that, whereas it puts less emphasis on abstraction, rights, utility and duty, and more stress on loving and caring for those we know and care about, it does not say much about how we deal with those we do not care about or those who do not come within our immediate intimate and friendly relationships. Furthermore, in nursing you are taught to value all patients not just those you know well. In fact health professionals are not encouraged to be too involved in the care of their own relatives when in hospital. The close family relationship may be frowned on as being far from objective and may even be viewed as too involved emotionally. Pence (2004, p. 24) puts the new ethics of care philosophy into perspective when he writes:

> One might view the ethics of care as a corrective to the previous emphasis in ethical theory on abstract, semilegalistic concepts . . . Reflecting a modern turning inward to the family and to those around one, fighting battles close at hand and letting far-off concerns such as world hunger take care of themselves. [It is a] . . . modest, minimalist approach to morality – a kind of within-my-circle-of-relationships approach.

Gilligan's care approach to ethics contrasts with Kohlberg's (1980) philosophy of moral development in which he proposed that moral reasoning and development operate on six hierarchical levels, and take into account 'universal ethical principles', such that actions are seen to be right only when they are taken based on these principles. Female ethical reasoning and decision making have certain overlaps with, and attributes of, 'narrative ethics' (with emphasis on case details), 'communitarian ethics' (with emphasis on importance of discussion) and the 'ethics of care' (Hope *et al.*, 2003, p. 12) although care ethics is viewed as an offshoot of feminist ethics.

How can the theoretical conceptualisations about ethics and ethical theories above help me in my nursing decision making?

It is pointless just reading and memorising the ethical theories, concepts and principles outlined above, and in the preceding chapter, without being able to say how such theories can guide me in my work as a nurse. This is a very big question that probably needs a chapter on its own. However, you have learned about the notions of principlism – *autonomy*, *justice*, *beneficence* and *non-maleficence* – in a preceding chapter. So in undertaking nursing care you should aim to make sure you respect such values when making nursing decisions: value patients' autonomy and right to participate in the decision making; be fair, considerate and equitable in caring for patients and clients, attempting always to be non-prejudicial; demonstrate equality and respect diversity, treating patients justly and fairly irrespective of their socio-cultural and economic backgrounds. Always aim to do good for your patient/ clients, attempting always to make sure they benefit (beneficence) rather than being hurt by your care.

In respect to the ethics of teleology, especially utilitarianism, and the ethics of deontology (and there are many different deontological notions described above) perhaps the best advice one can give you is to make sure that your ethical decision making takes on board as many as possible of the various ethical principles, since no one is complete itself and without weakness. Moreover, a combination of ethical principles seems to offer the best recipe for caring ethical decision making. Be conscious always to ask yourself whether your ethical decision making as a nurse is in line with legal expectations and principles. You must practise within the parameters of the law of the country you are nursing in. Most critically, be sure to follow the guidelines laid down by your professional bodies, which will no doubt have followed certain ethical and legal principles in laying down those professional guiding principles.

Whatever our religious and philosophical beliefs, there is a very strong case for valuing the virtues identified above under the notion of *virtue ethics*. It is true that moral values and virtuous characteristics are sometimes challengeable, depending on the context and the situation we are dealing with. It is also true that as society moves forwards (perhaps backwards, others may argue) we do tend to change or alter our moral reasoning, at times changing and adjusting our ethical values. A point of example is how today young people in particular seem to be less 'God-centred', less church minded than hitherto, with fewer people going to churches and other places of religious worship. It would still be difficult to argue that they are any less virtuous in their thinking even if we describe them as more secular.

Summary and conclusion

This chapter:

- introduced you to the ethical theories of teleology, deontology, virtue ethics and the feminist and care ethics;
- made links with the notion of ethical principlism;
- looked at these theories in terms of definitions and meanings and implications for ethical decision making in healthcare;
- focused critically on limitations of these theories in healthcare decision making;
- has shown you how you can use the various ethical theories, concepts and principles to inform your ethical decision making in nursing.

The conclusion may be drawn that it would be very difficult for a nurse, or any other health professional, to rely solely on any one of these theories to inform, support and justify ethical decision making. Therefore an eclectic approach seems the best option.

12   Record keeping

Objectives of this chapter

After reading this chapter you should be able to:

*   describe a health record and distinguish between different types of health records and systems;
*   talk confidently about the purposes, values and importance of good health record keeping;
*   describe what your professional body and the law require from you in the context of record keeping;
*   discuss the implications of good and poor record keeping;
*   demonstrate ability to find useful information sources regarding health record keeping.

Introduction

Record keeping is especially important in healthcare and nursing particularly, and can impact various aspects of our lives. Relating to the notion of record keeping impacting our daily lives, you may recall that on the day of your interview for nurse training you may have been asked to provide evidence of who you are, evidence such as a birth certificate, a driving or marriage certificate or a passport. You may even have been asked to provide original evidence of your academic attainment, for example your GCSE and A Level certificates. If you were, hopefully the process has demonstrated to you that record keeping, including keeping records on those patients/clients you care for as a nurse, is rather important. In healthcare generally, and nursing particularly, effective record keeping is essential for effective nursing care. As we have been focusing on *law*, *ethics* and *professional code of conduct principles* throughout this book, it is important to recognise, too, that these three dimensions of professional practice also have major influence on record keeping. We will see how as the chapter develops.

NMC pre-registration education standards and Code requirements for record keeping

In its publication *Standards for Pre-registration Nursing Education* the NMC (2010a, p. 11) talks about the *standards for competence* that your programme or curriculum must address to enable you to become a registered nurse. The document states: 'Competence is a requirement for entry to the.. register. It is a holistic concept . . . defined as the combination of skills, knowledge, attitudes, values and technical abilities that underpin safe and effective nursing practice and interventions'. Good record keeping in nursing requires all these factors and more. Under the Competency Domain 'Communication and interpersonal skills' the NMC also states: 'All nurses must maintain accurate, clear and complete records, including the use of electronic formats, using appropriate and plain language' (2010a).

The NMC 2008 Code requires nurses to:

- keep clear, accurate records of discussion had, assessments made and treatment and medicines given and how effective these have been;
- complete records as soon as possible after the related event;
- not tamper with original records;
- ensure entries made in paper records are clear, signed, dated and timed;
- ensure entries on patients' electronic records are clearly attributed to the maker of the entries;
- ensure records are kept securely.

So important is effective record keeping in nursing that the NMC (2009a) has further developed and published *Record Keeping Guidance for Nurses and Midwives*. You can locate these guidelines on the NMC website at http://www.nmc-uk.org. A professional advisor on record keeping to the NMC, Martine Tune, said in an interview (see NMC News 29, 2009): 'the quality of a registrant's record keeping is a reflection of the standard of their professional practice'. This point helps to augment the criticality of maintaining good health records in respect to your nursing practice.

Just to further highlight the importance of nurses keeping good records, I must make the point that nurses have been known to have been suspended from practice by the NMC for poor record keeping. In the interview referred to above, Martine Tune makes the point that 'We see record keeping consistently in the top three reasons why people appear before [NMC] Fitness to Practise Panels'.

NMC Conduct Committee Cases in relation to poor record keeping

In 2002 the NMC reports a case where a nurse from Coventry was removed from its professional register after she was found guilty of failing to keep accurate records of patient care. Ms Tune reports how in August 2008 a nurse was suspended from practice for six months after an independent panel of the Conduct and Competence Committee of the NMC found her guilty of failure to maintain accurate records. Whilst being employed at Peartree Care Centre in Sydenham, Kent, the nurse was found guilty of failing to record that a dose of antibiotic had been administered to a patient. She also failed to complete a wound chart and a body mapping chart after examining a wound on the patient's leg. The NMC (at http://www.nmc-uk.org/Documents/FTPOutcomes/Reasons%20CCCSH%20Stephenson%20 20100331.pdf) notes how in March 2010 a registered adult E-grade staff nurse received a suspension order for, amongst other failings, a failure to record that a drug, OxyContin, had not been administered to a patient. Note that in this case the nurse's record-keeping weakness was omission, not commission.

Wood (2003) notes that nurses are under increasing scrutiny over their record keeping, and statutes such as the Human Rights Act 1998 and the Data Protection Act 1998 have increased the profile of, and access to, health records. It seems that the problem of poor record keeping by nurses has been occurring for some time. Wood (2003) comments that nurses' record keeping was the 'second most common category of hearing brought before the UKCC in 2001'; the UKCC being the nurses' registration body that was superseded by the NMC. What is even more striking is the view that 'law courts adopt the attitude that if something is not recorded, it did not happen and, therefore, nurses have a professional and legal duty to keep records' (Wood, 2003). If nurses fail to maintain proper records then their hands-on care could fall down since proper record keeping and good hands-on care constitute an holistic picture of caring. None of us have memories that will not at some time fail us, even a little, and so to rely on memory for the nursing care given many weeks, months, years and decades ago is not a smart thing to do. Proper record keeping is essential for both our patients and ourselves as health professionals, and these records are also going to be helpful to other healthcare professionals caring for the patient. So what is a health record?

A health record

The Data Protection Act 1998 defines health records as 'information about the physical or mental health condition of an identifiable individual made by or on behalf of a health professional in connection with the care of that patient' [c. 29 S 68 1 (a) and 2 (a), (b)]. Taking this definition a little further, we could say that a health record may be in electronic or paper format. It is a recorded evidence of the investigations, results of investigations, care planning and implementation and documentary results of the care given to a patient. Health records can be found in various places or locations, for example contained in hospital data base locations, in GP practices, kept by a dentist, an optician, a district nurse, health visitor or midwife, a physiotherapist, occupational therapist, clinical psychologist, osteopath, chiropodist, speech and language therapist, psychotherapist, music therapist, pharmaceutical chemist; in fact such a record may be kept by anyone registered as a therapist under the Health Professional Order 2001. Good record keeping therefore is the responsibility of the multiprofessional team, including not just clinical but also administrative staff. The data controller is the person/agent responsible for processing the record, including keeping, making, destroying, transferring and so on.

Personal data are data about a living individual that enable him/her to be identified from the data alone, or with support from other information in the data controller's possession. Personal data include such things as the person's name, address, age, race, religion, gender, physical, mental and social health. As a student you may have to write patient care studies. If you are required to do so you will need to ask patients' permission to write about them, ensuring all confidentiality principles are accorded. As well as seeking the patient's consent, you must remember always to make sure none of the materials you record in your case study can identify the patient.

Data controllers, such as the NHS, process data. As a nurse you may be part of that processing procedure. Make sure your records are accurate, readable and up to date. The Department of Health (DoH, 2006) states that processing data means everything that is done to the information, for example holding, receiving, recording, using, disclosing, disposing, transferring, destroying, sharing or archiving. As a nurse you must remember that the Department of Health Records Management: NHS Code of Practice requires:

- each NHS organisation to have an overall policy statement on how it manages all its records;
- that in the above sense the record policy statement should be made readily available to all staff at all levels, through induction and regular updating;
- that all staff, clinical or administrative, must be trained/educated about their personal responsibility in record keeping;
- staff to know that as per the Public Records Act they are responsible for any records they create or use in their duties; all such records as stated above are public records that may be subject to legal and professional obligations.

The DoH (2006, p. 6) states that 'All individuals who work for an NHS organisation are responsible for any records which they create or use in the performance of their duties' and that such records are 'a public record' subject to both legal and professional obligations.

As a nurse you should know your right to be properly trained by your employer to become aware of your personal responsibilities in respect to record keeping and records management (DoH, 2006, paragraph 31). Clearly, as a student nurse, you cannot learn on your pre-registration degree programme all that you need to know in order to function effectively as a registered nurse for the rest of your professional life. Professional development is a life-long process and so when you obtain your first post as a registered nurse you must make sure you receive updating from your employer about record keeping. The records you help to create are a testament of fact about the care planned and given to the patient and the effects of the care, and as such could be called upon by a court of law in any dispute about care. Good record keeping is about good nursing care standards.

Sensitive nature of patients' records

Whatever format the patient's record is in, paper or electronic, it is an individual document, a sensitive, confidential personal file that must be handled with great care and sensitivity. Every attempt must be made, therefore, to ensure that patients' confidential files are kept safely and securely. A patient's record may be anything from medical and nursing notes to pathology reports, radiography reports, hand-written clinical notes, relevant emails, notes and letters whether handwritten or printed from one health professional to another, printout from data-gathering equipment such as an electrocardiogram (ECG machine) or a machine for recording patients' temperature, pulse and blood pressure, and incidents reports such as when a patient falls or has any mishaps affecting his/her care. A health record may also involve a photograph taken of an ulcer on the patient's body, a video recording, tape recording of a telephone conversation about the patient's care.

Confidentiality of records

As a student you have a responsibility to ensure that patients' records are kept safely with confidentiality in mind. In fact, in relation to confidentiality in respect to patients' records, the NMC record-keeping guidelines requires nurses to:

1. ensure they understand legal requirements and guidance regarding confidentiality, and ensure their practice is informed by local and national policies;
2. ensure they understand the rules relating to confidentiality appertaining to the supply and use of data for secondary purposes;
3. follow local policy guidelines when using records for research purposes;
4. refrain from discussing patients'/clients' care in places where they may be overheard;
5. not leave patients' records, electronic or paper, where they may be seen by unauthorised personnel, including other staff or members of the public;
6. not take photographs of any person that are not clinically relevant, and take them only with the consent of the person concerned.

Only persons involved with the patient's care and therefore having a right to access care-related documentation should be allowed to do so. Patients must be told that their record could be accessed by all the professionals who are involved in their care. Having said this, 'People in your care have the right to ask for their information to be withheld from you or other health professionals. You must respect that right unless withholding such information would cause serious harm to that person or others' (NMC, 2009a).

In relation to point (1) above, in respect to local and national policies, as a nurse you need to find out what your local trust policies are, but also look at the national picture; for example, visit the Department of Health website on 'Records Management' at http://www. dh.gov.uk/en/Publicationsandstatistics/Publications/PublicationsPolicy. At this point, carry out Student activity 12.1 in Box 12.1.

Good record keeping is integral and essential to effective and safe care. It is an essential nursing responsibility, not an optional one, and so if a nurse's omission or action falls short of the standard of record keeping expected (s)he could be disciplined by an employer or the NMC. Patient records must be clear, complete and accurate because a patient's life may depend on it. Nurses also work within a multidisciplinary context, in which case other health professionals may rely on the completeness and accuracy of the records made and kept by nurses.

The purpose of record keeping

Good record keeping, whether it is in hospitals or community care settings such as GP practices, NHS or private care agencies, at individual or team level, has a number of important functions, including *clinical*, *administrative*, *research* and *educational*. The record is fundamentally about having evidence of the investigation, treatment and effects of treatment of the patient. It forms the basis for future comparison of changes in a patient's health status, thus allowing progress and deterioration of patients' conditions to be carefully monitored, and treatments adjusted as appropriate. Without proper records we would be unable to tell one patient form another, thus complicating treatment, for example by giving a particular patient the treatment intended for another. Without records we are unable to make decisions about the next phase in the patient's care. Good record keeping is an essential and effective support tool to clinical practice and decision making, ensuring good communication, continuity, consistency, efficacy, efficiency and professional standards of care. It also promotes the professional image of the nursing profession. In the case of *Sanders v Leeds Western HA* [1993] 4 Med LR 355, a four-year-old child suffered heart failure and brain damage during surgery. The theatre staff claimed that the child's pulse had stopped suddenly. The court rejected this claim, however, because there was no systematic and sequential written evidence in the child's notes to indicate or support what the staff had claimed happened. This case goes to show you that you must ensure you record important happenings in your nursing care, sequentially, in sufficient detail. If there is no record the court will simply take the view that it did not happen. In the above case the Health Authority was held to be negligent.

BOX 12.1 Student activity 12.1

Use a section of your portfolio to record and summarise:

1   types of health records;
2   the purpose of keeping health records;
3   the NMC's views about health record as far as the responsibility of the nurse goes.

The Department of Health (DoH, 2006) notes that healthcare records and the principle of good record keeping:

- underpin delivery of high-quality evidence-based care;
- are of most value when defined by accuracy and accessibility when needed;
- support patient/client care and continuity of care;
- support day-to-day business that underpins care delivery;
- support sound administrative and management decision making, as part of the knowledge base for NHS services;
- meet legal requirements, including patients' requests for information under the Data Protection Act or the Freedom of Information Act;
- assist clinical and other types of audits;
- support improvement in clinical effectiveness through research;
- support archival functions by granting access to historical data that allows judgement to be made of the importance of such data and whether future research is indicated;
- support patient/client choice and control over treatment and services.

Proper legal, professional and ethical footing of records

Records provide evidence of whether or not care has been given to the correct standard and within required legal framework. The record is intended to demonstrate what the care was, who had given the care, the time it was given, chronological order of the care, the effects of the care, and whether any complications had been noted. It must be reinforced here that law courts tend to adopt the belief that if no record is made then care was not given; in which case a nurse could be on weak and tenuous grounds in trying to defend his/her nursing care in a court of law.

Dedicate record keeping time

Nurses need to make time to compile clear, accurate and factual accounts of their care. The investment of time in recording things close to the point of their occurrence could be well worth while in terms of quality of patient care and the quality of the evidence one can call on in a legal suit that challenges the quality of patient care.

Importance of records being on correct legal footing

Even before a legal case comes before a court of law, the patient's record will have been read and studied by legal people on both sides of the legal divide, and by potential expert witnesses. Therefore, if the records are of poor quality the legal professionals have already had time to form an opinion of the quality of the professionalism that has put those records together. Thus by the time of a formal legal hearing your reputation as a 'sloppy record marker' or in fact a 'very good record maker' will have preceded you. My experience as a student gaining experience in obstetrics had led me to conclude at that point in my professional development that, compared with nurses, midwives seemed to me then to be more meticulous at record keeping. They seemed to be more involved with what I would describe as an orderly, systematic and chronological recording of patient care, in respect to the progress of labour. They seemed rather methodical and systematic in terms of their real-time entries into the patient's record. Maybe what I observed reflected more on the relatively short period of a typical labour compared with the longer time a patient may spend in a typical general surgical or medical ward, in which case the comparative conclusion I had form about record keeping in the two professions may not be an entirely fair one. Chronology of events and real-time entries can be critical because care must always be prioritised, in which case chronology and real-time entry of details can be critical.

Given the *legal* applicability of records and their possible admission in court hearing, whether on negligence or criminal matters, it is imperative that documents be clear, accurate and properly signed. The patient's records are a legal document which a court of law can subpoena as and when required. In spite of the confidential nature of the patient's records these must be produced to the court when demanded. Under Rules of the Supreme Court order 24 any patient record can be demanded by the court, which takes precedence over our employers' and professional body demands. Courts can be suspicious of unclear records especially if they appear to have been tampered with. If you must inevitably make a correction to your earlier entry in the patient's note, it is crucial that even the old material crossed through remain readable. Moreover, it must be clearly signed and dated, and, in the case of a student making the changes, I strongly recommend that you get a senior member of the nursing staff to witness it and even agree to the change before it is done. Given that a nurse's record may be his/her saving grace in a court hearing in which his/her nursing care is in question, it is in his/her best interest to make sure the record entries are clear and accurate. You may wish to use your records to show that you gave the best care, on the right occasion, on the correct day and at the right time and to the right patient.

Importance of records on correct professional and ethical footing

We can use records to judge if the care given was in fact given on the proper *ethical* footing and also whether the proper professional standards and procedures of care had been followed. The NMC (2009a) summarised *important functions* of health record keeping as:

- helping to improve accountability;
- demonstrating how decisions about patient care were arrived at;
- supporting delivery of patient services;
- supporting clinical judgements and decisions;
- supporting patient care and communications between all concerned;
- making continuity of care easier;
- promoting communication between members of the multidisciplinary care team;
- helping to identify risks, enabling early detection of complications;
- supporting clinical audit, research, resource allocation and performance planning;
- helping to address complaints and legal processes.

Principles of good record keeping

Some of the principles outlined below have been guided by NMC recommendations.

- Clarity: records must clearly say what is intended to be said and must be accurate, consistent, objective, factual and unopinionated. Handwriting must be legible. Avoid nebulous, unhelpful statements such as 'had a good day'. What does this mean? That the patient was quieter today than yesterday? Did not make as many demands on the nursing staff as yesterday? That (s)he slept all day? That (s)he ate today, whereas (s)he did not eat yesterday? Be clear about what you are reporting. Sometimes nurses should use patients' direct words to describe their feeling. This can be more helpful than a nurse's opinionated statement, 'had a good day'. What about: the patient reported she was 'not in any pain today', where the words in quotation marks are those of the patient? Use quotations to reflect the fact of what the patient told you (s)he felt, saw and thought. Nurses often seem reluctant to quote their patients' direct words as a measure of the patient's own evaluation of their care and response to it. In the case in Box 12.2 the Court of Appeal held that health professionals have a duty to write clearly and legibly so that it can be read by careless and busy staff.

- All entries to the record must be signed, timed and dated. The NMC (2009a) requires that in the case of written records, 'the person's name and job title should be printed alongside the first entry'. Avoid initials. Wood (2003) suggests you follow the SMART model: *Specific*, *Measurable*, *Achievable*, *Realistic* and *Time-based*. This is particularly helpful when you and your patient are working together to set goals and targets and also when measuring these.
- The NMC advocates following local policy; however, it recommends that a valid and critical principle involves putting the date and time on all records, in real time and in chronological order of how the care was carried out.
- Accuracy: all records must be accurate, with clear unambiguous meaning. Use your professional knowledge and skills and work with the patient to ensure this objective.
- Record must be factual and not include unnecessary abbreviations. I am aware that nurses often abbreviate, although I will not accept this in an academic nursing paper, unless of course the abbreviated words are first written out in full with the abbreviated version(s) juxtaposed in brackets. Subsequently, the abbreviated format may be used. This way everyone is clear what the abbreviations mean. In practice, however, some abbreviations have clear interpretations, for example B/P for blood pressure and TPR for temperature, pulse and respiration. Dimond (2008) points out, however, that PID can be misleading because it could easily be interpreted as 'pelvic inflammatory disease' when in fact its writer meant 'prolapsed intervertebral disc'; MS can be taken to mean 'multiple sclerosis', when in fact its writer meant 'mitral stenosis'; and so on. Where abbreviations are to be used there should be agreement in the ward, clinic or department what the abbreviations mean so that everyone has the same (correct) understanding. I personally hate abbreviations. I do not recommend their usage in health records, but I would be a liar if I said I did not know it goes on.
- What is recorded should be a matter of the writer's professional judgement, but if you are a student it is best to ask for guidance and to observe good record-keeping and reporting practices before you take responsibility to make entries in the nursing notes.

BOX 12.2 Case showing injury to patient due to lack of clarity in handwriting

The case of *Prendergast v Sam and Dee Ltd* [1989] 1 Med LR 36 is the classic example of transcription error that led to harm to the patient. In this case a doctor's handwritten prescription for the antibiotic Amoxil was misread by the dispensing chemist. As a result, a toxic dose of the drug Daonil (glibenclamide, a diabetic drug used to reduce blood sugar) was dispensed to be taken three times a day. This dose exceeded the normal 15 mg daily dose by some 50 times. The patient, Mr Prendergast, was not a diabetic and from taking the drug sustained permanent brain damage and symptoms of hypoglycaemia. The GP concerned (Dr Miller) was found to be 25 per cent liable for the harm caused by his poor, unclear handwriting, and the pharmacist was held to be liable for 75 per cent of the harm.

Always follow 'best practices'. However, your record must be in sufficient detail to provide evidence that you have done your job. If your record is sparse and incomplete it can seriously undermine you and your employer in a court case or official enquiry. See the case of *Sanders v Leeds Western HA* referred to above.

See Box 12.3 for the value of good record keeping. The case of *Reynolds v North Tyneside HA* [2002] Lloyds Rep Med 459 also demonstrates that good records stand the test of time. In this case a 21-year-old woman argued that negligent management of her birth had caused her to have cerebral palsy. One must emphasise that this case came to court more than 20 years after the event the woman claimed was responsible for her condition. The records were intact and well written, showing that the staff followed the hospital's policy. In this case therefore it was not the record that let down the hospital side, but the hospital policy itself. Thus Reynolds was able to win her case.

- Record, clearly, details of all observations, assessments, findings and the plan of care implemented, ensuring there is reasoned rationale for decisions taken and recorded. Results of care implementation, reviews and evaluations must be recorded. The NMC (2009a) requires you to 'provide clear evidence of the arrangements you have made for future and ongoing care', including details of information about care and treatment.
- Record details of information you provided the patient about his/her care. This should include any risks or problems you pointed out, against which the patient still consented to the care and treatment. Clearly, where there are major risks or procedures involving internal examinations, patients should have consented to these in writing. Evidence that the patient consented to treatment is critical.
- In your multiprofessional line of work your records must show where you communicated with other professionals and your patient and his/her significant others about the people in your care.
- Do not destroy or alter records without proper authority. If you alter any record you must give your name and job title, signing and dating the original documentation, and ensuring that the alterations made and the original records are clear and audible.

BOX 12.3 Case showing that good records stand the test of time

In the unreported case of *O'Keeffe v Cody* (March 11, 1994) (HC (Irl)) the plaintiff alleged negligence on the grounds that, amongst other things, the hospital staff did not observe and alleviate adverse neurological symptoms which she alleged manifested after an epidural injection and following child birth. The operation took place 10 years before the trial by which time hospital staff who gave evidence had no recollection of the patient. Gaps in the plaintiff's memory were also evident; for example, she claimed that her bowels had not moved during the 10 days she was a patient in the hospital after the birth of her daughter. The nursing records (bowel movement charts) showed, however, that the patient had had bowel movement and in fact even had laxative to assist her in the early days following delivery. 'The judge had no doubt that the patient was completely wrong in her recollection that her bowels had not moved during the ten days that she was in the hospital' (Muldowney, 1999, p. 86). The patient lost her claim for negligence because these records stood the test of time and were able to confound the plaintiff's recollection of the care she had received 10 years earlier.

- Write up your notes as soon as possible after the event. Memory can let you down if you leave your recording for too long.
- Avoid using jargon; use clear English where your meanings cannot be misconstrued.
- Your record should be readable when photocopied or scanned.
- Do not use coded language, sarcasm or humorous abbreviations to describe your patients/clients. (I recall as student a consultant physician writing 'Fyffe syndrome' in a patient's medical notes. I tried for quite a few days to understand its meaning, consulting many medical books to do so, but to no avail. When I asked the ward sister of the meaning of this syndrome, she did not know either. So we both asked the senior house officer. He replied that Fyffes were a major shipping company for bananas coming into England and that he thought the consultant was sarcastically saying he thought the patient was mad – Fyffe being allied to the figurative expression 'going bananas'. I reflected on that situation even up to today and wondered what a court of law would have made of such unprofessional entry into a patient's record, had a law suit involving this patient had been brought. Professionals need to keep it professional. Avoid sarcasm in your patient's notes.
- You must not falsify records; it could get you struck off the register and sacked from your employment, costing you your daily bread. (Please refer to the cases in Box 12.4 below.)
- If you have notable objections to the care given, you should record this. As a registered nurse you are responsible and accountable for your practice, professional judgements and decision making. You may have a very strong and well-reasoned view about care differing from other health professionals, and may not agree with the approach taken. If this is the case record your objections.

The case in Box 12.4 demonstrate that fraudulent practices by healthcare professionals are very much in evidence, and involve not just nurses but other health professionals such as midwives, physiotherapists and doctors, to name only some. The practices range from unqualified staff, such as student nurses and midwives, to qualified and very senior health professionals such as managers and senior doctors. As a student nurse, aspiring to qualify and gain professional registration, you must not only maintain a steely and professional determination to be honest in all your dealings with respect to records and record keeping, in private and in public, but must also strive to wipe out fraudulent practices from amongst your colleagues and peers, for example overtly or by whistle-blowing practices reporting those you suspect of committing fraud. Do not alter records illegally and without proper authority. It is important also to remember that the principal UK statutory requirement for health professionals' compliance with record management principles is the Data Protection Act 1998. It regulates the processing of all data, whether they be held on computers or manually.

Disclosure and transfer of records

Apart from the Data Protection Act there are a range of other statutory provisions that regulate, limit, prohibit or set conditions for the transfer or disclosure of records to third parties. There is insufficient space and scope in this book to go into all of these. However, if you are interested to know more about the law in such matters, please refer to Annex C of the DoH (2006) publication: *Records Management: NHS Code of Practice, Part 1*, online at: www.dh.gov.uk/publications, or obtain it from the DH Publications Order-line,

**BOX 12.4 Case evidence of fraudulent use of records by nurses/other
health professionals**

Trainee midwife lied about qualifications

A student midwife faked her qualifications to get a full-time post. In November 2003
and September 2006, during her training at Southampton University Hospital she
forged her mentors' signatures on her portfolio of clinical skills to claim she was fully
qualified to become a midwife. She had claimed to be present during certain procedures
and that she had in fact carried them out herself. At Southampton Magistrates' Court
she pleaded guilty to forgery and deception and was ordered to pay £250 compensation to the NHS and £100 prosecution costs, and sentenced to a 32-month jail term,
suspended for 12 months, and ordered to carry out 200 hours' unpaid work. Source:
Clare Kennedy, *Daily Echo*, 15 October 2007, online at http://www.dailyecho.co.uk/
news1760149, accessed 12 February 2011.

Mental health nurse jailed for fraud

A mental health nurse from Essex was jailed for nine months for defrauding the NHS
of £65,000. This 32-year-old nurse fraudulently obtained NHS training bursaries,
training and NHS employment with a false birth certificate. In August 2005 Basildon
Crown Court heard how she used the NHS bursaries to fund her living expenses whilst
a diploma mental health student nurse at South Bank University. Source: Steve Ford,
Nursing Times.net, 20 December 2010, online at http://www.nursingtimes.net/nurs-
ing-practice/clinical-specialisms/mental-health/essex, accessed 12 February 2011.

Nursing graduate jailed for fraud

A nursing graduate was jailed for eight months by Liverpool Crown Court for defrauding the NHS of £27,697. She had used forged documents to obtain a NHS student
bursary whilst she did a three-year operating department practitioner course at Edge
Hill University between 2006 and 2009. Source: Nursing Times.net, 21 August 2010,
online at http://www.nursingtimes.net/whats-new-in-nursing/news-topics/ethics-and-
law-in-nursing, accessed 12 February 2011.

Practice manager jailed for fraud

An NHS practice manager was jailed for 15 months and ordered to repay £48,000
after he swindled a West Country surgery out of £70,000, between 2003 and 2007.
The 52-year-old manager was found out after a doctor checked financial records and
noticed that a large amount of petty cash had gone missing. Source: Nursing Times.
net, 29 September 2009, online at http://www.nursingtimes.net/whats-new-in-nursing/
primary-care/practice-manager-jail, accessed 12 February 2011.

Physiotherapist struck off after fraud conviction

In this case a physiotherapist fraudulently claimed £2,825 in benefits then tried to hide
details of her conviction from her boss. The court gave her a 12-month conditional
discharge in 2008, but she hid the fact from her manager at Leicester Partnership
Trust. A Fitness to Practice Panel of the HPC ordered removal from the HPC register

of physiotherapists. She admitted that she knew claiming the benefit was unlawful, and that after conviction she felt so ashamed she said she 'didn't want to tell people anything that would make them think I was a dishonest person'. Source: *Leicester Mercury*, 6 October 2010, online at http://www.thisisleicestershire.co.uk/news/Physio-struck-fraud-conviction-revealed/article-2725953-detail/article.html, accessed 12 February 2011.

Doctor struck off for fraudulently obtaining drugs for his schizophrenic brother

The GMC struck off this 68-year old GP after hearing that for at least nine years he had faked prescriptions for sedatives and antipsychotic drugs, which he sent to Egypt for his brother. His fraud came to light in 2008 when Sunderland Teaching Primary Care Trust conducted an audit of the practice's computer records. He had been writing prescriptions for four of the health centre's patients claiming they were exempt from changes, but deleted all mention of the prescriptions and the drugs from the computer records. Source: http://www.journalLive.co.uk/north-east-news/todays-news/2010/11/18/, accessed 13 February 2011.

PO Box 777, London SE1 6XH, email dh@prolog.uk.com, quoting the reference 270422/1/ Records Management: NHS Code of Practice Part 1. This document provides a comprehensive range of the statutes involved, and some of the ways they relate to, control or limit, transfer of records.

For the purposes of this book I have picked out what I believe are some useful pieces of information, from a maze of statutory and organisational provisions available relating to record keeping and disclosure or non-disclosure of information. You will also find some of the information interesting. Hopefully the information in Table 12.1 will help you answer some of the sorts of questions that your patients may well ask you in relation to record keeping, sharing, disposal and so on.

Reflection exercise

As a nursing student, I implore you to revisit your profession's *The Code: Standards of Conduct, Performance and Ethics for Nurses and Midwives* (NMC, 2008a) that guides your professional standards, conduct, performance and ethics. See the Nursing and Midwifery Council website at http://www.nmc-uk.org/Nurses-and-midwives/The-code/. Please note particularly those Code standards relating to aspects such as *respect for patients, patients' rights to confidentiality, privacy, dignity, protection of personal information* and *entitlement to continuity of high standard of care through sound record keeping*. In Chapter 1 of this book you were introduced to the fact that there are other health-regulating bodies apart from the NMC (for example the GMC and HPC). So, for comparison and deepening of your knowledge, read and reflect on the codes for these professions by visiting their websites: for the GMC see http://www.gmc-uk.org/about/register_code_of_conduct.asp; for the HPC code of conduct and ethics for all its registrants and prospective registrants, including physiotherapists, visit http://www.hpc-uk.org/assets/documents/10001BFBSCPEs-cfw.pdf. Reflect on the information, addressing yourself to the question: how can I help to provide and maintain the highest standard of record keeping for my patient, my profession and myself?

Table 12.1 Legal and professional provisions relating to permitting, limiting, prohibiting or setting conditions in respect to disclosure of records to third parties

Primary law sources, e.g. relevant statutes, Health Care Professionals' Code of Conduct and DoH (2006b)	Purpose/functions of the instruments in the left hand column
Abortion Regulations 1991	Doctors who carry out terminations must inform Chief Medical Officer within seven days and retain the certificate for at least three years
Access to Health Records Act 1990. See http://www.dh.gov.uk/ assetRoot/04/03/51/94/04035194. pdf	Relates to records of deceased patients since 1 November 1991 Access: (a) deceased personal representatives, to carry out their duties; (b) persons having a claim resulting from the death Limiting rights: deceased's wish that information not be disclosed; if disclosure would physically or mentally harm any living person; if disclosure would identify third party (not health professionals) not consenting to disclosure
Access to Medical Reports Act 1988	Allows individuals to see medical reports about them for employment or insurance purposes. Patient approval needed for report to be written. Allows patient to disagree with report, withdraw consent, refuse its supply, correct inaccuracies or append points of disagreement Limitations: patient may be prevented from viewing all/part of report if doctor thinks viewing may cause patient serious harm; where disclosure may disclose third-party information without consent
Blood Safety & Quality Legislation, as amended by Quality (Amendment) Regulations 2005 and Blood Safety & Quality (Amendment) (No. 2) Regulations 2005). See http://www.opsi.gov.uk/ si/si2005/20050050.htm	Implemented Directive 2002/98/EC on retention periods for data on human blood. Blood establishments must retain certain data on donors and their establishment's activity and testing of donated blood, for 15 years. Hospital blood banks must retain data for traceability for 30 years from receipt of blood. Controls confidentiality, except to Court Orders and Secretary of State inspection; enables traceability to donors and recipients
Caldicott Guardians	These or their support staff should be involved in proposed disclosure of confidential information, informed by DoH (2003)
Census (Confidentiality) Act 1991	Makes it a criminal offence to unlawfully disclose census information Defences: genuine belief one was acting with lawful authority; information disclosed not personal census States penalty for conviction of unlawful disclosure
Civil Evidence Act 1995	Allows use of records to be admitted as evidence in civil legal proceedings
Common Law Duty of Confidentiality. See: Confidentiality: NHS Confidentiality Code of Practice: http://www.dh.gov.uk/ assetRoot/04/06/92/54/04069254. pdf Not statute based, but based on previous court judgements (precedent)	Information given where it is expected duty of confidence applies, cannot normally be disclosed without the information provider's consent. (See Chapter 6 on confidentiality in this book; look especially at exception to confidentiality). All patients' records must normally be held in confidence. Lawful disclosure: (a) person whom the information relates to consent to disclosure; (b) overriding public interest; (c) legal duty to disclose, e.g. a Court Order

Primary law sources, e.g. relevant statutes, Health Care Professionals' Code of Conduct and DoH (2006b)	*Purpose/functions of the instruments in the left hand column*
Computer Misuse Act 1990	Creates three offences of unlawfully gaining access to computer records: (a) unauthorised access; (b) unauthorised access with intent to commit further offences; (c) unauthorised modification of computer materials
Consumer Protection Act (CPA) 1987	Allows persons who suffered damage/injury to themselves or private property to claim compensation from manufacturers/suppliers of products. Not necessary to prove negligence, just damage Under the Limitation Act 1980, limitation period on start of action is three years from date of damage/knowledge that a cause of action had accrued. When the person dies, limitation of three years starts to run, or from three years of the deceased's representatives' knowledge that a cause of action has accrued
Congenital Disabilities (Civil Liability) Act 1976	Allows a child born disabled owing to negligent treatment of the mother to bring civil action for damage. Limitation starts to run from the child's eighteenth birthday. Period may be extended where material facts unknown
Control of Substances Hazardous to Health (COSHH) Regulations. See http://www.hse.gov.uk/coshh/index.htm	Specify a number measures employers must follow to limit/prevent employee exposure to hazardous substances: (1) risk assessment; (2) prevent/control exposure; (3) precautions; (4) control measures ensured/maintained; (5) monitor exposure; (6) health surveillance; (7) plans/procedures to deal with accidents/incidents/emergencies
Criminal and Disorder Act 1998	Provides for anti-social behaviour order by police or local authority against people 10 years and over. The Anti-Social Behaviour Act (2003) amends the 1998 Act to include Strategic Health Authorities, NHS or Primary Care Trust
Data Protection Act (DPA) 1998	Enough said above about this Act, but essentially it regulates processing of personal data, including health records held manually or on computer. Defines personal data and health records widely. Demands compliances with eight key principles: fairness; data obtained for lawful purpose; personal data adequate, relevant, not excessive for purpose; accuracy and updated records; not kept for longer than necessary for purpose; data processed in line with rights of data subjects under the Act; measures against unauthorised/unlawful processing, loss, destruction, damage; none-transference of data to non-EU countries. Places no restriction on the Court accessing records
Data Protection (Processing of Sensitive Personal Data) Order 2000. See http://www.opsi.gov.uk/legislation/about_legislation.htm	Amends DPA 1998 and provides that personal sensitive data, e.g. on physical and mental health, may be lawfully processed without explicit consent in substantial public interest in disclosure, e.g. crime prevention, malpractice/incompetence and mismanagement
Disclosure of Adoption Information (Post-Commencement Adoptions) Regulations 2005	Requires adoption agencies to keep records on adopted children they have placed for at least 100 years; places limits on what can be disclosed

Table 12.1 (continued)

Primary law sources, e.g. relevant statutes, Health Care Professionals' Code of Conduct and DoH (2006b)	Purpose/functions of the instruments in the left hand column
DoH and GMC agreement re ethical obligation to relatives of deceased persons in terms of maintenance of confidentiality	There are no clear legal obligations of confidentiality to deceased persons (DoH, 2006b). However, the DoH and the GMC agree that there is an ethical obligation to surviving relatives to continue to maintain confidentiality. Disclosure permitted to assist: (a) Coroners/other officers re inquests/ fatal accident injury; (b) national confidential enquiries; (c) provision of death certificates 'Deceased persons records are public records under the Public Records Act and it has been argued that they should be accessible under the Freedom of Information Act 2000' (DoH, 2006b, Annex C)
Electronic Communications Act 2000	Designed to increase confidence in electronic transactions by providing legal admissibility for digital signatures; registration of cryptograph services providers
Freedom of Information Act (FOIA) 2000. See http://www.foi.gov.uk and http://www.ico.gov.uk	Requires public bodies, e.g. local authorities, NHS, to keep and make information available on request. Signals public recognition and interest in openness about government. Additional to other access rights such as the DPA 1998
Gender Recognition Act (GRA) 2004	Gives transsexuals the right to live in their new gender. Establishes Gender Recognition Panels with authority to issue Gender Recognition Certificates. Protects information under certain conditions
Gender Recognition (Disclosure of Information, England, Wales & N. Ireland) (No. 2) Order 2005	Not an offence to disclose 'protected information' under GRA 2004 if disclosure is for medical purposes to a health professional; if the person disclosing reasonably believes the subject concerned has given consent to disclosure, or is unable to consent
Health and Safety at Work Act 1974	Imposes duty on employers to look after employees' health, and obligation on employees to comply with employer's health and safety measures
Health and Social Care Act 2001	Section 60 empowers the Secretary of State for Health to make regulations that require or allow patient information to be shared for medical reasons, including improvement of care, and for public interest purposes

Primary law sources, e.g. relevant statutes, Health Care Professionals' Code of Conduct and DoH (2006b)	Purpose/functions of the instruments in the left hand column
Human Rights Act 1998	Covered elsewhere in this book, but essentially: incorporates the European Convention on Human Rights into UK law 1998, commencing October 2000, allowing people to assert their Convention rights in UK courts and tribunals rather than going to the European Court in Strasbourg. Such rights as right to life, privacy and confidentiality, respect for one's home and correspondence, and not to be subject to torture, inhumane and degrading treatment all have implications for nurses and other health professionals Right to respect for private life puts obligation on public bodies to meet subjects' request for information held on/about them. Denial of access could be seen as breach of Article 8. Legislation must be read in ways that are compatible with the Human Rights Act Human Rights Acts are 'qualified rights', so under certain circumstances can be lawfully set aside by the state, e.g. in the interest of national security; public safety; protection of health or morals; crime prevention; economic well-being of the country; protection of rights and freedoms of others
Limitation Act 1980	Sets time limits within which actions for personal injuries and death may be brought. See the Consumer Protection Act (CPA) 1987 and the Congenital Disabilities (Civil Liability) Act 1976, above
NHS Trusts and Primary Care Trusts (Sexually Transmitted Diseases) Directions 2000	Section 2 repeals Regulation 2 of the NHS (Venereal Diseases) Directions 1991 and Annex B Part 1 of the NHS Trusts (Venereal Diseases) Directions 1991 The NHS (Venereal Diseases) Regulations 1974 (S1 1974/29) imposes on health authorities an obligation to treat confidentially information obtained by their officers on sexually transmitted diseases. The 1991 Directions impose similar obligations on trustees and employers of an NHS Trust The new Directions (which apply in England only) impose the same obligations of confidentiality on members and employees of both NHS and Primary Care Trusts
NMC (2008a) Code. Also see NMC additional advice on confidentiality principles at http://www.nmc-uk.org/Nurses-and-midwives/Advice-by-topic/A/Advice/Confidentiality/	The Code states that nurses: must respect people's right to confidentiality; must ensure people are informed about how and why information is shared by those who will be providing their care; must disclose information if they believe someone may be at risk of harm, in line with the law of the country in which they are practising
Public Health (Control of Diseases) Act 1984 and Public Health (Infectious Diseases) Regulations 1988	Imposes duty on doctors in England and Wales to notify a 'Proper Officer' of a local authority of awareness of patients suffering from one of the notifiable diseases. These can be found on the Health Protection Agency's website at http://www.hpa.org.uk/infections/topics_az/noids/menu.htm

Table 12.1 (continued)

Primary law sources, e.g. relevant statutes, Health Care Professionals' Code of Conduct and DoH (2006b)	Purpose/functions of the instruments in the left hand column
Public Interest Disclosure Act 1998	Allows a worker, e.g. a nurse or any employee for that matter, to breach confidentiality towards his employer by 'whistle blowing', e.g. in circumstances of criminal activity; breach of civil law; miscarriage of justice; compromised health and safety; damaged to the environment; or evidence that any of the above are being concealed
Public Records Act 1958	Makes all NHS records and those of NHS predecessor bodies public records under the terms of the Public Order Act 1958 The maximum period for holding records prior to transfer is usually 30 years. If an NHS body feels it needs to hold records for longer before transfer it must consult with the National Archives (DoH, 2006b, Annex C)

Time limits on patient claim for injury and records destruction

As is clear from the Limitation Act 1980, time limit of three years from the cause of action arising, or date of knowledge of the cause of action arising, is placed on clients/patients bringing cases for personal injuries. However, judges can use their discretion to vary time limits, so that a judge may decide to allow a case to proceed even though it is outside the time limitation zone. The issuing of the claim form starts the court action. If a patient did not know (s)he was injured by a health professional's negligence in the time allowed, then the time limit does not apply until that patient has that knowledge. As pointed out in Table 12.1, a minor under 18 years who has been injured by the negligence of the practitioner does not have his/her time limit running until (s)he reaches 18; only then do the three years start to run. Equally, people with learning disability are not statute barred by time unless their disorder ceases.

To learn about *preservation, retention and destruction of GP general medical services records relating to patients,* see the Department of Health (1998) publication of the same name in *Health Service Circular HSC 1998/217.* Hopefully you will have been convinced by this chapter that the NHS has clear policy for the management of records; please read the DoH (2006b) policy document *Records Management NHS Code of Practice, Parts 1 and 2.*

Minimum retention periods are given for certain documents; you can read up on these at your leisure. It should be clear, however, that keeping documents is an expensive business and so at some time certain documents will be destroyed as per the DoH policy, whilst others may be archived. What is critical is that the destruction of records must be legal, authorised and done with their confidentiality preserved. Destruction may be by shredding or incineration or other appropriate means. The DoH makes it clear that where contractors are used to destroy documents the Trusts who contract with them must make sure that all stages of the process (handover, transport and destruction) use proper safeguards against loss and disclosure.

If you want to find out more about the role of the *Keeper of Public Records* and the *Public Records Office* please consult the *National Archives* website at http://www.nationalarchives. gov.uk. It will be apparent, therefore, that some records are archived for medical and historical research. Clearly, if proper procedures are not followed to preserve records for the appropriate recommended time, patient care could be undermined.

Chapter summary and conclusion

The chapter has established that nursing records are essential to good-quality care and can be the nurse's saving grace at a legal hearing where the nature and quality of his/her care is being challenged. We focused on record keeping, health record and personal data definitions and the purposes, importance and principles of good record keeping. The NMC's requirements and competencies standards for good record keeping by nurses were also examined. The examination not only considered good principles of record keeping but demonstrated what can happen to nurses who fall short of the professional, legal and ethical principles of record keeping. The situation of the data controller was examined in relation to the record making, keeping and disposal and transfer of record process. Although patient's records are confidential, the law does stipulate, through various Statutes and the common law, how and when healthcare records may be shared, kept, disposed of, transferred and archived. An important reality is that patients do have a right to know what is being kept about them. Even after their death what they had in life wished for in relation to the confidentiality of their records must be respected. Under certain conditions, however, the law allows records to be disclosed contrary to patients' wishes. There is no doubt that the law relating to confidentiality plays a big part in relation to health records. Nurses have a very critical part to play in helping to ensure that patients' record keeping is of the highest standard.

13 Caring for older people

Objectives of this chapter

After reading this chapter you should be able to:

- talk confidently about ageism, discrimination and abuse in older people;
- discuss legal, ethical and professional issues in caring for older people; including using the NMC (2009b) *Guidance for the Care of Older People*;
- distinguish between *advanced directives/living wills* and *lasting and enduring power of attorney*, saying how they can help older people;
- say how the Court of Protection and the Mental Capacity Act 2005 can help older people;
- discuss *end of life* issues relating to older people, including *resuscitation/'not for resuscitation'*, *withdrawal of medical treatment*, *permanent vegetative state* and euthanasia, together with implications for nursing;
- discuss how nurses can use the National Service Framework for Older People single assessment process to further the interests of older people;
- discuss the place of covert medication when nursing older people;
- use knowledge gained from this chapter to further develop your portfolio, being able to critically address the problems within the student activities set.

Introduction

If you are wondering why I have written a separate chapter on *caring for older people*, when in fact English law does not necessarily distinguish between the older and younger adult, then your thoughts are along the right lines. However, there are a number of reasons for this particular chapter. First, in the UK and indeed in many developed and developing countries older people are living longer. In the UK older people are utilising considerable health and social care resources (Royal College of Psychiatrists, 2005; NMC, 2010b). Along with this trend is the issue of *ageism*, seen as a *process* of *systematic stereotyping* of, and *discrimination* against, old people. Ageism sets up a fear and denigration of the ageing process, giving legitimacy and credibility to the use of chronological age as a systematic way of denying resources and opportunities to elderly people (Bytheway and Johnson, 1990).

With increasing longevity, many nurses will be faced with looking after an increasing number of older people in hospitals and the community; a real twenty-first-century challenge to the nursing, medical and other health and social care professions to *provide high-quality care to old people* (Wheeler, 2011). This has to be done *within a sound legal, ethical and professional framework*. Research has demonstrated a number of problem issues surrounding care of older people; for example, *negative attitudes* reflecting *ageist stereotypes*, and 'knowledge deficits about ageing that significantly influence the practice of registered nurses and the quality of care older patients receive' (Courtney, Tong and Walsh, 2000, p. 62). Additionally, longevity is the 'greatest risk factor in developing cancer, with 60% of all cancers diagnosed in the over 65s' (Kearney *et al.*, 2000, p. 599). Yet oncology health professionals demonstrate 'persistently negative attitudes' towards elderly patients (Kearney *et al.*, 2000, p. 599). These researchers also found that in acute care settings older patients experience *reduced independence*, *reduced decision-making opportunity*, *little consideration of their age-related needs*, *increased social isolation* and *limited health education*. Moreover, there is evidence that registered nurses have negative attitudes towards geriatric nursing as a clinical specialty, owing to the perception of working with elderly patients as having a low status. Furthermore, geriatric nursing is perceived as an unpopular specialty by student nurses (Slevin, 1991; Snape, 1986; Stevens and Crouch, 1995; Treharne, 1990). Older people are often perceived by policy makers as 'problems', draining resources and demanding considerable attention (Palmer and Short, 1994); and as being 'marginalised', 'oppressed' and 'relegated to a lower status in the acute care setting' (Higgins *et al.*, 2007, p. 225). Interestingly, age stereotypes and discrimination are not confined to sick people. Indeed in a study by Chiu and colleagues (2001) which looked at age discrimination and stereotypes of older workers in the UK and Hong Kong, two different socio-political cultures, it was shown that stereotypes 'were related to discriminatory attitudes' towards old people, for example seeing them as 'less adaptable' (p. 629). Moreover, stereotypical beliefs were found to significantly affect attitudes towards the training, promotion and retention of older workers, younger people's willingness to work with older people and the former's support for positive discrimination against older people. These findings in the work place seem to have parallels to health professionals' attitudes towards older patients in the healthcare setting, a significant reality given current government policies for older people to remain at work for longer, and any attitude nurses, and other health and social care professionals might have towards helping older people to fight discrimination in care and work place settings.

It is therefore important to see how law relates to and protects the older person from unfair discrimination and prejudices. Although many aspects of law that apply to the younger adult apply equally to the older adult, there are some areas of law and professional guidance that appear to have particular relevance and applicability to older people. Nurses need to understand these to be able to make a useful contribution to the health and social care of older people. For the purposes of this chapter the legal and professional areas of major concern are:

- ageism, discrimination and elder abuse in various strata and levels of society;
- mental competency and the Mental Capacity Act 2005 and people's ability and capacity to take mentally and legally competent decisions about their care;
- the issue of autonomy linked to consent and confidentiality linked to notions of privacy and dignity for older people;
- anticipated lack of capacity and actual incapacity to consent due to, among other things, age-related incapacity, diseases and senility;
- the law in relation to end-of-life decision making for older people, including resuscitation and not-for-resuscitation issues; euthanasia and assisted suicide;
- the Nursing and Midwifery Council's *Guidance for the Care of Older People* (NMC, 2009b);
- the relevant sections and standards of the NMC (2008a) Code that require nurses to challenge inequality and discrimination, such as *ageism*, which Age Concern (2007) says is the most common form of discrimination in the UK;
- the European Council Directive 2000/78, which makes age discrimination in employment illegal;

- the law relating to legal instruments such as *advanced directives (ADs)* or *living wills*, and *lasting powers of attorney (LPA);*
- the NHS Framework for older people;
- the English common Law relating to caring for people in a permanent vegetative state;
- the Human Rights Act 1998, which establishes fundamental human rights not only for the young but also for the elderly.

The above are the key elements of this chapter, because they indicate that nurses have an important role in caring for older people, ensuring that they advocate in their best interests, needs and welfare. Some older people will have lost their capacity and ability to champion their own causes, thereby relying on health and social care professionals to advocate for them. Many old people have contributed and are still contributing much to society and the economy particularly. Some are still working and paying taxes; others are paying taxes through the pension funds they have built up in their working life. Some are contributing in being friends, parents and grandparents to many younger people, many of whom depend on them for social, psychological, emotional and, in some cases, financial help and support. Old people deserve to enjoy the healthiest lifestyle that nursing can help them to achieve, not only for themselves but for the benefit of relatives, friends and the wider society. When their time on earth is up, old people are entitled to a peaceful and dignified death, and the law and our ethical and moral values have a significant role to play in making this happen.

NHS failing to deliver good care to the elderly

As I write I am reading in the *Daily Mail* online, Tuesday 15 February 2011, the disturbing headline 'Exposed, neglect of the elderly on wards of shame'. This article claims that the NHS is 'failing' to meet the most basic standards of care of older people, and that patients are 'left so dehydrated on wards [that] they cannot even cry out for help'. The paper refers to setting up a campaign called 'Dignity for the Elderly'. Similarly, on 21 February 2011 the *Daily Telegraph* online (http://www.telegraph.co.uk/health/healthnews/8326299/No-NHS-workers-disciplined-over-neglect-of-elderly.html) claims 'No NHS workers disciplined over neglect of elderly' including failure to provide elderly people with the most basic standard of care. On this same date *The Independent* online (http://www.independent.co.uk/life-style/health-and-families/health-news/hungry-thirsty-unwashed-2215119.html) reports that in the NHS patients are left 'hungry, thirsty, unwashed, in soiled clothes, without adequate pain relief or an emergency call button to reach'.

The shocking claims above are a sad indictment of nurses, doctors and other healthcare workers. By implication the reports call the law into question: how does the law fail so badly to protect vulnerable old people from neglect and abuse? Just in case you the reader are thinking that these sad newspaper headlines are sensationalising the reality for emotional overreaction, I would ask you to think about two issues. First, even if some of these papers are regarded as tabloids, there are some well respected broadsheets amongst them also making the same claims. Second, what is more important is the fact that these papers were responding to some shocking stories detailed in an official investigation by the well-respected Parliamentary and Health Service Ombudsman (NHSLA, 2011). This report has accused NHS staff of an 'ignominious failure' to care for older people.

Taking the Parliamentary and Health Service Ombudsman's report to be accurate, an additional point that must be raised is the question of what is the purpose and usefulness of the Department of Health's policy called the *National Service Framework for Older People* (NSFOP) (DoH, 2001). This central policy advocates patient assessment being individual person-centred, matched to individual circumstances and free from biases. Is it not working? This single assessment process was designed so that patient assessment findings could be shared by the multiprofessional and other carers of older people. This single seamless assessment process implies that where one profession fails another should compensate; where for example nurses fail, doctors should pick up and vice versa; where healthcare fails, social services should pick up; where health and social care professionals and official care policy fail, family and other informal carers should pick up. Such an objective depends on corporation between the services, families and other service user groups. This appears not to be happening. Above all, the *single assessment process* means that all those involved in caring for older people should pool resources to identify and address possible risks, plug loopholes and carry out seamless care to the highest standard for the benefit of vulnerable older people. Yet we read these disturbing newspaper and NHS Ombudsman's investigation reports. The UK's legal framework appears to be failing the elderly patient.

Commenting on the NSFOP, Norman (2011) points out that the NSFOP assessment framework requires nurses to play their part in taking a full and comprehensive patient history, gathering and sharing the old person's assessment information, ensuring that their assessment document takes into account: the patient's full name, date of birth, address, NHS number, GP and care coordinator; patient's main language and availability of interpreters if necessary; preferred medium of communication, such as written language, verbal discussion, pictures, listening to tape recordings; medical conditions/impairment; needs being met by others (professionals, family, friends etc.); details of others involved in the patient's care; time table of care; contact details (e.g. telephone details in/out of hours); and finally medication patient is taking. It is important that the single assessment findings be shared between carers to guarantee that all those involved in caring for the elderly actually play their part.

Ageism, age discrimination and elder abuse

Age Concern (2007) says that ageism is the most common form of discrimination in the UK. It is a type of prejudice and stereotyping that pigeonholes elderly people into homogeneous little boxes, for example the wrong assumption that they are a drain on society, they drain NHS resources and so on. Help the Aged (2002) defines *ageism* as pre-judgement, stereotyping and making assumptions against people on the basis of age. Age discrimination is institutionalised in official policies and in everyday health and social care practices (Norman, 1985; Roberts, 2000; McDonald and Taylor, 2006). With so many older people using the health services, there are particular issues nurses have to deal with, such as helping the increasing number of older people combat negative attitudes, discrimination and age-related prejudices; assisting them with rehabilitation; helping older people achieve/maintain healthy lifestyles as far as it is possible to do so; creating recreation; and caring for older people through terminal illnesses, assisting them, where appropriate, to achieve a peaceful death.

Although older people are the highest consumers of acute NHS services (Norman, 1985; Roberts, 2000; McDonald and Taylor, 2006; Wheeler, 2011) many old people have made huge contributions to the national wealth and indeed to the NHS and are therefore entitled to the best NHS provisions. Even if they had not, on ethical and humanitarian grounds it would be difficult to deny them the best NHS care. Indeed one of the premises on which the NHS was established is people's entitlement to care on the basis of needs, rather than on their ability to pay. Old people should not be discriminated against. Nurses have an important part to play at two levels: (a) being strong advocates for the welfare of the aged, in the everyday clinical operations, and (b) at the higher-up strategic care-planning level, putting the case of the elderly to the strategic planners who are responsible for allocating scarce resources to make sure the needs of the elderly are met. If as a nurse you fail to champion the cause of the elderly you may find health and social care resources being distributed unfairly against elderly people. You may, through your silence, also perpetuate the negative stereotypes around old people as hopeless consumers of health resources.

Employment law and the elderly

There is no law in the UK that introduces 'cut-off' points for medical and nursing interventions for the older person. Furthermore, Wheeler (2011) has made the point that legally, ethically and professionally nursing care cannot be withdrawn or withheld from a person on the basis of age. Even in the province of employment the European Council Directive 2000/78 makes it illegal to discriminate in employment on the basis of age up to 65. In 2006 the Employment Equality (Age) Regulations implemented Directive 2000/78 in the UK. Prior to 1 October 2011, Employment Equality (Age) Regulations (October 2006) applied in the UK, to employment and vocational training up to age 65. A worker could have been compulsorily dismissed by virtue of achieving age 65, although the employee had the right to request working beyond 65 and the employer an obligation to consider such a request. However, since 1 October 2011, the UK government has abolished the default compulsory retirement age of 65 years. This means that an employer can no longer compulsorily retire an employee at the previous default retirement age of 65; a policy aimed at removing work-based age discrimination. The policy should also boost the economy and people's earnings and savings at a later retirement age. (For further information about the new employment regulations and removal of the default retirement age of 65, see BIS 2011.) This point should hopefully alert a nurse that (s)he may well find herself in a position to advise elderly persons seeking employment of their right under the law.

There is limited legislation militating against age discrimination, for example the EU legislation against age discrimination in employment. Article 14 of the Human Rights Act, 1998, militates against discrimination against any person and naturally the elderly are included here. Article 8 also supports the idea of the person having a right to private family life. This is very crucial to older people who are sometimes deprived of their right to personal privacy and dignity (Whitehead and Wheeler, 2008). The Disability Discrimination Act helps older people too, since many of them are registered disabled and can draw on this Act to protect them against discrimination due to their disability. Of course younger people too can become disabled but with increasing age and frailty the elderly are more likely to suffer from major disablement.

NMC *Guidance for the Care of Older People*

As a nurse, familiarise yourself with the NMC (2009b) *Guidance for the Care of Older People*, which identifies key principles of caring for the older person against standards set out in the NMC (2008a) Code. In particular, note the NMC policy statement that requires nurses to:

* challenge negative attitudes to older people;
* promote healthy lifestyle for older people;
* value and respect older people as individuals;
* respect older people's dignity;
* show kindness and compassion towards older people;
* communicate effectively and respectfully; and
* be committed to equality and diversity.

Moreover, the NMC asks nurses to make sure they consult with older people and involve them as equal partners in decision making about their care and treatment. Within this, nurses are asked to actively challenge poor care at all levels and in all settings. As a nurse you should aim to provide compassionate and dignified care. A reflection on the statistics in Box 13.1, based on some figures provided by the NMC in 2011, should give you a realistic

---

BOX 13.1 Older people in society

Older people in society

- 2008: 20.5 million people aged over 50 years (up 690,000 since 2002).
- 2009: More pensioners in UK than children under 16.
- 2005: Royal College of Psychiatrists, predicts in next 20 years number of over-85s in England will double; number of people over 100 years old will quadruple.
- By 2050 there will be around 250,000 people aged over 100 in comparison with 2008 figure of 10,000.
- By 2031 there will be close to 27 million people aged 50 and over.

Care of older people

- 2006/7: estimated 2.5 million older people in England with some need for care/support.
- 2006: 70 per cent of those aged 75 and over have long-standing illness; 50 per cent said long-standing illnesses limit their ability to carry out daily activities.

In hospital

- Two thirds of NHS beds occupied by people aged 65 or over.
- 60 per cent of NHS patients will have pre-existing mental health problems, or develop these whilst in hospital, depression, dementia and delirium accounting for 80 per cent of these.
- 2007: 20 per cent of hospitalised older people needing help to eat said they did not get enough support.
- 2004: 20 per cent of older people (aged 50 or more) attended out-patient department or A&E three months prior to interview. Ten per cent were in-patients in the previous 12 months. The number of older people with long-term illness or disability increases with age. Just over 25 per cent of men and women aged 50–64 in Great Britain report such disability compared with two thirds of men and three quarters of women aged 85 and over in 2001.

Within care homes/the community

- End of March 2008: 373,000 places in care homes for older people.
- April 2007: 420,000 people in UK living in care homes, whilst 346,700 people in England received local authority-funded home care each week.
- Majority of older people live in the community well into later life.
- Just under three quarters of those aged 90 and over living in private households in 2001.
- 2006: 150,000 older people purchasing care at home privately; 118,000 older people were purchasing places in care homes privately.

Source: based on figures provided by the NMC (2011).

picture of the size of the challenge, to be able to plan and care adequately for older people, and the increasing trend in the number of older people who will need health and social care in years to come.

After you have done the exercise in Box 13.2 refer to Table 13.1 for some ideas of how I believe the NMC principle statements above could be achieved in practice.

Abuse: the Bournewood case

Age UK (2010a) points out that older people who lack mental capacity are particularly exposed to abuse, which may be *financial*, or *not being consulted* and *informed about medical treatment,* or *being treated without their consent*, or being admitted to and detained in hospitals without proper safeguards in respect to their human rights. You may be familiar with the case of *HL v UK* (2004) ECHR 720, otherwise known as the *Bournewood* case.

In this case the European Court of Human Rights concluded that a 49-year-old man with autism, who lacked capacity and was admitted informally to Bournewood Hospital out of 'necessity' (that is, for his own benefit, or in his *best interest*) had been deprived of his liberty. He had been an in-patient but had not been detained under the Mental Health Act (MHA) 1983. He was admitted under the common law doctrine of 'necessity' in his best interest. As he was not detained under the MHA he could not take advantage of the facilities provided by the Act, for example to seek a review of his in-patient status with the Mental Health Review Tribunal. The patient brought legal proceedings against the hospital claiming unlawful detainment. The UK High Court rejected the claim, saying he had not been detained and that any detention would have been in his best interest and so lawful under the common law doctrine of necessity. The Court of Appeal disagreed, saying that the patient had been detained and that such detention would have been lawful only under the MHA 1983. The House of Lords reversed the decision, agreeing with the original High Court decision. The case went to the European Court of Human Rights, which agreed with the Court of Appeal that the patient (Mr L) was in fact detained and that under Article 5 of the European Convention on Human Rights (ECHR) his liberty had been breached. The ECHR also ruled that Mr L's detention under the common law was incompatible with Article 5 of the ECHR because it was too arbitrary and lacked sufficient safeguards such as those allowed patients detained under the MHA 1983.

BOX 13.2 Portfolio exercise 13.1

Reflect on how you personally could work to achieve the NMC five key principles for caring for the older person. To do this just take each statement, write it out in an appropriate section of your portfolio and note beside or underneath each one what you feel you could do when caring for older people to achieve the principle statements above. Use other reading and communication/people sources as you see fit to help your reflection.

Now, write a personal reflection on what you perceive you have learned, and the extent to which you feel you have developed professionally and academically by undertaking this portfolio reflective exercise.

Table 13.1 Suggested examples of how the NMC principle statements in relation to caring for older people could be achieved

Challenge negative attitudes to older people	Assume old people's capacity, autonomy and ability to participate in care, making worthwhile contribution; assume older people's ability and need to maintain active lifestyles; promote healthcare professionals' knowledge and understanding of the aging process; promote culture of respect, acceptance of diversity, rejection of discrimination, prejudice and negative stereotyping and abuse; promote inclusion rather than social isolation, independence rather than dependency. Be knowledgeable, confident, assertive, empathetic and competent to challenge negative attitudes/stereotypes toward old people. Challenge poor practice which condones prejudice towards old people. Ensure own professional standards are above reproach in the first place, so have a powerful platform from which to challenge poor care riddled with negative attitudes, stereotypes and discrimination against old people
Promote healthy lifestyle for older people	Health educate patient about the bio-psychosocial nature of healthy living. Increase work, social and recreational opportunities and resources as appropriate. Promote independence, healthy eating, drinking, exercise and rest in good balance. Provide social and recreational resources, facilities and opportunities. Create a culture that supports the philosophy of equal opportunity and non-discrimination against elderly people. Promote appropriate recreational, occupational therapy opportunities in hospital and community social and health care settings. Undertake individual assessment of health needs, leading to appropriate treatment, including rehabilitation; disease prevention programmes
Value and respect older people as individuals	Promote a culture that respects and values individuality in terms of people's interests, needs & aspirations. Recognise individual autonomy and right to privacy, confidentiality, consent, personal space. Promote effective individual assessment; find out how the patient wants to be cared for, particular likes/dislikes. Respect fairness and dignity. Inculcate and demonstrate positive, caring, friendly attitudes to older people. Project a sense of valuing older people as valid members of the caring partnership and the wider society, having potential for active participation and control over their own lives
Respect older people's dignity	Respect the old person's personal space, privacy and individuality. Promote independence rather than helplessness. Promote the awareness amongst the staff of old people's right to a sense of personal pride and self-respect. Promote equality in the health promotion and care setting. Respect the old person's rights under the Human Rights Act 1998, especially Articles 2 (right to life), 3 (right not to be subjected to inhuman/degrading treatment), 8 (right to respect for private and family life). Promote the five UN Principles for Older Persons: *independence, participation, care, self-fulfilment, dignity*. Respect older people's right to their beliefs, freedom from exploitation, physical, psychological, financial, sexual, institutional and discriminatory abuse. Protect them from neglect
Show kindness and compassion towards older people	Be empathetic: having sense of what the patient is going through, putting yourself in the person's place, imagining how you would feel in the person's situation. Be pleasant, kind, sincere and compassionate, always willing to go the extra step to meet the person's needs without prejudice and off-handedness, caring enough to want to help to make the person's situation better. Be reliable and dependable, keeping your promises to the patient without fail, showing willingness to help amidst any major obstacles; this necessitates assessing your patient and knowing him/her well. Show kindness in your communication, e.g. not just talking clearly using appropriate vocabulary to promote understanding, but also listening effectively. Be reliable and punctual in meeting their needs. Be thorough in your care, documentation and disengagement from the therapeutic relationship when the caring partnership comes to an end

Table 13.1 (continued)

Communicate effectively and respectfully	Communicate effectively, verbally and non-verbally, using appropriate vocabulary to aid understanding and being a good listener too. Eye contact maintenance; communication aids & interpreters if necessary. Talk to patients on their physical height level as necessary; do not be in a hurry, looking at your watch whilst speaking to the patient; pay attention; correct tone of voice, not shouting at partially deaf people; simple, clear language; adequate information for informed patient decision making; using communication opportunity to make valuable observation/assessment of patient, e.g. of progress; in communication find out what the person's needs are, what is troubling him/her and how you can help; using appropriate body language, including appropriate facial, hands, eye movements. A smile can be reassuring. Make allowances for older people's possible failing sight and hearing, cognitive failure and loss of speech. Make appropriate referrals to appropriate services, e.g. to speech/language therapists, ophthalmologists, opticians. Inform patients why information about them is shared with other health professionals; respect confidentiality and right to consent. Communicate up as well as down in relation to all category of staff involved with the person's care. Give constructive honest response to patients. Address patients by their preferred title/what they would like to be called
Be committed to equality and diversity	Be prepared to care for people in appropriate diverse settings, taking into account their individual needs: caring in hospital, patient's own home, sheltered housing, hospices, prisons, care homes etc. Be non-judgemental, fair, non-discriminatory, non-prejudicial and respectful. Put the patient at the centre of care, attending to needs with appropriate urgency, to the correct standard of practice. Demonstrate expectation that patients will contribute to decision making about their care. Value patients' autonomy – e.g. right to say no, right to consent, confidentiality and respect. Meet each person's specific needs rather than treating them as a homogeneous group. Respect the diversity older people come with – e.g. different levels of education, understanding, degree of physical, social and psychological functioning, experience (e.g. of caring contexts) and capacity to look after self, different cultural and social class backgrounds, belief systems, gender differences, sexuality, race, ethnicity; making the necessary professional adjustments to bring about the best patient care outcomes. Value the criticality of an individualised approach to the old person's care amidst the array of differences just mentioned. Value, embrace and accept individual and collective differences amongst people; ensure the service is equipped to meet diverse needs of your service users but in an individual way. Do not discriminate against your patients; treat them with equal respect, right to the best available and affordable diagnostic, assessment, care planning and implementation facilities. Do not discriminate on the grounds of age, race, ethnicity, social class, gender, sexual orientation, religion, disability, ethical and philosophical beliefs

Older people's rights per se under the Human Rights Act 1998

Like any younger adult, older people have the following rights under the Human Rights Act 1998:

- Article 2, schedule 1, right to life;
- Article 3, schedule 1, right not to be tortured or subject to degrading and inhumane treatment;
- Article 8, schedule 1, right to private and family life;
- Article 9, schedule 1, right to freedom of thought, conscience and religion;

- Article 10, schedule 1, right to freedom of expression;
- Article 14, schedule 1, right not to be subjected to discrimination;
- Article 17, schedule 1, right to freedom from abuse of their human rights; and
- Article 18, schedule 1, a right to the protection of their property.

Consider them in Box 13.3.

These rights under the Human Rights Act can be invoked against the state, although in extreme situations some of them (e.g. under Articles 9 and 10) may be temporarily suspended in the interest of public peace, to stop destruction of the economy, to prevent crime and terrorism. This makes them 'qualified' rights. As a nurse you should be alert to the possibility that some of the elderly patients you care for may have lost some or all their ability to maintain their privacy and dignity and fight for other fundamental human rights. Therefore they rely on you to do this for them. Some may be confused and not too aware of their environment, restless and agitated, perhaps stripping off their clothes in public places, maybe wandering the ward and hospital corridors aimlessly and in danger of stumbling and falling, or at risk of losing their privacy and dignity. It is your duty to protect the patients, making sure they are safe and not in danger of falling, slipping on wet floors, walking along dark corridors and recesses. Make sure suitable *reality orientation* programmes are devised to help combat unawareness, disorientation and confusion when present in old people.

Some elderly patients are confused and restless because they are in a new environment; others are very restless, agitated and confused because they are in pain, and/or may be constipated, distressed, lacking social stimulation, lacking appropriate occupational and recreational stimulation and activities that are within their capability. It could be helpful for a nurse to enquire of the elderly, restless and confused patient if (s)he wishes to be taken

---

BOX 13.3 Portfolio exercise 13.2

Using your developing professional portfolio, take in turn, each of the Articles above from the Human Rights Act, and against each one write down in an appropriate section of your portfolio what you feel nursing, including yourself, can do in the practical context of caring for older people to make these articles into practical realities. To do this:

- Think about caring for elderly patients in appropriate settings of your choice and focus on each article in turn.
- Address yourself to the questions:
  - What can I do for the elderly patient to ensure my nursing care complies with this Article?
  - What have I seen happen in clinical practice that has been out of keeping with this Article?
  - What can be done to address the above weaknesses I have observed in practice?
  - Which reflective model can I use to help me reflect on how best to achieve the objectives of this Article and how do I use this model in this particular context?
  - Is there any sense in which the reflective model I have chosen and used in the present context falls short in terms of enabling me to undertake the reflection necessary?

for a little walk out in the gardens of the care home or hospital where (s)he is being cared for, provided of course his/her medical condition, state of physical fitness, and mental and psychological condition permit these therapeutic interventions. Be sure to always assess your patient carefully, working with the patient, their family and other appropriate health and social care professionals, becoming aware of any bio-psycho-social problems they have. Nurses cannot do it all! Each professional group has its limitations, and this is why the multidisciplinary team is so crucial. Nurses cannot be expert at everything and every patient need. As a nurse you need to work with other members of the multiprofessional team to address the needs of patients, taking on board their holistic needs and wishes. If your elderly patient has lost mental capacity it is not sensible to sit back expecting him/her to assert his/her rights under the various articles of the Human Rights Act. You have a legal, professional, ethical and moral obligation to think, act and advocate in the interest of the elderly confused patients.

Severe memory loss, abuse and Alzheimer's disease

Some elderly patients will be suffering from major recent and distant memory losses, from illnesses such as Alzheimer's disease, severe depression, varying states of senile dementia, or in some cases late-onset paranoid psychoses. They need constant observation and safety measures put in place. Always remember that under the Mental Capacity Act 2005, as a health professional looking after patients who have lost their capacity and mental competence, you are legally and professionally obliged to act always in the patient's best interest. You will be as shocked as I was to read below, and online, of the care assistant who, instead of feeding her confused patient suffering from Alzheimer's disease, actually sat there and consumed the patient's food herself. What food she did not want or could not eat herself she discarded in the bin, leaving her 70-year-old patient to starve. She did this not once, but repeatedly. One can only hope the court will punish her suitably to the crime, suitably to her wicked and unkind act.

Research findings of significant common forms of abuse of older people

As a student nurse, aspiring to become a qualified nurse, you must be alert to common forms of abuse that patients may face, for example physical cruelty from staff and visitors, psychological, drugs, alcohol and sexual abuse. In a study by Homer and Gilleard (1990) it was found that few patients admitted to being abused; 45 per cent of carers admitted to some form of abuse, with alcohol consumption by the carer being the most significant risk factor in physical abuse. Other significant risk factors identified by this research were previous abuse over several years, plus long-term relationships of poor-quality care. In other words, institutional poor care can become so 'institutionalised', so deeply embedded and accepted as 'normal', that it becomes unrecognisable by its perpetrators after a while. As a nurse, therefore, you must be alert and not become complacent about poor-quality care, given by you or by others. You must learn to speak out against poor quality care, however greatly the odds seem to be stocked against your doing so. You are there to champion the cause of the patient. *Whistle blow* if you have to. As Wheeler (2011) has pointed out, under the Public Interest Disclosure Act 1998, nurses can expose poor care – in fact any form of patient abuse, cruelty or illegality especially if they have pointed these out and management have failed to act. You may safely whistle blow against individuals and management. Abuse of patients is not an option, whether such abuse comes from health professionals or from informal carers, including family members. It can come from visitors too; be alert.

As alluded to above, on 24 January 2011 BBC Northern Ireland (http://www.bbc.co.uk/news/uk-northern-ireland-12264415) reported on the sad case of a 70-year-old patient with Alzheimer's disease having her daily dinners eaten by her carer, who was filmed in the act unknown to her by the patient's family. The patient's relatives had noticed for some time that their elderly relative was losing weight and looking rather thin. They were suspicious she was not being properly fed in the healthcare setting and decided to set up a secret camera to observe her care. The 54-year-old carer admitted in court to abusing the patient, eating her food and throwing away what she did not want or could not eat herself. She was found guilty of abuse and will be sentenced appropriately by the court in due course. The NHS Trust concerned – Northern Ireland's South-Eastern Health Trust – apologised to the family for the abuse. This type of unprofessional behaviour must be stamped out and you as nurses can help to do it.

Competency and the Mental Capacity Act 2005

The law asserts that older people have the capacity to make personal decisions. Yet at the same time it provides for vulnerable old people who lack the capacity to take personal healthcare decisions. For example, under the Mental Capacity Act (MCA) 2005 old people in England and Wales, like any other competent adult, are deemed to have mental competence/capacity to make personal decisions unless circumstances prove otherwise. This means that being an old person does not automatically imply a lack of capacity. So long as the older person has capacity, no other individual has a right to assume their autonomy to make decisions on their behalf.

Family and friends do not normally carry legal responsibility for their competent young adult relatives and friends, so why should they do this for an elderly competent relative or friend? An important implication here for nurses is to always assume competence on the part of the older person, until you can prove otherwise. In this way address all enquiries to the patient, in confidence, rather than assuming that because the person is elderly you talk to his/her visitor or escort instead of him/her. I have seen this disrespect played out in hospital on many occasions: nurses and doctors talking about the competent old person as though they were not present. This is not acceptable. Besides, if you address questions that should be aimed at an older person to their friends or visitors, instead of them, you are breaching their human right to confidentiality, privacy and dignity. You are also disrespecting the patient and failing to do what your code of conduct says: put the individual patient at the centre of care, respect their autonomy, privacy, dignity and right to confidentiality.

Advanced decision

The law allows a mentally competent adult to make an 'advanced decision' (AD), otherwise called, variously, a 'living will', 'advance healthcare directive', 'personal directive', 'advance directive' or 'advance decision', all interchangeable terms. Advanced decisions are instructions given by individuals specifying what actions should be taken in respect to their health and treatment in the event that they are unable to make decisions on account of illness or incapacity. Crucially, this AD must be taken when the person has capacity, otherwise it is invalid. The purpose of an AD is to indicate refusal of a particular treatment in the future should the person lack capacity. The person cannot demand the treatment option (s) he would prefer, but can rule out certain treatment options. If an elderly incompetent patient needing care has not made a living will whilst (s)he had capacity then under the MCA 2005, section 5, (s)he must have decisions made for him/her in their 'best interest'.

In the UK, planning for mental incapacity through making ADs is something many older people are reluctant to do (McDonald and Taylor, 2006), even though making ADs is encouraged (Age UK, 2010b). By contrast, in the USA up to 70 per cent of elderly people in 'community dwelling' have made ADs (Silveira *et al.*, 2010; Teno *et al.*, 2007). In the USA the popularity of ADs has grown despite debate about their effectiveness (Fagerlin and Schneider, 2004). In fact, up to the year 2007, 41 per cent of Americans had made a living will (http://en.wikipedia.org/wiki/Advance_health_care_directive).

Advanced decisions and resuscitation

A patient whilst possessing capacity may make a living will stating that (s)he does not under any circumstances, or under specified circumstances, wish to be resuscitated if the need arises. This is perfectly acceptable in law, and so, as a nurse, you must find out in good time whether the elderly person you are caring for has made such a provision for his/her future healthcare. It would be careless, reckless and incompetent to be artificially resuscitating an 85-year-old lady who had a valid AD in her nursing or medical notes that indicates very clearly that she does not wish to be resuscitated. You would have perhaps needlessly broken a few of the elderly patient's ribs, bruised parts of her body, perhaps giving her what she regards as undignified cardiac massage and mouth-to-mouth resuscitation. Always check beforehand if your patient has made a living will and exactly what it rules out. You should also remember that a 'living will' or AD is not the same as an ordinary will that the patient has made allocating her worldly goods to name benefactors. For further information on the 'resuscitation' and 'not-for-resuscitation' debate, go to the section below on 'End of life issues and the older person'.

An AD does not have to be written. It can be from the patient's lips, so long as it is witnessed, preferably by a senior member of the medical staff. However, my advice is that *written* ADs are safer and surer grounds for the nursing staff to act on. For further advice and guidance about ADs visit http://www.direct.gov.uk/en/governmentcitizensandrights/death/preparation/dg_10029683.

Common law influence

Always remember your obligation under common law to respect the competent patient's wishes to refuse treatment, food, water, medicines, blood, blood products and so on (*Re T (An adult: refusal of medical treatment)* [1992] All ER 649). However, an important point I must impress on you is the fact that an AD cannot rule out basic nursing care of an incapacitated patient; neither can it demand an illegal treatment.

Lasting power of attorney (LPA)

Having said earlier that relatives and friends do not normally assume legal responsibility for an older person, the law, under the Mental Capacity Act 2005, does provide legal instruments such as a *lasting power of attorney*, which an older person can have set up, for example by a lawyer, sign it and have it witnessed, empowering another competent adult to look after their property, possession and personal welfare when (s)he becomes unable to make such decisions for him-/herself. Whoever formally agrees to carry such a duty of care to an older person or to any person for that matter, the law will recognise as having such accountability. The person who holds the power of attorney (the *donee*) must carry out that responsibility with due diligence, acting always in the 'best interest' of the elderly person who donated the power (the *donor* of the power).

An older legal instrument known as an *enduring power of attorney (EPA)* gives delegated power only in relation to the person's property and affairs, whereas the new LPA can give delegated power relating to decisions about personal welfare, including health issues. From 1 October 2007 an EPA can no longer be set up. However, those that were in use up to this date can remain. An LPA relating to management of property and affairs empowers the donee to act even whilst the donor still possesses capacity. With respect to personal welfare the donee can act only if the donor lacks capacity.

The MCA 2005 does not apply in Scotland; instead the Scots have an equivalent Act known as the *Adults with Incapacity (Scotland) Act 2000*. Northern Ireland is currently working on equivalent legislation; you can follow its development online at http://www.northernireland.gov.uk/index.htm.

Mental capacity, autonomy and consent

The MCA defines *mental capacity* as cognitive ability to understand information, recall information when required, believe in the information, weigh it up in arriving at a decision, and communicate that decision. The decision need not be a wise one. The MCA (section 1) says that the Act operates on the following principles:

- that every adult has capacity unless proved otherwise;
- that all help must be given to the person to make decisions and such a person must not be regarded as lacking capacity until all the help given has failed;
- a person must not be regarded as unable to take decisions simple because he makes an unwise one; in other words we are all capable of making unwise decisions (so do not criticise your patient and judge him/her unfairly if his/her decision does not agree with yours or contradicts your faith and belief system);
- any decision made by others under the MCA on behalf of another must be done in the person's 'best interest';
- before the decision is taken on another's behalf, regard must be had to whether the purpose for which it is needed can be as effectively achieved in a way that is less restrictive of the person's rights and freedom of action.

Under the law the older person has autonomy: right to self-determination. As a nurse you must remember, for example, that you have no right to touch the elderly patient without his/her consent, unless under conditions such as emergencies, incapacity as in unconsciousness and the like, where you act out of necessity, in the patient's 'best interest'. So long as patients have capacity they can refuse to be hospitalised unless their situation is so grave that legal instruments such as the Mental Health Act need to be employed to stop them being dangers to themselves and others, on account of their mental state. A person suffering from a mental illness can still have mental capacity to decide what is best for him/her. However, sometimes elderly patients are unwilling to accept even a temporary transfer to hospital where they can be cared for till their rationality has returned and their safety and that of others are better assured. In these cases the health professional needs to persuade the patient to accept hospital or social care/community provisions to help him/her through his/her difficulties. When an elderly patient refuses to drink, eat or take his/her medication you have to decide if the refusal is from a position of possessing capacity or from one of mental confusion and lack of capacity. If the patient is lacking capacity, again decisions have to be made in his/her best interest.

As Wheeler (2011, p. 47) has pointed out:

> As nurses, we may feel that we want to persuade the patient to have the treatment that the best evidence indicates would benefit the patient. However, that mentally competent older person has the right to refuse treatment and cannot be forced to accept treatment simply because professional staff believe that they should.

Some practical nursing implications of ADs and LPAs

Will you as a nurse ever likely to be involved with LPS and ADs? The first point to make is that you should be aware of their existence. An AD can influence the nursing care decisions you make and take regarding a patient's care; for example see the section above on 'Advanced decisions and resuscitation'. Second, do not get into the habit of trusting verbal statements and assertions; for example, a relative or friend may just casually say in passing, 'Mrs so-and-so did make a decision that in the event of her suffering a cardiac arrest nurses should not resuscitate her.' It is always a more sound practice to find out from the competent patient if what you are being told is in fact the case. Furthermore, look in the patient's files/notes for written LPAs and ADs to confirm the verbal statements you hear. In my clinical role as a student and later as a newly qualified member of staff I recall being asked by patients to phone their lawyer or other legal representative for them, asking him/her to pay the patient a visit. I usually respond positively. I have also been asked by patients if I would write out an AD for them. As a nurse you should not get involved with such matters. Advise patients in these circumstances to get either their legal representatives or appropriate members of their family in, or ask senior administrative and managerial staff within the caring establishment to advise the patient. You may also have to guide patients' legal representatives to where they are in the hospital ward. Do not sign LPAs and ADs, or it could compromise your position and that of your employer.

Beware of fraudsters and trickery: I recall a man coming into the ward asking me if I would persuade his mother to sign a piece of paper that would allow him to sell her house and put the money into a bank for her so that when she moved into the nursing home she would have the money to pay her keep and otherwise live off. I suggested to him that if his mother was refusing to sign the paper it was probably for a good reason; I refused to get involved. A couple of days later an argument broke out on the ward between this son and the lady's eldest daughter. Why? She was in fact the patient's LPA who had the right to make such decisions in consultation with her mother, who incidentally at that point was perfectly capable of taking such decisions herself. Hence perhaps the reason she refused to accede to her son's request. She had capacity. The altercation brought home to me the fact that the lady's son was trying to dupe his mother and undermine her and her daughter with the bona fide LPA. Further information revealed that the son had recently got out of prison after serving five years for theft and fraud. He was ripe for defrauding another person; his own mother!

As I have stated in a previous paper (Wheeler, 2011, p. 50) if as a student nurse:

> you have reasons to think that your patient who lacks capacity is being abused by anyone, relatives included, it is your responsibility and professional obligation to act. You must advocate on your patient's behalf by pointing out irregularity to a senior member of staff. If . . . in doubt about the credibility of a document in the patient's notes that says [for example] this patient is not for resuscitation,... question it. All questionable documents are worth questioning.

Ethics and some realities in nursing older patients

Nurses need to remember first and foremost that their elderly patients are individuals. They have the right to what Beauchamp and Childress (2008) define as the right to:

- The ethics of *autonomy* and self-determination – being able to decide for themselves; being able to act independently, with self reliance and self power. This implies not taking away an elderly patient's ability to be independent by doing for him/her what (s)he can and would rather do for him-/herself. Do not teach what the psychologist calls 'learned helplessness'.
- The ethics of *beneficence* – to benefit from the good the nurse does for them. This implies that as nurses you are there to do things that will benefit the patient, not harm him/her.
- The ethics of practising *non-maleficence* – doing your patient no harm. Harm can be physical, psychological, social and emotional. (Reflect on how a nurse could cause any of these types of harm to their elderly patients.)
- The ethics of *justice* – being fair, non-discriminatory, non-prejudicial and respectful to your patient.

The inevitable vulnerability of the ageing person and your duty of care

It is true that because of the normal ageing process, which in time erodes all the body systems, the brain included, it is natural that elderly people are more likely to become disorientated in new care environments, for example hospitals and care homes, than younger competent adults. Nevertheless, as a nurse you must always assume competence, but at the same time be on the alert for the patient who is seriously lacking awareness, orientation and is utterly confused, such that his/her capacity is seriously undermined. Your duty then is to work with the medical staff, the family and possibly other health professionals to establish whether or not the patient is truly lacking capacity. If (s)he is, then clearly you are obliged to act in his/her best interest. Sometimes patients are so confused that they forget to eat their meals. You will need to remind them, and feed them if necessary. Do not leave food on their locker uneaten, then throw it into the swill bin when dinner time is over, pretending the patient has eaten it.

Patients have been known to be underfed and undernourished whilst in hospital. You owe it to your patient to maintain your duty of care in feeding the elderly patient who cannot feed him-/herself. By the same token, if an elderly competent patient refuses to eat, you should encourage him/her to do so, or encourage him/her to have nutrition by other routes. However, one overriding principle exists; you cannot force a mentally competent adult to eat. Even if (s)he is bent on starving him-/herself to death you cannot in law force him/her to eat. You do however have a professional obligation to find out the reason for the refusal of food. Ascertain what is troubling the patient, making him/her depressed and refusing to eat. You owe it to the patient to persuade him/her to take adequate nutrition, but you cannot force him/her to eat.

Another approach is to find out what the patient likes to eat and see if it can be provided. If you cannot persuade the patient to take in adequate nutrition, can someone else in the team do so? Would another member of staff or the patient's relative be more successful than you in persuading the patient to eat or take nutrients in other acceptable forms?

A nurse who enters into a professional caring relationship with an older patient, for example by virtue of being an employee of an NHS Trust, carries a legal, ethical and professional duty of care to that patient. You owe your patient a duty of care to safely undertake competent assessment of his/her needs, implement an appropriate plan of care to meet his/her holistic needs, cooperating and liaising as appropriate with other members of the multi-disciplinary team, including members of the patient's family.

As a nurse you have a duty of care to communicate with the patient, providing him/her with all the information necessary to help him/her make decisions relating to his/her health and wellbeing. Your commitment is to the older person, not his/her daughter or son, although as family members their interrelated and interdependency needs will have to be considered and taken into account. However the patient is your primary responsibility. If that person has lost capacity and is therefore unable to take personal decisions then the person(s) holding the lasting power of attorney can make decisions on his/her behalf, but only in his/her best interest. Under the tort of negligence, if as a nurse you carry out your duty carelessly and hurt your patient, you and your employer could be sued by the patient or his/her representative for compensation for any injury caused. The reader is referred to Chapter 7 on negligence for more information on how patients can sue for compensation.

Patients' statutory right to care

As healthcare professionals our statutory obligation to look after our patients comes mainly from the NHS Act 1977, which imposes powers and duty on NHS Trusts, and therefore on its employees (such as nurses) the obligation to provide health and social care to patients. McDonald and Taylor (2006) argue that the state's obligation to provide health and social care is based on needs, disability and mental health status. Thus, care intervention is embedded in 'the general law', which confers elderly patients' rights on them and gives nurses obligations to care for them.

Social care

Health authorities (NHS Trusts) and Local Authority care agencies have to work closely to provide social and healthcare, thus creating if possible a seamless health and social care package. The Local Authority social services are empowered by the Local Authority Social Services Act 1970. Under this Act, from time to time, to make for smooth caring operations, the government uses *statutory instruments* to effect care and changes in caring procedures easily. For example, in 2004 the Secretary of State for Health issued the *Community Care Assessment Directives* forcing Local Authorities to establish partnerships with service users and carers to effectively carry through a single assessment process in determining service users' needs. (See reference to the NSFOP above.) It is an advantage to the older person that health and social services work together because as people get older there is a greater possibility they may need both services, and clearly if both agencies work in collaboration the older person is less likely to get missed. However, nurses and social workers can do much collaboratively to ensure elderly patients are properly looked after. Nurses are in a very good position to coordinate many of the services the elderly patient is likely to need, for example, physiotherapy services, ambulance, occupational therapy, speech and language therapy in conditions such as strokes, dieticians, podiatrists and orthotists, orthodontists, ophthalmologists, dentists, orthoptists, orthopaedic surgeons, GPs in after-care situations, district/community nurses, and so on.

The elderly and consent and confidentiality

As with younger people, the law regards the older person as entitled to consent, refuse to consent and withdraw consent. Equally the law accords the elderly the right to confidentiality, privacy and dignity. Statute law (e.g. the Data Protection Act 1998; Article 8 of the Human Rights Act 1998; Access to Medical Report Act 1988) grants rights of confidentiality. Being old does not remove one's right to confidentiality, privacy and consent or refusal/withdrawal of consent. Ethically too, the elderly person is entitled to justice, autonomy, beneficence and non-maleficence. As a nurse you owe it to the older people in your care to maintain their right to confidentiality by virtue of respect for them as people, their right to autonomy, the obligations put on you by nursing code of conduct, and obligations under common and statute law principles. Your breach of an older person's confidence can be punished professionally, legally and through an employer's disciplinary code.

Under the Access to Health Records Act 1990 an elderly patient has the same right as any other adult person under Section 3(1) to demand that in certain situations their health records must not be accessed after their death. Refer to Table 12.1 to refresh your memory on the deceased's right to protection of their confidence even after their death, under the Access to Health Records Act 1990. Also see the Department of Health policy guidance online at http://www.dh.gov.uk/assetRoot/04/03/51/94/04035194.pdf.

It should never be taken that simply because a person is old (s)he has lost his/her rights with regard to consent issues, confidentiality, autonomy and self-determination, respect, dignity and privacy. Moreover some old people maintain their mental capacity right up to the point of their death. Some of them also have sharper brains than some young people. Do not take them for granted.

Court of Protection and the elderly

The MCA 2005 has set up a new *Court of Protection* empowered to take decisions with regard to people's property and finance; whereas the former Court of Protection could only make decisions regarding *property and affairs*. Where a person had not set up a LPA with provisions for the person holding the LPA to make decisions relating to serious medical treatment and accommodation, for example, the MCA 2005 makes it possible for 'independent mental capacity advocates' to be appointed if necessary.

Such a person is regarded as an *independent mental capacity advocate* with authority to report on *best interest of the patient*. An *independent mental capacity advocate* could be asked to make decisions or recommendations in respect to patients transfer from hospital to accommodation at home or in community facilities. Although nurses are not expected to do such things as sign patients' wills, or hold patients' power of attorney, they certainly have responsibility to make assessment in determining whether patients are mentally competent/have capacity. If nurses have doubt about patients' capacity then the rest of the multidisciplinary team is there to work with: senior nurses, doctors, clinical psychologists, psychiatrists, the NHS Trust's legal team, social workers, appropriate members of the family who know the patient well, and so on. On the issue of nurses being advised not to get involved in signing patients' wills, we have to recall the case of Dr Harold Shipman, who failed to observe such considerations. In fact he went so far in the wrong direction that he forged patients' wills, making himself the patient's beneficiary. A poor role model by any account, never to be emulated.

End of life issues relating to the elderly

'Do not resuscitate' (DNR) or not for resuscitation (NFR)

We would be unrealistic and naive, if not hypocritical, to cover the topic of legal issues and the older person in this book, or any other book for that matter, by just talking about the wonderful, positive and enduring aspects of ageing or being old. The fact is that we will all die at some point and it is a reality that owing to the ageing process older people are more likely to die before younger ones do. Therefore it is important to address issues such as *cardiopulmonary resuscitation* (CPR) and *not for resuscitation* (NFR), *euthanasia* and issues around *permanent vegetative state* relating to *the quality of life*. This section of the chapter addresses these issues.

Definition of CPR

First, let us define CPR. In a joint statement on CPR from the BMA, the RCN and the Resuscitation Council (RC) (UK) (RCN, Resuscitation Council (UK) and BMA, 2007), CPR is defined as 'an attempt to restore breathing (sometimes with support) and spontaneous circulation in a patient in cardiac and/or respiratory arrest'. It is invasive as it involves chess compression, attempted defibrillation with electric shocks, injection of drugs and ventilation of the lungs. During your training, especially if you are pursuing adult branch nursing, you are likely to observe or even be involved in a CPR. In my three-year psychiatric training I participated in CPRs at least four times, and in this branch of nursing the need for CRP arises comparably less often than in adult branch nursing. As a student doing general nursing (now called adult nursing) I took part in CPRs many, many times. As a staff nurse, charge nurse and senior nurse manager my involvement in CPRs has been numerous. As an adult nursing student you are bound to observe and/or be involved with CPR at some point, sooner rather than later. As a student pursuing children's, mental health and learning disability nursing you are also likely to observe and be involved with CPR. There are some complex legal and ethical issues tied into the subject of CPR; for example, who should have CPR, patients' legal and ethical rights to CPRs, who makes decisions about giving CPRs, patients' views and decision making in CPR. There has been considerable debate and much research into CPR and we look at some of this below.

Who decides?

I recall my early days as a student (in the early 1970s) when it was not unusual to find medical and senior nursing staff making almost arbitrary and subjective decisions about which elderly patient should be resuscitated in the event of a cardiopulmonary arrest. When very elderly patients were admitted (often to 'geriatric wards', where I gained some of my clinical experience during my training) and were seemingly in a poor physical and mental state of health, one of the first questions I recall the nursing staff asking the medical staff was whether the patient was for resuscitation. I recall doctors responding by asking: 'How old is the patient?' On reflection the latter question implied that some 'not-for-resuscitation' decisions were based on age only. Yet the RCN, Resuscitation Council (UK) and BMA (2007, p. 7) statement states that CPR decisions must not be prejudicial or discriminatory and 'must not be made on . . . assumptions based solely on factors such as the patient's age, disability, or on a professional's subjective view of the patient's quality of life'.

Moreover 'blanket policies' that deny CPR to groups of patients, including those in hospices and nursing homes, run counter to sound ethics and law. What is more, 'age' is also a state of mind, in the sense that one is as old as one believes and feels. Chronology of age is an objective concept that has very little meaning outside a dictionary's number-focused definition. Some people really feel 'old' when they are in their fifties and sixties, whereas some people feel relatively young in their seventies and eighties. A person you may consider old may feel far from ready to give up the ghost! 'Age' may also be a state of mind for the health professional making a decision of NFR. A person may be in his/her seventies or eighties and still feel and think relatively 'young' in his/her mind. Such people may even feel they have the physical and emotional strength to support their feeling and conceptual view of themselves. They may regard the quality of their life as good and feel they are ready to continue to live on for a long time to come. It is therefore not for health professionals to make arbitrary decisions, often based on the chronology of ageing, about whether people ought or ought not to be resuscitated. It is a fact, however, that health professionals also need to consider the quality of life of the individual being appraised, in terms of whether or not resuscitation is a questionable issue. Most important of all, the competent patient is the person with whom the issues of resuscitation should be explored, taking into account his/her medical condition, outlook, attitudes to life, quality of life and so on.

Research evidence in relation to CPR and NFR: the picture

The issue of cardiopulmonary resuscitation (CPR), especially controversies surrounding it, is widely debated and researched (Cobbe *et al.*, 1996; Willard, 2000; Costello, 2002; Laakkonen *et al.*, 2005; Vandrevala *et al.*, 2006). Most elderly patients die with 'DNR' or 'NFR' orders in place, yet global evidence demonstrates that many elderly patients across the world want to be resuscitated (Cherniack, 2002), even though they lack knowledge about the resuscitation issue and what is involved, and wish to be involved in the decision making (Pfeifer *et al.*, 1994; Rosenfeld *et al.*, 2000).

Older patients are more likely to be given 'DNR' orders than younger ones (Meyers *et al.*, 1990). Many patients prefer their physicians to initiate discussion around resuscitation and prefer to rely on the physician's judgement in the end (Agard *et al.*, 2000). Yet patients are often excluded from the decision making about CPR and their preferences are not asked for (Costello, 2002), even though the RCN, Resuscitation Council (UK) and BMA (2007) argue that 'communication and the provision of information are essential parts of good quality care' (p. 3). I advise you to visit the RCN/Resuscitation Council (UK)/BMA policy guidance on resuscitation online (http://www.resus.org.uk/pages/dnar.htm) for a comprehensive account of the policy. In a nutshell their main recommendations about grounds for CPR are summarised below:

* CPR must be based on individual assessment of patients.
* Advance care planning and early decisions about CPR in respect to those at risk of cardio-respiratory arrests are essential and part of good clinical care.
* Communication, including provision of information, is essentially part of good care.
* It is not a good practice to initiate discussion about CPR with patients not at risk of cardiopulmonary arrest.
* Where there is no explicit decisions, for example ADs, about CPR, there should be a presumption in favour of CPR.
* If CPR would not restart the heart do not attempt it.
* Where the expected benefits of CPR would be outweighed by the burden, the patient's informed views are paramount.
* If the patient lacks capacity his/her closest relative or legal representative (e.g. someone holding a relevant LPA that gives power to make such decisions) should be involved in discussions exploring the patient's wishes, feelings, beliefs and values.
* Where patients with capacity refuse CPR, or where those without capacity have valid ADs to refuse CPR, this should be respected.
* A NFR does not override clinical judgement in the unlikely event of a reversible cause of the patient's cardio-respiratory arrest that does not match the circumstances envisaged.

Background and purpose of CPR and DNR/NFR

Cardiopulmonary resuscitation came about from the need for cardiac surgeons to restart the heart during cardiac surgery, whereas the purpose of a DNR order 'is deliberately to with-hold life-saving measures when a patient's cardiac or respiratory function suddenly ceases' (Costello, 2002, p. 1). The *usefulness and efficacy* of CPR have been questioned (Mello and Jenkinson, 1998) with arguments supporting the relatively low survival rate after CPR for cardiopulmonary arrest (RCN *et al*., 2007). Other arguments raise concerns about the futil-ity of CPR given the high cost and the morality and economic wisdom of routine use of CPR particularly for elderly patients with serious co-morbidity. There is a poor survival rate after CPR (De Vos *et al*., 1999; RCN *et al*., 2007), particularly among elderly, frail, hospitalised patients (Baskett, 1990).

Since patients tend not to be consulted about CPR, especially when they are well, the reason for the CPR seems to lie somewhere in the perceived *medical beneficence*, linked to historical paternalistic attitudes of hospital doctors; although there is evidence of CPR being done to improve the quality of the patient's life (Costello, 2002). The primary goal of health-care is to benefit patients, in the process maximising benefit whilst minimising harm and risks. Prolonging life must be positively linked to the ethics of *beneficence*. However, we should not prolong life at serious costs to the patients, or where the benefits of prolonging life are eaten up by the burdens and disadvantages. So then if a treatment fails or is strongly believed to be heading for failure there cannot be justification to continue giving it or to start it respectively. In giving CPR, therefore, we must balance *value* over *disvalue, ben-efits* weighed against risks and burdens, with full consideration of valuing the individual's wishes, values, feelings and other concerns.

Nurses' and patients' position

There is evidence that suggests that many nurses are often uncomfortable and concerned about DNR/NFR orders (Payne *et al*., 2000). Moreover, health professionals per se are aware of the sensitive and distressing nature of discussions about CPR. The RCN, Resuscitation Council (UK) and BMA (2007) note that some health professionals do not find it easy to discuss CPR with patients, although this should not stop discussions involving informing patients and involving them in CPR decision making. Nurses need to be aware of the key issues surrounding the debate about CPR and NFR orders, especially as they spend more time with patients than any other health professional groups. Yet discussions about resusci-tation rarely take place in UK hospitals (Landon, 2000), because medical professionals do not want to cause patients emotional distress, and do not want to be bearers of bad news (Marik and Zaloga, 2001).

Failure to discuss the issue of CPR and NFR orders seriously undermines patients' autonomy and right to self-determination. If failure to discuss the issues is what patients are faced with in hospital, then they would be best advised to formulate living wills and discuss their wishes around CPR and NFR orders with their lawyer, their GP and their family before they become ill and are taken into hospital. On the other hand, why should nurses and doc-tors who claim to provide holistic care fail to, or be reluctant to, discuss sensitive issues with patients? Either the care is holistic, meaning full, whole or total, or it is not. There can be no compromises and half-measures. Discussions and decision making about CPR and NFR are essential to good-quality healthcare. It seems to me that we in Britain still regard certain aspects of our lives (e.g. CPR and NFR and even praying with patients) as major taboo subjects to be avoided. If we as health professionals do this we are shirking our professional responsibilities.

The Human Rights Act 1998 and CPR

Since the Human Rights Act 1998, Article 2, guarantees patients life protection, it is of concern that health professionals should not want to discuss CPR with patients. Yet Article 4 guarantees freedom from inhuman, degrading treatment. From the writer's professional experience CPR can be intrusive, degrading and belittling of human dignity, privacy and respect. If a patient has made an AD stating (s)he does not wish to have CPR and through professional unawareness and carelessness it is mistakenly given to the patient, it could be argued that such an action or omission of the patient's expressed wishes would be in contravention of Articles 4 and 8 of the Human Rights Act 1998. Why should we not want to communicate with patients on matters involving CPR and NFR when Article 10 of the Human Rights Act guarantees freedom of expression, including the right to hold opinions and to receive information? It seems to me that health professionals who fall short in carrying out this obligation lay themselves, their employers and their country wide open to legal challenges under the relevant Articles of the Human Rights Act. Indeed Article 14 guarantees freedom from discrimination in relation to the rights under the Act.

Patients' views on CPR and NFR orders

Ebrahim (2000) argues that DNR/NFR orders without patient consultation are 'barometers for unethical and inadequate care' (Costello, 2002, p. 2). Yet many patients are never consulted about these issues. Moreover, the majority of research surrounding patients' preferences in relation to *end of life* care decisions have been conducted on hospitalised patients. Therefore, little is known of the views of older healthy people. Vandrevala and colleagues (2006) articulate the *dilemmatic* nature of resuscitation decision making, citing the two reasons for the dilemma as, on the one hand, the *quality of life issues* (e.g. medical condition and fitness, mental versus physical incapacity, age and ageing and burden as to who takes the decision) versus, on the other hand, the question of *patients' loss of autonomy*. The main problem about involving other people in what is after all a very personal decision for the patient is the danger of a loss of autonomy to the patient concerned.

To summarise this section it is reasonable to state that age by itself should not be a criterion in CPR decision making. After all, age is only a chronological event in one's life and so one can have a fit old person and a very unfit, unwell and sick young person. Every older person is a unique individual, enjoying varying qualities of life, independence or dependency. Each case must be judged on its own merit. The quality of life for an older person depends on many things: degree of interaction with others or degree of loneliness, unhappiness and isolation; state of physical and mental health and well-being; financial status and monetary ability to provide for one's self, for example in terms of appropriate nutrition, quality of housing, recreation and entertainment; mental capacity and ability to make personal decisions; level and quality of bio-psycho-social support and whether one is suffering from diseases and disability; one's perception and outlook as to one's quality of life, degree of mobility, dependency and independency; and so on. All these things must be weighed up with the most important consideration, which is the patient's feeling about his/her life and especially about issues in his/her life such as CPR and NFR orders. Moreover, individuality is the singular most critical overriding factor in decisions about CPR and NFR measures. No two patients are exactly alike. To decide on CPR and a NFR order on the basis of chronological age alone is highly discriminatory, illegal, unethical and unprofessional.

Withdrawal of medical treatment in permanent vegetative state

The case of *Airedale NHS Trust v Bland* [1993] 1 All ER 821 demonstrates that medical interventions may be withdrawn when patients' prognoses are hopeless and the quality of their life equally hopeless.

The case of Tony Bland

Tony Bland, a young Liverpool football supporter survived the Hillsborough football stadium disaster of 15 April 1989. Too many fans had entered the stadium (the home of Sheffield Wednesday Football Club) and a crowd surged forward, crushing people, 96 of whom died, all Liverpool supporters. Bland survived but with brain death and having no chance of recovery. He could breathe and digest food, but could not hear, see, taste, communicate, or smell. He was described as being 'brain dead' and in a *permanent vegetative state*, facing a hopeless prognosis and a equally hopeless quality of life. He did not, however, require a ventilator. The question for the doctors and his family was whether the patient should continue to be artificially fed and watered since the care was perceived to be not benefiting him and certainly not likely to benefit him in the short or long term. His quality of life, far from improving, would actually deteriorate. The House of Lords was required to decide whether Bland's artificial feeding and watering could be stopped. The Court ruled that it was not illegal to withdraw artificial feeding and hydration as feeding and hydrating him in this way was *not in his best interest*. The court made no distinction between withdrawing food and water and other life-sustaining treatment. Withdrawal of medical intervention in cases of *permanent vegetative state* does not amount to deprivation of life under Schedule 1, Article 2 of the Human Rights Act 1998 (*An NHS Trust v M*; *An NHS Trust v H* [2001] 2 FLR 367). This case decision, however, would not preclude basic nursing care such as keeping the patient clean and comfortable until he finally dies. As a student I would ask you to read the case of *Airedale NHS Trust v Bland* [1993] 1 All ER 821. It is the all-important (landmark) English case that sets out the conditions and principles under which medical intervention may be correctly legally withdrawn without risk of prosecution or professional liability in the law of negligence.

Euthanasia

Euthanasia comes to mind when discussing such issues as *permanent vegetative states* and *prolonged suffering from intractable, painful disease processes* that many patients often endure. For these reasons I will say something here about euthanasia. The first point I wish to make is that euthanasia is sometimes referred to as 'mercy killing', which is regarded as helping someone to die in a merciful way, because of an incurable, painful condition or some other seriously debilitating illness that progressively erodes the quality of the person's life. The *Oxford Paperback Dictionary* (1979) describes euthanasia as 'the bringing about of a gentle and easy death for a person suffering from a painful incurable disease'. The second critical point I must make is that at present (March 2011) euthanasia is illegal in the UK. Therefore, should you as a nurse attempt to assist a patient to die by any means whatsoever you are committing a crime, most probably assisted murder or assisted suicide. Taking a patient's life should never be the intention or objective of any nurse. We know that sometimes some of our patients suffer from intensely intractable pain due to forms of incurable disease, for example cancer, especially of bones with metastases to other sites in the body. We must do our best to relieve their pain, cure it if possible, but as English law stands we simply cannot do anything to end the patient's life. If we end a patient's life for him/her we have committed a serious crime, most probably murder.

If you aid, abet, counsel or procure the suicide of another person you also commit a crime, punishable by a maximum of 14 years in prison [Suicide Act 1961 Section 2(1)]. It is true that as we age we move closer to death. We are also more likely in old age to suffer from serious illnesses that can take our lives, for example conditions such as strokes, heart attacks and incurable cancers. Bone cancers can and often cause intense and severe protracted and intractable pain. In these conditions I have on many occasions been faced with patients asking me to help them end their lives. It is not a pretty situation for any doctor, nurse or other health professional, or for the patient him-/herself. By reiteration, although as a health professional you must do all you can to legally and safely relieve a patient's pain, you should do nothing to end his life.

Consider the case study in Box 13.4. Interestingly, by contrast, in another case (that of Dr Bodkin Adams, in *R v Bodkin Adams* [1957] Crim LR 365) the court decided that a doctor who correctly prescribes pain relief cannot be guilty of murder if that pain relief happens to shorten the patient's life. This is because the drug would not have been prescribed with the intention to kill the patient; it just incidentally had the side effect of hastening the patient's death. There is a difference. Here is an example of how this situation could happen in reality. Morphine is one of those drugs that can be very effective against severe pain. However, as a side effect, morphine could, over time, depress the patient's respiration, thus shortening his life. Provided the primary or sole intention of giving the morphine is to control the patient's pain, and not to kill him, the health professional cannot be guilty of murder if that drug happens to hasten the patient's death. If incidentally the morphine shortens the patient's life this is not the same as deliberately trying to kill him.

Euthanasia: can a sick person legally secure his/her own death under UK law?

Under UK law no individual has a legal right to secure his/her own death. Whereas Article 2 of the Human Rights Act 1998 affirms a right to life, the House of Lords (in *Pretty v DPP* [2002] 1 All ER 1) and the European Court of Human Rights (in *Pretty v UK* [2002] 2 FCR 97) ruled that a 'right to life' does not mean a right to die by assisted suicide (Box 13.5). By implication, just as Diane Pretty's husband, Brian, could have been tried for murder had he assisted his wife, Diane, to die, so could nurses or relatives who deliberately assist patients

---

BOX 13.4 Case study

Dr Nigel Cox, a rheumatologist, was convicted of attempted murder for administering a dose of potassium chloride to a 70-year-old patient (suffering from rheumatoid arthritis, gastric ulcer and gangrene – all intensely painful conditions) after heroin failed to control his pain. Dr Cox was sentenced to one year in prison, suspended for 12 months. He faced disciplinary inquiry from his employers, Wessex Regional HA, but was luckily not sacked. The GMC's professional disciplinary committee also admonished him but did not remove him from the medical register, having taken the view that he acted in good faith.

BOX 13.5 The case of Diane Pretty

Mrs Diane Pretty, a mentally alert woman, suffered from motor neurone disease. This is a progressive, degenerative disease for which there is currently no cure. She wanted to die by a means and at a time of her choosing but was physically unable to kill herself. She petitioned the Director of Public Prosecutions (DPP) (in *Pretty v DPP* [2002] 1 All ER 1) for an undertaking that if her husband, Brian, helped her commit suicide he would not be prosecuted under sestion 2(1) of the Suicide Act 1961. (This section of the Act makes assisting suicide a criminal offence.) Not surprisingly the DPP refused. Mrs Pretty challenged the refusal in the Divisional Court and later in the House of Lords, arguing that prohibition of her suicide under English law infringed a number of her rights under Articles of the Human Rights Act. [The Act, as you may know, arose out of the European Convention on Human Rights (UCHR) and was adopted into English law in 1998, effective from October 2000.] The House of Lords dismissed her application. In other words her husband had not been granted immunity from prosecution should he assist her to die. Mrs Pretty then petitioned the ECHR in Strasbourg (*Pretty v UK* [2002]2 FCR 97). The ECHR ruled against her, saying that 'a right to life' does not mean a right to die by assisted suicide.

---

to die. At least you would be charged with assisted suicide, a criminal offence. In spite of the legal restrictions, there are cases where UK citizens who want to put an end to their own miserable lives on account of serious incapacitating illnesses have actually travelled to places outside the UK, for example the Dignitas (Euthanasia) Clinic in Switzerland, to seek euthanasia.

In the UK, nursing philosophy is still about promoting health and social welfare and not promoting euthanasia. We often refer to Virginia Henderson's definition of nursing. It reads:

> The unique function of the nurse is to assist the individual, sick or well, in the performance of those activities contributing to health or its recovery (or to peaceful death) that he would perform unaided if he had the necessary strength, will or knowledge.
>
> (Henderson, 1960, p. 15)

'Or to peaceful death' does not mean doing anything to end the patient's life, however merciful that 'anything' is. Virginia Henderson is referring to things such as making the patient comfortable, or perhaps giving them their pain-relieving drugs as medically prescribed. UK nursing philosophy embodies provision of the best quality of care regardless of age. UK nursing philosophy is also about helping the elderly patient to be comfortable and pain free when dying. This does not mean actively killing the patient, because that would be murder! I must reiterate that it is illegal to knowingly give a patient a lethal dose of morphine. Yet any patient in pain is entitled to pain relief. If that pain relief then gives rise to a life-shortening side effect such as respiratory depression, which eventually could lead to the patient's relatively early death, this is not euthanasia. Some people may disagree, arguing that this is 'passive' euthanasia. Not in my book! There is no such thing as passive euthanasia. Euthanasia is about a conscious and deliberate, active attempt to end the patient's life to relieve him/her once and for all of his/her pain and suffering. In the UK euthanasia is a criminal offence. If you give it as a nurse, it is murder. Do not do it!

Analysis of the Diane Pretty case using the Human Rights Act

How do Articles under the Human Rights Act apply to Mrs Pretty's case?

Article 2(1) provides: Everyone's right to life shall be protected by law; no one shall be deprived of his life save on an order of the court.

Diane Pretty's argument was that Article 2 protected not only her right to life but her freedom to choose whether or not to go on living. The courts disagreed.

Article 3 provides: No one shall be subject to torture, inhumane or degrading treatment/ punishment.

Diane Pretty argued that the UK government, by denying her wish, had subjected her to unfair, degrading and inhuman treatment. (In fact her disease caused her much suffering and although she wanted to kill herself she did not have the necessary physical strength to do so.) The courts did not agree with Diane Pretty's line of reasoning. In fact her disease had caused her suffering, not the British government.

Article 8 provides a right to respect for private and family life. There will be no interference with one's right to privacy by a public body, save in accordance with the law; for example for the provision of interest of national security, public safety, economic stability of the country, prevention of disorder and crime, protection of health and morals and the protection of the right of others.

Diane Pretty argued that she had a right under Article 8 to self-determination, including the right to decide where, when and how to die. The court thought Mrs Pretty had a tiny point here, but went on to say that Article 8(2) justified interference with Article 8(1) right. It agreed that it was legitimate for the criminal law to protect potentially vulnerable people by law, such as section 2(1) of the Suicide Act, which might at times affect Article 8(1) rights of some people in the same society. So once again Mrs Pretty lost out.

Article 9 provides everyone with the right to freedom of thought, conscience, religion and the right to change religion, beliefs and the like.

Diane Pretty argued for her belief in assisted suicide, which the court denied her. The ECHR disagreed, on the grounds that a belief in assisted suicide was different from a belief in, say, religion or freedom of thought and conscience.

Some implications arising from the Diane Pretty case

- Patients will from time to time suffer from diseases so crippling, disabling and painful that they may seek help from nurses to end their lives. Please do not get involved in such an illegal activity.
- If you as a nurse help a patient to commit suicide you have committed a crime under UK/English law, and could be jailed for it.
- If Diane Pretty's husband had helped to kill her he would have been charged with at least assisted suicide, or possibly murder.

Reflect on what the above means for you as a nurse.

As I have argued in a previous paper (Wheeler, 2011), nursing is about caring competently, knowledgeably, compassionately, diligently and sensitively for healthy as well as sick people, including those who are dying. This does not stretch to assisting suicide or engaging in mercy killing – or euthanasia.

Following the case of Debbie Purdy (Box 13.6), in February 2010 the DPP published a final policy statement, which has fundamentally not changed the law. It is still a crime

---

BOX 13.6 Euthanasia and assisted suicide: the case of Mrs Debbie Purdy

After the Diane Pretty case the law relating to assisted suicide still appeared unclear to some people. In October 2008 Mrs Debbie Purdy, a sufferer from progressive multiple sclerosis, brought a high court action against the DPP. She claimed that the DPP infringed her human rights by failing to clarify and make very clear the law relating to assisted suicide. Her situation was almost the same as Mrs Pretty's. She wanted the DPP to provide her with assurances that if her husband, Omar Puente, assisted her suicide, for example by escorting her to the Dignitas Clinic (in Switzerland) to die (euthanasia), he would be immune from prosecution. Mrs Purdy argued that if her husband would be prosecuted she would make the journey by herself earlier, presumably when she could travel by herself. Both the High Court and the Court of Appeal gave no clear ruling in favour of Mrs Purdy. In fact the Court argued that it was up to Parliament to change the law related to assisted suicide.

In July 2009, the House of Lords heard Mrs Purdy's appeal and unanimously backed her call for the DPP to make clear when someone might be prosecuted for helping a loved one to accept euthanasia abroad. Accepting that there was a real need for clarification, the Law Lords ordered the DPP to end the uncertainty by issuing a clear policy. (It is worth noting that around this time it became public knowledge that a number of UK citizens had been travelling abroad to secure euthanasia.)

---

to assist someone to commit suicide. Contrary to what some had hoped, the DPP policy statement has not opened the gate to euthanasia in the UK. Indeed the DPP (2010) states:

> Nothing in the policy can be taken to amount to an assurance that a person will not be prosecuted if he or she does an act that encourages or assists the suicide or the attempted suicide of another person.

Nursing implications

The NMC's policy takes the view that assisted suicide is illegal, and 'the law on assisted suicide has not changed'.

Similarly, the BMA (2010) states that:

> The law on attempted suicide has not changed. Helping or encouraging another person to end his or her life remains a criminal offence and all cases are referred to the Crown Prosecution Service [CPS].

The BMA further notes that among the DPP guidelines on the public interest factors in favour of prosecution for assisting suicide are circumstances under which the person accused of assisting suicide 'was acting in his or her capacity as a medical doctor, nurse . . . other health professional' (BMA, 2010). It is worth reading the DPP guidelines because they spell out the *discretionary power of the CPS* to prosecute or not to prosecute, taking into account all the circumstances of each individual case. It will be useful for you to read and consider the implications of some of the factors within the policy that militate against prosecution, for example:

- where the victim had a clear spontaneous decision to kill himself;
- where the suspect was wholly motivated by compassion and had reported the suicide to the police and shown a willingness to assist with police inquiries.

The published and known discretionary powers available to the DPP could influence whether or not he decides to prosecute UK citizens who escort their loved ones abroad for euthanasia. It is also worth reading the 16 factors in favour of prosecution for assisted suicide. Where suspects are found to have been paid for their involvement they stand a very high chance of being prosecuted. As a health professional you must understand that, even if the person escorted to die had a terminal illness, an incurable physical disability or severe degenerated physical illness, these will not necessarily militate against prosecution. The guidelines focus more on the motives of the suspect and less on the health status of the victim.

For ethical, moral, legal and professional reasons, it inadvisable to help, encourage, assist or in any way facilitate your patients to commit suicide, including telling them they can go abroad to end their life. It is ill-advised to tell patients what constitutes the fatal dose of a drug if you know they are contemplating suicide by drugs overdose. You should not provide them with information about how they may commit suicide. It is clear then that in the UK no one has a legal right to get another person to kill him/her even if this be for the purposes of putting the victim out of a miserable disease state. No one has the right to assist another to commit suicide.

Covert medication, the law and the older person

It is worth looking at the issue of covert medication whilst talking about care of older people, since this is where the issue is most likely to prove a problem. Covert medication means that a person has not consented to taking the medication (s)he is given. However, covert medication may be essential when nursing some people, for example to save life. Some incapacitated patients may not wish to take medication that is essential to them. The United Kingdom Central Council (UKCC, 2001) developed a policy on covert medication for nurses. In 2006 its successor, the NMC, in its A-Z Advice sheet, *Medicines Management* (NMC, 2006), confirmed the essence of the previous UKCC policy, which basically states that:

> The covert administration of medicines is only likely to be necessary or appropriate in the case of patients or clients who actively refuse medication but who are judged not to have the capacity to understand the consequences of their refusal.
>
> (UKCC, 2001, p. 5)

The policy takes the view that:

- In covert drug administration the interest of the individual patient is critical.
- Covert medication is essential for the patient's benefit, welfare and the safety of others.
- Covert medication must not be taken lightly, routinely or ritualistically, but after careful consideration and as a contingency measure, based on needs.
- The decision must be taken only after careful discussions with patients' carers, relatives and the multidisciplinary team, including the pharmacist, with whom the method of administering the medication must be agreed.
- Careful documentation and review of procedures is critical.
- Covert medication is not the 'be all and end all'; constant effort must be made to encourage the patient to take the medication.
- Written local policy on covert medication is necessary.

Exploring covert medication using the NMC (2007) policy 'Covert administration of medicines: disguising medicine in food & drinks'

For a guide to the above policy please visit the NMC website. Nurses are likely at some time to find themselves administering covert medication to older confused and mentally incompetent patients. They need to follow established protocols. As a nurse always remember your professional obligation to act always in the patient's best interest, never, as Kant says, treating people as means to an end but as ends in themselves. As the NMC (2007) covert drugs administration policy says:

> The best interests of the patient or client are paramount. The interests of the registrant, team, or organisation should not determine any decision to administer medicines.

The NMC policy acknowledges that covert administration of medicines is a complex issue that must be carefully thought through. There should be local policies in place to guide nurses. These policies should be backed by considered legal advice from Trusts' legal advisors. There needs to be a framework within every clinical setting for 'open multi-professional discussion and access to legal advice if necessary' (UKCC, 2001, p. 2). Actions from these discussions must be documented in the patient's care plan. Local policies on covert medication must be in line with the principles of the NMC Code.

Important principles about covert administration of medicines include:

- Administration of the medicine cannot be against the will of the competent adult patient who has capacity, unless such a patient is being treated legally under, say, mental health legislation, in which case such a patient can have his/her right to consent to medication suspended.
- To disguise medication for patients with capacity is to erode patients' right to informed consent, autonomy and self-determination, which epitomises deception and fraudulent nursing practice.
- With respect to patients who lack capacity, distinction should be made between those for whom no disguising is necessary because they are unaware they are being given medication, and those who would be aware if they were not deceived into thinking otherwise.
- In making a decision to participate in administering medication covertly, the registrant must make sure what (s)he does is defensible; does not erode public trust and confidence in nursing practice; acknowledges professional obligation to provide high-quality care; reflects professional responsibility and accountability; and demonstrates practice that is open and collaborative in terms of cooperation with patients, their relatives and other professionals involved in the patient's care. Ensure you do not act alone and in splendid isolation, but that you have the support of the multidisciplinary team.
- In disguising medication in food and drinks the patient/client is being led to believe (s)he is not receiving medication, when in fact (s)he is. The nurse must therefore be sure (s)he is acting in the patient's best interest, and thus can justify his/her actions.
- There are instances when administering medication against someone's will/consent/agreement is lawful, for example where patients are detained under the Mental Health Act 1983 for treatment. This context is not the same as administering medication in disguise or deception.
- High-quality record keeping is essential, demonstrating how the original decision for covert medication was arrived at, that all known risks had been considered and that alternative approaches had been weighed and balanced against all known important variables.

- The aims and objectives of administering medication covertly must be established and be clear; for example to save life, prevent deterioration or achieve improvement in the patient/client's mental and/or physical condition.
- The aims and objectives mentioned above must be taken in recognition of the patient's legal rights, for example to give, withdraw or refuse to give consent; not to be subject to inhumane, degrading treatment or torture; to privacy, dignity and confidentlality; not to be discriminated against; and of course the patient's ethical right to beneficence, non-maleficence, justice, autonomy and self-determination.
- The possibility of seeking the approval of the court must be borne in mind, where doubt exists in professional decision making and contemplated actions.
- In terms of the consent issues and the MCA 2005, in covert medication management, one must remember the following critical principles:
    - Every adult is presumed to have capacity to consent or refuse treatment, including medication unless unable to take in and retain information, understand information and weigh it up as part of their decision making.
    - Assessment of capacity is primarily the responsibility of the treating clinician, who is expected to participate in discussions about the assessment.
    - Where an adult patient is competent to give or withhold consent to treatment, no medication should be administered against their agreement, saving where the law overrides.
    - The consent must be informed by appropriate correct information about purpose, risks, side effects, possible outcomes.
    - A competent adult can refuse treatment even if to his/her peril, although no health professional should administer a drug knowing it will kill the patient.
    - To give treatment such as medicines to mentally competent people (not obliged by law to accept such treatment) is to run the very strong risk of being sued for in civil law for trespass, or in criminal law for criminal battery/trespass to the person.
    - Where patients are suspected of being incompetent to consent to medication or other forms of treatment, a comprehensive, objective assessment of their mental, physical and psychological state and need for treatment is required.
    - Before giving medications covertly or overtly it must be known whether the patient during capacity had made an advanced decision (AD) living will ruling out that therapy.
    - No one, not even a spouse, can consent for or on behalf of an adult, competent person to accept or refuse treatment including medication, although the views and of family and close friends may be sought to ascertain the patient's wishes, feelings, values and so on in arriving at decisions about his/her 'best interests'.
    - 'The administration of medicines to patients/clients who lack capacity to consent and who are unable to appreciate that they are taking medication (unconscious patients/clients, for example) should not need to be carried out covertly. If such patients/clients recover awareness, their consent should be sought at the earliest opportunity' (NMC, 2007, p. 4).

Communication and time issues: give old people extra time

One final critical piece of advice I want to give to all nurses is to always remember that older people, because of the normal ageing processes and consequential decline in mental faculties and physical condition, may be slower than younger people to absorb new information and respond appropriately. They need a little more time, patience, empathy and understanding. As a nurse you need to demonstrate sensitivity, always aiming to provide explanation in an appropriate format, for example in simple language and using appropriate audio-visual aids where necessary. Direct eye contact is critical in communication, especially when communicating with old people who may have defective faculties such as hearing, sight, smelling and feeling. Help them make adjustments as necessary for their limitations. Give them the respect they are entitled to and acknowledge their achievement in arriving at a ripe old age, something many nurses may not be able to attain. Avoid shouting at old people who are hard of hearing. Avoid startling them, for example through surprise and unannounced visits. Provide them with artificial aids if required. Advocate and champion their cause in respect to other facets of their care.

Summary and conclusion

This chapter:

- Set out to identify the extent to which UK law defines and caters for healthcare needs of older people.
- Argues that there is no specific body of law that defines older people, or advocates cut-off points at which health and social care interventions for them could be justified.
- Concludes that there is very limited human rights and employment legislation that militates against discrimination, prejudice and negative stereotypes that affect older people.
- Argues that there are deep seated age discrimination and prejudices in institutional health and social care policy provisions for older people, and that although the NSF for older people is making a difference progress is slow.
- Identifies a number of legal instruments, such as ADs/living wills and LPA, that older people can use to influence their lives in terms of, for example, ruling out certain care interventions in future. The conclusion is drawn that nurses have important roles to play in caring for older people. However, they should never compromise their position and that of the patient by, for example, signing and witnessing patients' personal legal documents.
- Concludes that age is only chronologically defined, saying nothing of significance about individuality of the older person. Therefore nursing care of the elderly must be on the basis of individual assessment and care, provided in safe legal, ethical, moral and other professional frameworks. Nurses need to work in partnership with patients/ clients, their significant others, social services, and other health and social care agencies to care effectively for older people.
- Examines euthanasia, assisted suicide, the withdrawal of treatment in permanent vegetative state and the notion of resuscitation and NFR.
- Considers the question of administering medication covertly, the debate showing that this is a very complex area of care that requires considerable analysis of the issues involved, skilled, competent and highly reasoned decision making, as well as clear local policies that acknowledge the NMC code principles, the law and ethical reasoning. Finally the conclusion was drawn that administering medication covertly must respect patients' rights, individuality and best interests.

Draw together the elements of the chapter in Student portfolio activity 13.3 (Box 13.7).

BOX 13.7 Student portfolio activity 13.3

Reflection questions

1 Use your portfolio to analyse this chapter in terms of what you think you have learned from it. Within this, discuss how you feel studying this chapter has helped your academic and professional development.
2 The Mental Capacity Act 2005 addresses the concepts of *capacity* and *incapacity*. Identify a tool which you feel nurses and others could use to assess the *mental capacity* of older patients in your care; within this, offer an argument that evaluates the credibility and validity of your chosen assessment tool.
3 Obtain a copy of the National Service Framework for older people. Select one of the standards and analyse the extent to which you believe that any of your student nurse placements has addressed this standard to the patients' benefit.
4 Identify the extent to which you feel that older patients are still being discriminated against on the basis of age. What strategies could the multiprofessional team use to outlaw discrimination based on age?
5 From your knowledge and experience, is there evidence that older people from the black and minority ethnic groups are discriminated against, more so than older people from the indigenous white population?
6 You are working in a clinical setting of your choice but specifically designated to care for mentally confused older clients/patients. As a nurse what would you do to promote favourable attitudes, a positive philosophy and the right ethical values that would benefit the older person being cared for in a social and/or healthcare setting?

Case study using a problem-based learning (PBL) portfolio approach

1 Write a short problem-focused patient scenario based on your memory of an older patient you have helped to care for (or conceptualisation of caring for an older patient if you have not had that opportunity yet). Working collaboratively with this PBL group analyse the scenario, identifying all the issues and problems within it, and draw up a plan of care to resolve the problems.
2 Write up the exercise at (1) above in your portfolio; adding to it your thoughts and feelings about your learning, growth and professional development having read and worked through this chapter.

14 Child protection
Legal, ethical and professional issues

Objectives of this chapter

After reading and working through this chapter you should be able to:

- give a legal definition of a *child* compared with an *adult*;
- define child abuse and describe different types of child abuse;
- describe how each type of child abuse may be manifested;
- discuss nurses' and other health and social care professionals' responsibilities in protecting children from child abuse;
- describe how the 1989 and 2004 Children Acts and special safeguards within the Mental Health Act (MHA) 1983 (as amended by the MHA 2007) protect children from abuse;
- discuss how the NMC code and standards for pre-registration nursing education and practice relate to nurses' role and responsibilities as advocates in safeguarding children and young people from abuse;
- use your portfolio to critically reflect on your learning in this chapter;
- identify common law cases to support discussion on child abuse;
- identify agencies that the Children Act 1989 (as amended by the 2004 Children Act) charges with the responsibility to make provisions for the care and welfare of children, including protecting them from harm;
- discuss legal, ethical and professional issues arising from the scenario in Box 14.10 below.

Introduction

As a healthcare professional you are very likely at some point to work with and care for children and young people. If you are a registered children's nurse you obviously care for children and this chapter is of particular relevance to you. As a student nurse you will at some point in your training work with and care for children and young people. It is therefore critical that you have some understanding of the law as it relates to children, particularly in respect to protecting children from abuse and neglect. I want to start by defining what the law regards as a *child* compared with an *adult*. Under English law, a *child* is a person or 'minor' under 18 years of age. (Before a child is born it has no legal identify under English law; legal identify commences with a live birth.) At 18 years and above the person has become a 'major' or an *adult*. As children are a society's future we need to take care of them and the law aims to achieve this, but only in so much as it identifies legal processes and agents with particular responsibilities in this regard; nurses have a part to play. Children are perhaps the most vulnerable group in society and every childcare professional has a responsibility to protect them. Not only do nurses have a part to play but so do many other professionals, including doctors, physiotherapists, Local Authority social care workers, the police, teachers, other healthcare professionals, organisations such as the National Society for the Prevention of Cruelty to Children, and any other organisation that deals with children. Recognition of the need to protect children has resulted (in the UK, at any rate) in over a century of legislation aimed at child protection (Batty, 2004).

NMC requirement for nurses

For a nurse, the NMC *Standards for Pre-registration Nursing Education Competencies* for entry to the register of Children's Nursing states that:

> Children's nurses must understand their role as an advocate for children, young people and their families, and work in partnership with them. They must deliver child and family-centred care; empower children and young people to express their views and preferences; and maintain and recognise their rights and best interests.
>
> (NMC, 2010a, p. 40)

In order to achieve the above NMC objectives, nurses need an understanding of law as it relates to children, particularly child welfare and protection from abuse. One would point out that the above responsibility towards children and young people is not the exclusive province of registered children's nurses or of students aspiring to registration in children's nursing, but for any registered or student nurse who comes into contact with children and young people during the course of their work. As a student nurse aspiring to become an *adult*, *learning disability* or *mental health* nurse you are likely to find yourself working with children and young people in different care settings: hospitals, children's nurseries, schools, GP practices to name a few. You have the same responsibility as the child branch student to protect and care for children and young people. In fact in its December 2007 'Guidance for Nursing Staff' document entitled *Safeguarding Children and Young People: Every Nurse's Responsibility*, the RCN makes clear that:

> This guidance is for all nurses, not just those whose work focuses on safeguarding children. Whether you work directly with children and young people or with adults whose lives impact on children, what you see – and what you do about it – can make a difference.
>
> (RCN, 2007, p. 2).

Section 1.1 of the *Field standards for competence* (see NMC, 2010a), in respect to children's nursing, states that nurses must have a clear understanding of 'the laws relating to child and parental consent, including giving and refusing consent, withdrawal of treatment and legal capacity'.

General rule of consent and specialist mental health law to protect children

We have already, in Chapter 5 on Consent, looked at consent issues in relation to children and adults, including children who have capacity within the terms of the Mental Capacity Act 2005 and the Family Law Reform Act 1969 and by being 'Gillick/Fraser' competent within the framework of the Common Law. Chapter 15 of this book on the Mental Health Act (MHA) 1983, as amended by the MHA 2007, also points out added safeguards for admission and detention of children under the MHA Act, in particular the fact that 16- and 17-year-olds 'with capacity' cannot be admitted to mental health hospital 'informally' without their consent. In fact under a new section 131(2) to (5) of the MHA 2007, a competent child (under 18) cannot be admitted 'informally' to a mental health hospital on the basis of the consent of the person with parental responsibility. This replaces the common law rule established in *Re C (Detention: Medical Treatment)* [1997] 2 FLR 180. Yet parents can still consent to their *mentally incapable* child of any age being admitted 'informally' to hospital. Under the amendments of the 1983 MHA by the 2007 Act, section 57 provides that intrusive treatments such as electro-convulsive therapy (ECT) cannot be given to any *competent* patient (i.e. patient having mental capacity) (competent children included) without their consent. Moreover, a new duty is introduced by the MHA 2007 s. 131A(2) putting obligation on hospital managers to ensure that children under 18 who are admitted to mental health hospitals, *formally* or *informally*, are placed in suitable environments, having regard to the child's age and needs. In discharging such a duty the hospital management must consult a person with suitable knowledge of cases involving children [a new section 131A(3) of the MHA 1983 as amended by the MHA 2007].

The key purpose of this chapter is to alert you to the various ways in which children and young people may be put at risk of abuse and neglect. Indeed the chapter aims to alert you to the possibility that children in your care may be abused by adults and therefore of your responsibility and obligation in relation to detecting, reporting on and helping to remove children from actual abuse or risk of it. Under the Children Act 1989 and your professional code of conduct you are expected to refer suspected cases of abuse to an appropriate authority so that the children concerned can be protected. The chapter therefore identifies legislation and other measures that are available to protect children from abuse.

The NMC states that 'Children's nurses must recognise that all children and young people have the right to be safe, enjoy life and reach their potential' (NMC, 2010a, p. 40). By knowing what the law advocates about ensuring child safety you will become more adept at helping to ensure child protection. Indeed Article 19 of the *United Nations Convention on the Rights of the Child* puts the UK government under the obligation to consider, and as required legislate to protect, the fundamental rights of children (United Nations, 1989). As a healthcare professional you have a responsibility to help children to achieve their rights. For example, in respect to children, as well as adults of course, you have a responsibility to challenge inequality, discrimination and exclusion from access to care and 'must practise in a way that recognises, respects and responds to the individuality of every child and young person' (NMC, 2010a, p. 40). Each child is an individual human being who deserves respect, inclusion and freedom from discrimination and abuse. So, apart from the MHA 2007 special safeguards of children under that Act, how does the law protect children under other Acts, example the 1989 Children Act?

Before reading what is written below about 'child abuse' and the law, see Box 14.1 for Student reflective exercise 14.1.

Child abuse and need to safeguard and protect children

The need for child protection arises because of the actual existence and potential manifestation of child abuse. So how do we define *child abuse*? What is it? The World Health Organization (WHO, 2011) defines child abuse as follows:

> Child abuse or maltreatment constitutes all forms of physical and/or emotional ill-treatment, sexual abuse, neglect or negligent treatment or commercial or other exploitation, resulting in actual or potential harm to the child's health, survival, development or dignity in the context of a relationship of responsibility, trust or power.

BOX 14.1 Student reflective exercise 14.1

Write down in a section of your portfolio what you think 'child abuse' means. Also as a nurse how would you be able to recognise child abuse?

Reflection: How does the above WHO definition compare with your own as written in your portfolio?

The National Society for the Prevention of Cruelty to Children (NSPCC, 2011a) simply defines child abuse as 'when an adult intentionally harms a child', in any of the following ways:

- *neglect*, for example parents or carers persistently failing to provide for a child's basic needs – such as food, warmth shelter, safety and access to medical attention;
- *sexual* – when a child is used sexually by an adult or young person, for example by having sex with the child, touching the child in a sexual way, or making a child look at pornographic materials;
- *physical* – includes hitting, kicking, punching, butting, burning, scalding, poisoning, drowning, smothering, or using other ways to inflict pain on that child;
- *emotional* – when we undermine a child's confidence and self-esteem, for example constantly putting him/her down, verbally, ignoring him/her, giving degrading treatment, constantly threatening and humiliating him/her;
- *domestic violence* – when a child constantly witnesses domestic violence, which can be physical, emotional, social, financial or other domination;
- *bullying*, for example name calling, threats, insults, hitting, kicking, depriving the child of his/her property.

Reflective pause

From what you know about child abuse so far, use your portfolio to record indicators that may lead you to suspect that a child in your care was the subject of abuse. Say what you would do in this situation and why. [You may wish to draw on one of the reflective models mentioned in this book, for example Gibbs (1988)].

Prevalence and incidence of child abuse and neglect

The problem is major. The exact number of child abuse cases in the UK is unknown (NSPCC, 2011b), for obvious reasons. Not all cases come to light, especially in situations where children's abusers take every opportunity to cover up their abuse and neglect of children. Some abusers do everything possible to further heap up abuse on top of abuse by threatening children with further hurt and punishment if they speak out. However, the NSPCC (2011b) reports that as at 31 March 2010 approximately 46,700 children in the UK were known to be at risk of abuse. One in four young adults (25.3%) was severely maltreated in their childhood. The UK does not publish statistics on the number of proven cases of child abuse recorded annually (NSPCC, 2011b). Even if we know the number of children on child protection registers who are subject to child protection plans, this still does not give us the real figure of the number of those who are abused, because some cases investigated will have proved to be the case, and others not. Moreover, not all cases of child abuse are reported.

Indeed child abuse and neglect are 'under-reported and under-recorded' (NSPCC, 2011b). The NSPCC also reports that, of the 46,709 children on children protection registers in the UK as at 31 March 2010, the breakdown figures per country is as follows:

- England: 39,100;
- Northern Ireland: 2,361;
- Scotland: 2,518;
- Wales: 2,730.

In order to put some significance to the above figures you may wish to work out the relative percentage for the population of child abuse in each country for a more useful comparison, since taking the raw figures by themselves, as supplied by the NSPCC, does not seem particularly useful given the huge disparity in the size of the population of the four countries cited. In any case a single incident of child abuse is one too many.

It should be apparent especially to those of you studying to become children's nurses that given the above NSPCC figures the problem of child abuse is real and should not be taken lightly. Sometimes healthcare professionals have a suspicion from a child's behaviour, appearance and what the child tells the professional that that child is being abused. If you have the slightest suspicion that a child in your care is being abused, you should bring your suspicion to the attention of a proper authority. If you are a student nurse you could discuss your suspicion with your mentor, named nurse, doctor, or another appropriate senior member of the care team. Sometimes a healthcare professional's suspicion is awakened by a less than favourable interaction observed between the child and his/her guardian. Your suspicions may prove to be founded or it may prove to be groundless, but at least you will feel satisfied that you tried to protect a vulnerable child from abuse/further abuse. It is better to be safe than sorry!

Personal reflection

I recall a child abuse case that was discovered on a paediatric ward I had worked on as a student. A very experienced paediatric ward sister had told the nursing staff of her suspicion that a particular four-year-old child could be the subject of abuse. Sister had pointed out to the nursing team evidence of what she thought were cigarette burns on the back of one of the child's hands. She also pointed out the fact that the child, on admission, looked particularly dirty and unkempt, was evidently undernourished and appeared extremely fretful. Sister's suspicion was proved correct when the child's 17-year-old mother was caught in the ward, two days later, shaking the child violently. The police and social workers were notified and the child was eventually put into protective custody and eventually made a ward of court. A less observant person than that ward sister might have missed that case. However, on reflection I think that with such conviction and almost certainty on sister's part, from her long experience and skill at making such observations (she had been correct before with reference to other cases) she could still have acted immediately to remove the possibility of the child being shaken and sustaining further injury two days later. Another sad reflection is that, with respect to child abuse by adults, little has changed in the intervening years. The relatively recent horrific child abuse cases of Victoria Climbie (Laming, 2003) and, even more recently, 'Baby P' (real name Peter Connolly), who were both killed by the adults who should have protected them are testament that little has changed in the intervening years since I was a student. The case of Victoria Climbie is described in Box 14.2.

BOX 14.2 The case of Victoria Climbie

Victoria Adjo Climbie was a black child born on 2 November 1991, in Abobo, Ivory Coast, Africa. She died in London from child abuse on 25 February 2000, aged just eight years. She was actually murdered by her guardians, her great-aunt, Marie-Therese Kouao, and her great-aunt's boyfriend, Carl Manning. Victoria had left her country of birth with Kouao, for an education in France. They travelled about France and arrived in England in April 1999. Both Kouao and her boyfriend abused Victoria, over some period of time, doing such cruel things to her as burning her with cigarettes, tying her up for periods of more than 24 hours, hitting her with wires and bike chains. Victoria's death led to a public inquiry that resulted in Lord Laming's (2003) Report, which advocated significant changes in child care protection in England.

The case of Baby P

'Baby P', real name Peter Connolly, was a 17-month-old English boy who died in London on 3 August 2007 from horrific child abuse injuries inflicted on him by his mother, her boyfriend and her boyfriend's brother. All three were convicted of causing or allowing the death of Baby P. The mother had pleaded guilty to the charge. Over an eight-month period Baby P had suffered more than 50 injuries. His post-mortem revealed that he had swallowed a tooth after being punched. Other injuries included a broken back, broken ribs, finger tips sliced off and nails pulled out.

Some sad realities emerged from this case with serious implications for child care services in this country. For example, in December 2006 a GP had noticed bruises on Baby P's face and chest. His mother was arrested and Baby P put into the care of a family friend, but returned home to his mother in January 2007. In the succeeding few months Peter was admitted to hospital twice with bruises, scratches and swelling of the side of the face. In May 2007 the mother's boyfriend was arrested for crimes related to baby Peter. In June 2007 a social worker reported to the police marks on Peter indicating abuse; a medical examination confirmed abuse. On 4 June Baby P was placed with a friend for safeguarding. On 1 August 2007 Baby P was taken by ambulance to St Ann's Hospital, in north London, after a locum paediatrician had referred him. On 3 August 2007, at about midnight Baby P died in hospital after attempts to resuscitate him failed.

From the above sketch of the case it is clear that there were many slip-ups in the case by professionals who should have better protected the child. Clearly a catalogue of errors led to his continued abuse and his eventual death, which could have been prevented. (Use your portfolio to reflect on how you think Baby P's case could have been better dealt with to stop his abuse and his eventual untimely death.)

As a nurse working with children you must be vigilant about protecting them, not of course to the point where you go around the ward or community placement deliberately and obsessively *looking for* signs of child abuse. That sort of preoccupation, though it may prove fruitful, may not be healthy for you the observer as it may lead to prejudgement, prejudices and a closed mind. However, be alert to unusual scratches and bruises and to other physical and psychological signs of child abuse such as those indicated in Boxes 14.3, 14.4, 14.5, 14.6 and 14.7.

Prejudging good parents and other child guardians could be problematic, interfering with any good relationship you as a healthcare professional may otherwise have built up with

BOX 14.3 General and principal guidance points and indicators of child abuse

You should be aware that:

- Children may be abused in family, institution or community settings by those who know them or, rarely, by a stranger (HM Government, 2006).
- Abuse may be physical, emotional, sexual, neglect, domestic violence, bullying (NSPCC, 2011a).
- Presence of just one sign may not be conclusive but calls for watchfulness.
- Children typically receive bruises at play/other physical activity, on particular parts of the body – knees, defensive hand grazes in falling, on elbows, forearms, sometimes foreheads – so not every bruise or graze indicates abuse.
- Injuries from abuse may be internal and not obvious – e.g. to eyes, brain injury, internal damage to abdominal structures, internal swelling, pain, tenderness and even vomiting. These are not always visible to the observer.
- Abusive injuries to the head may result in brain tissue oedema causing dizziness, headaches, blackouts, retinal detachment and even death; so not all abuse signs and symptoms are obvious.
- Some children are more prone to abuse than others, for example children with disablement, learning disability, hyperactivity, infants, premature infants. [Death from severe physical abuse is 10 times higher in babies than children aged one to five years (RCN, 2007)].
- All types of child abuse and neglect inflict lasting scars – physical, emotional, sexual and psychological. These can be detectable by the trained observer.
- Family and social factors may account for abuse, e.g. alcoholism, drug addiction, domestic violence, animal abuse, mental health problems, poverty, unemployment, family homelessness and gambling problems. Parents who have been abused as children stand a greater chance of abusing their own children than parents who as children were not abused/neglected.

a child and his/her parents/guardians. However, if you have the slightest suspicion a child is being abused, report it, because, whereas you may be able to rebuild a good, trusting professional relationship with the parents during the child's period of care, damage done to the child because of your carelessness and failure to be vigilant may never be able to be repaired. However, try to strike a balance between being keenly observant of children in your care, protecting them from harm, and the need to be fair and objective in your observation and reporting. Try not to make false accusations against parents. Having said this, remember that children must be protected. It would be ideal to do so within a framework that values parental and child needs. At the end of the day, however, the needs of the child in your care must take priority over the parents' as the legal guardians. Where you have good cause to believe a child is being abused by any adult, or that a child is at risk of such abuse, you must act fast.

A key UK legal cornerstone for UK child protection policies and procedures is the *Children Act 1989* (see this Act online at http://www.legislation.gov.uk/ukpga/1989/41/part/1). However, some parts of the 1989 Act were changed by the Children Act 2004,

BOX 14.4 Signs of physical abuse

- Unexplained burns, bites, bruises, broken bones, black eyes;
- child seems frightened of the parents and reluctant to go home;
- evidence of unexplained poisoning, shaking, malnourished and dehydrated states not explainable by medical illness/diseases;
- parents hitting, or slamming the child into objects, belting the child or using other physical objects such as sticks/whips to hit the child;
- fading bruises on the child after return to school following unexplained absence;
- child shrinks when adults approach, or lashes out with aggression and disruptive behaviour;
- relates injuries received at the hands of parents/guardians or some other adults;
- both child and parents offer unrealistic, unconvincing and conflicting explanations for the child's injuries;
- parents describing the child as 'evil', requiring harsh punishment;
- partially healed unexplained fractures, cuts and bruises;
- child reporting being hungry, starved, under-fed;
- parents insisting on and defending physical punishment as acceptable forms of child discipline;
- child destructive to self/others, shows fearless, extreme risk taking;
- child cheats, steals, lies;
- wears clothes that covers the whole body even in summer, without a cultural necessity to wear such clothing; covers for wounds/bruises;
- dislikes physical contact, shrinks from it, does not like to be touched;
- bald patches can be signs of intense stress at home/other places;
- expresses fear of abuser being contacted, fear of medical help.

BOX 14.5 A case of physical abuse of a baby by her young mother

R v Barraclough **[1992] 13 Cr App R.(S) 604**

In this case a young mother was given a custodial sentence of two years detention in a young offender institution, imposed upon her by the Crown Court at Leeds on 1 November 1991. She had pleaded guilty to an offence of cruelty against her own child contrary to section 1(1)(a) of the Children and Young Persons Act 1933. The young mother appealed against the sentence but it was upheld by the Appeals Court.

The court held: 'Cases of this kind engaged the consciousness of the Court, whose task on behalf of the public was to mark the wickedness of acts of violence to defenceless children by the administration of retributive justice. There were repeated acts of violence to a very small child which threatened the child's life, although the period over which they were committed was not very long. The gravity of the crime could not yield to the perceived interests of the appellant; public justice required that a sentence of this kind should be firmly and clearly upheld by the Court'.

BOX 14.6 Child sex abuse

Types of and signs/indicators of sexual abuse

Sexual abuse may involve forcing or enticing the child or young person to engage in sexual activities, including prostitution, viewing pornographic materials, whether or not the child or young person is aware of what is happening and the consequences thereof;

- physical contact including penetration of anus, vagina, mouth;
- non-penetrative acts, e.g. getting children to look at sexual acts, touching of sexual parts, encouraging children to behave in sexually inappropriate ways;
- getting or encouraging children to visit online sex sites to view sexual images or the act itself.

The problem may show up as:

- medical problems such as frequent cystitis, painful genitals, venereal diseases;
- drawing sexually explicit pictures; seductive behaviour incompatible with age; interest in sexual acts, pictures etc.;
- child being noticeably affectionate and cuddly in sexually inappropriate ways, taking into account the child's age;
- fear of a familiar person, not wanting to be alone with them; consciously avoiding them without obvious reason; this could be someone in the child's family or a baby-sitter/child minder, etc;
- expressed and physical worry and agitation at the removal of personal clothing;
- trouble walking, sitting or standing;
- reluctance to change clothing in front of others, taking into account the age of the child;
- pregnancy, especially under the age of 14 years;
- extreme behaviours such as sexual mutilation, wrist cutting, other forms of self-mutilation, suicidal behaviours, running away from home, taking drug overdoses, drug addiction, anorexia nervosa;
- personality changes, e.g. extreme introverted behaviours, insecure clinging, isolated and withdrawn behaviours;
- emotional disorders such as depression, anxiety states and poor concentration;
- regressive behaviours, e.g. return to bed wetting, thumb sucking, returning to previously abandoned teddy bears and other cuddly toys;
- oversensitive and aggressive behaviours, being unduly touchy.

Child sex abuse cases

R v MacKreth (deceased) [2009] EWCA 1849

The appellant was convicted on 23 counts of indecent assault and 10 counts of rape, committed between 23 and 27 years before his trial. His abuse was of teenage girls (in some sort of trouble) living in a residential home the appellant was in charge of. The trial judge in the trial court had rejected the appellant's application for a stay (suspension of a judgement) on the grounds of *abuse of process* (improper use of the legal process). The appellate court upheld the trial judge's rejection of stay and the conviction for indecent assault and rape was upheld (stood).

R v B [2003] EWCA (Crim) 319; [2003] 2 Cr App R 13

The appellant stood trial and was convicted for sexually abusing his stepdaughter between September 1968 and September 1972. In January 2002 an application was made *before the start of trial* that the trial should be stayed on *abuse of process* for reason of delay in bringing the case to trial. The judge refused the application. The appellant appealed on the ground that the evidence against him was unsupported and unreliable. The Court of Appeal allowed the appeal and quashed (cancelled/annulled and made void) the conviction on the grounds that the conviction was unsafe. The Court of Appeal said the trial judge was right in refusing to grant a stay. However, such applications should not normally be made before the start of trial, but at the end, all the evidence being heard. The 'best time to assess whether the process should be stayed on grounds of delay is at the end of the trial'. The appellant's case was prejudiced by delay. Given the time lapse between the offences and the trial, much happened; for example, people whom the appellant might have called on to testify had died.

which was passed on 15 November 2004. The Amending 2004 Children Act was largely a consequence of Lord Laming's Report, which came out of the Victoria Climbie inquiry (see Box 14.2). The 2004 Children Act is therefore the current basis for most UK government administrative policies designed to protect children.

The 2004 Act *aims* to improve and integrate children's services, promote early intervention and leadership, bringing different professionals together into multidisciplinary teams to achieve the best outcomes for children and their families. As you will see, whilst being powerfully centred on child protection, the 2004 Act favours professional efforts that, where possible, are aimed at *preserving the child's home and family links as far as it is possible to do so*. It puts Local Authorities at the centre, charging them with securing partners' cooperation in setting up children's trust arrangements. The 2004 Act encourages flexibility in how child care trusts are structured and operationalised to achieve a UK with better, safer child care measures for children of all ages, through:

- children-centred approaches including targeting specialist services to needs;
- early assessment and identification of children's needs, with timely and appropriate intervention;
- children keeping *healthy*, *safe*, being able to enjoy and achieve, make a *positive contribution*, as well as enjoy *economic* well-being;
- better integration of planning, commissioning and delivery of children's services;
- clearer accountability for children services through appointment of a Director of Children's Services, with a lead councillor for children's services;
- the creation of a legislative basis for better sharing of information;
- the creation of statutory Local Safeguarding Children Boards to replace non-statutory Area Child Protection Committees; and
- A Children's Commissioner for England.

BOX 14.7 Emotional abuse

This form of abuse is characterised by repeated and persistent emotional mistreatment of the child or young person, resulting to disturbance in the child's emotional development, mental health, social development and adjustments that leave permanent mental and emotional scarring. It may be recognised as follows:

- child expressing feelings of worthlessness, poor self-image, poor self-esteem and feeling of being unloved;
- being constantly tearful and emotional even over what appears to the un-abused as trite;
- evidence of a lag in physical, mental and emotional development;
- expressed feelings of being belittled by significant others such as parents, other family members and outsiders;
- sudden, unexplained speech disorders such as stammering;
- utterances of self-deprecation, words such as 'I have let everyone down', 'I am useless', 'am stupid, ugly and fat', 'am too short/too tall';
- negatively comparing self with others;
- sleeping disturbance, for example cannot get off to sleep, sleeping for short periods only, early waking and wondering of mind, screaming out in sleep from nightmares;
- overactive mind and difficulty concentrating or settling down at anything requiring concentration;
- hiding in corners and often 'sinking into the floor' when spoken to;
- self-punishment and self-deprecation, limited contact with others, refusing to give or receive hugs and kisses and other signs of affection;
- cruelty to animals, for example pets;
- extreme fear and over-reaction to little mistakes;
- utterances of 'I deserve what's happening to me';
- postural problems, for example curling up into the foetal position, rocking, head banging and other forms of neurotic behaviours.

The 2004 Act expects local authorities to achieve *cooperative partnership* working arrangements to improve children's well-being, being able to do so by establishing a range of partnership arrangements, from joint commissioning, through single service partnerships, to full integration of social care, education and health services. Hopefully the emphasis on cooperative partnerships and working will remove multiple entries on child care, where one child care agency does not speak to the other, keeping its own records in splendid isolation from those of other agencies relating to a particular child. This sort of fragmentation of important child care and child protection information largely contributed to Victoria Climbie's falling through the protective net. If there had been greater integrated working of all the child care agencies at the time, Victoria Climbie might have been alive today.

As the website http://www.surrey.gov.uk/ (Surrey County Council, 2011) points out, the 2004 Act is supported by an important strategic document for English authorities called the *Every Child Matters: Change for Children*. The document:

- stresses that there is no single integration and delivery model;
- provides an overview of the national framework for change;

- sets a framework of outcomes and aims that local authorities can use to work out their own programme to change child care services for the better, working to a national framework;
  - gives guidelines on the essential components of a children's trust and working approaches;
  - outlines requirements to achieve a Common Assessment Framework and multiagency working strategies;
  - explains the support structure the government provides; and
  - provides a timeline of statutory requirements and government expectation for local action, publication and dates for key documents.

The main measures in the 2004 Children Act are summarised below:

1. Children's Commissioner;
2. imposition of a duty on childcare agencies to *cooperate* to improve children and young people care and well being;
3. imposition of a duty to *safeguard* and *promote* children's *welfare*;
4. setting up of *new agencies' sharing databases* of information about children;
5. Local Safeguarding Children Boards;
6. children and young people *plans*;
7. Director of Children's Services and Lead member (sections 18 and 19)
8. framework for *inspection* and *joint area reviews* (sections 20–24);
9. new powers of *intervention* in *failing authorities* (section 50);
10. duty to promote *education* of *looked after children* (section 52);
11. finding out and meeting *children's wishes* (section 53).

Further information about the measures created by the 2004 Act can be found at http://www.everychildmatters.org.uk.

Law case putting child over parental needs

It must be remembered that as a childcare professional your duty and obligation are to act first and foremost in the child's best interest, for, as the landmark cases of *D v East Berkshire Community Health NHS Trust*, *Mak v Dewsbury Healthcare NHS Trust* and *RK v Oldham NHS Trust* [2005] UKHL 23 have demonstrated:

> Healthcare and other childcare professionals did not owe a common law duty to parents not to make negligent allegations of child abuse.
> (*D v East Berkshire Community Health NHS Trust; Mak v Dewsbury Healthcare NHS Trust; RK v Oldham NHS Trust* [2005] UKHL 23)

The judgement in the case of *D v East Berkshire Community Health NHS Trust & others* made it clear that a health professional's owing parents such a duty of care would amount to a *conflict of interest*; a healthcare professional is under an obligation to act in *the best interests of his/her patient*, the *child*, rather than the interests of the parent, and if the health professional was suspicious of child abuse he needed to act 'single-mindedly' in the child's best interests without regard to the possibility that a parent might sue on the basis that the health professional owed them a duty not to make unfounded allegations of child abuse. So, above all, this case demonstrates that the law will tend to be on the side of an honest, well-meaning child care professional (for example a nurse caring for a child) who genuinely believed at the time of making an allegation of child abuse that (s)he did so in the honest belief that the action was well founded. One may, however, question the ethics of a childcare professional who, maliciously and without any foundation whatever, actually goes ahead and castigates a parent, by making false allegations. Often such allegations leave indelible negative marks and suspicion. If could be argued, too, that such an allegation could permanently damage the relationship between the professional and the parent and child. On the other hand, one might take the view that it is better to speak up, if one has reasonable suspicion of child abuse, than to remain silent. (Use your portfolio to *reflect on the reasoning behind this last statement*.)

In any case, if a child is of an age at which (s)he possesses the mental competence to remember his/her interactions with his/her parents and in fact what had really happened between him/her and his/her parents with respect to a health professional's allegation that a parent was abusing a child, and the child thought that allegation to be false, then surely such an allegation would be unlikely to damage the child and his/her relationship with his/her parents. The parents may (like those in the case of *D v East Berkshire Community Health NHS Trust & others)* feel aggrieved that they have been falsely accused, but it is also likely that a good parent will in the end understand why an honest and well-meaning professional might have moved to protect their child. It is possible that a robust parent will recover from a false allegation, whereas an abused child may not recover from the abuse done to him/her. Baby P, Victoria Climbie and Maria Colwell are just three tragic examples of child abuse. As a nurse I would be inclined to operate on the basis of the decision in this landmark case of *D v East Berkshire Community Health NHS Trust & others*. The court had clearly struck down the parent's claim that the health professional had negligently diagnosed child abuse rather than the actual cause of the child's health problems, which the family claimed had disrupted their family life and caused them psychiatric damage. Moreover, this is what the House of Lords judgement in the *D v East Berkshire* case said at paragraphs 85, 86 and 87:

85. In my view the Court of Appeal reached the right conclusion on the issue arising in the present cases. Ultimately the factor which persuades me that, at common law, interference with family life does not justify according a suspected parent a higher level of protection than other suspected perpetrators is the factor conveniently labelled 'conflict of interest'. A doctor is obliged to act in the best interests of his patient. In these cases the child is his patient. The doctor is charged with the protection of the child, not with the protection of the parent. The best interests of a child and his parent normally march hand-in-hand. But when considering whether something does not feel 'quite right', a doctor must be able to act single-mindedly in the interests of the child. He ought not to have at the back of his mind an awareness that if his doubts about intentional injury or sexual abuse prove unfounded he may be exposed to claims by a distressed parent.

86. This is not to suggest doctors or other health professionals would be consciously swayed by this consideration. These professionals are surely made of sterner stuff. Doctors often owe duties to more than one person; for instance, a doctor may owe duties to his employer as well as his patient. But the seriousness of child abuse as a social problem demands that health professionals, acting in good faith in what they believe are the best interests of the child, should not be subject to potentially conflicting duties when deciding whether a child may have been abused, or when deciding whether their doubts should be communicated to others, or when deciding what further investigatory or protective steps should be taken. The duty they owe to the child in making these decisions should not be clouded by imposing a conflicting duty in favour of parents or others suspected of having abused the child.

87. This is not to say that the parents' interests should be disregarded or that the parents should be kept in the dark. The decisions being made by the health professionals closely affect the parents as well as the child. Health professionals are of course fully aware of this. They are also mindful of the importance of involving the parents in the decision-making process as fully as is compatible with the child's best interests. But it is quite a step from this to saying that the health professionals personally owe a suspected parent a duty sounding in damages.

Brief timeline of UK child protection legislation

Batty (2004) gives a nice timeline of the legal history of UK measures to protect children. The first Parliamentary statute of 1889 was a sort of 'children's charter' that was aimed at preventing child cruelty. It intervened between the child and the parent and gave the police power to arrest anyone found ill-treating a child. Under this law the police could use a warrant to enter a household if there was reasonable belief a child was in danger.

The 1894 Children Act amended the 1889 Act, allowing children to give evidence in court. It also recognised mental cruelty. It made denying children medical attention a crime. The Children Act 1908 set up juvenile courts and introduced registration of foster parents. Sexual abuse within families, for example incest, became a province of law and no longer that of ministers of religion. The 1933 Children and Young Persons Act widened the powers of juvenile courts and introduced supervision orders for children at risk.

The 1933 Children and Young Persons Act amalgamated all the then existing child protection laws. The NSPCC (2010) makes the point that, albeit one of the older pieces of legislation, the Children and Young Persons Act 1933 has parts that are still in force today; for example, it includes a list of offences against children, referred to as *Schedule One Offences*.

The Children Act 1948 set up a children's committee and a children's officer in every local authority. The Local Authority Social Services Act of 1970 unified local authority social work services, social work provision and child care services under social service departments. In 1973 a seven-year-old child, *Maria Colwell*, was killed by her stepfather (Scott, 1975). This tragedy was highly publicised and eventually led to a public inquiry. The inquiry report revealed a serious lack of coordination within child protection services. This stimulated the setting up of *Area Child Protection Committees* (ACPCs) with responsibility to coordinate all agencies responsible for the safety of at risk children. Before moving to what I call the 'giant' of child protection legislation (the 1989 Children Act, amended in parts by the 2004 Children Act), see Box 14.8 for a little more about the Maria Colwell case. Then reflect on the comparable scenario in Box 14.9.

The Children Act 1989 as updated by the 2004 Children Act

Current children protection systems have their foundation in the Children Act 1989, which was enacted to reform and clarify the plethora of laws relating to children. Indeed, the original Act indicates its purpose as:

> An Act to reform the law relating to children; to provide for local authority services for children in need and others; to amend the law with respect to children's homes, community homes, voluntary homes and voluntary organisations; to make provision with respect to fostering, child minding and day care for young children and adoption; and for connected purposes.

> (Children Act 1989, ch. 41, preamble)

BOX 14.8 The case of Maria Colwell: a critical turning point

Maria was born in March 1965 and fostered at an early age. Her foster parents reported her to be a happy, normal child (*The Times*, 23 October 1973). She returned to live with her biological mother, Pauline, on the Whitehawk council estate, Brighton. The child's biological father was no longer in the picture. Pauline was now living with a new man, William Kepple. He had children of his own and apparently looked after them well (*The Times*, 31 May 1973). He would give his own children enticing treats, for example buying them ice cream, and have Maria sit and watch them eat. How cruel! Although neighbours and teachers reported their concerns to various child protection agencies, nothing was done about the problem, and Maria was allowed to continue to live with Kepple and his own children, even though the child was by now skin and bone, 'almost a walking skeleton' (*The Times*, 11 October 1973). On the night of 6 January 1973 Maria was taken to the Royal Sussex County Hospital, Brighton, where she died from severe internal injuries, including cerebral damage.

BOX 14.9 Student reflection

As a student working in a hospital, a nursery or a community clinic you have encountered a child fitting the description of Maria at the time she lived with her mother and stepfather. What thoughts would have been running through your mind? What would you do about those thoughts? In terms of your thoughts and the resultant actions you would take, please draw on your knowledge of legal, ethical and professional considerations. Write your answer in a section of your portfolio, ensuring you include a justification in support of all the actions you feel you would take.

The Act has the following key principles:

1. *Paramount consideration of children's welfare,* meaning that the child's welfare is paramount when making decisions relating to his/her healthcare, upbringing, schooling and so on. Under the Act the court must always:
   - Ascertain the child's wishes and feelings (taking into account age and degree of understanding) and take these into account when making Orders in favour of the child. It shall not make an Order unless this is better for the child 'than making no Order at all' (section 1); taking into account:
   - The child's physical, emotional and educational needs;
   - Likely effects on him of changes in personal circumstances;
   - Age, sex, background;
   - Any harm suffered or at risk of suffering (courts not having to wait to see evidence of abuse or significant harm);
   - Capability of parents or guardians;
   - The range of powers at the court's disposal.
2. *Parental responsibility*: the Act defines parental responsibility (section 3) as 'all the rights, duties, powers, responsibilities and authority which by law a parent of a child has in relation to the child and his property'. Where the child's father and mother were married at the time of his birth they each have parental responsibility. Where they were

unmarried at the time of the child's birth, the mother shall have parental responsibility; the father shall not, unless he acquires it under provisions of this Act.

Legal, ethical and professional issues arising from Box 14.10

In considering the issues within the scenario in Box 14.10 please bear in mind that the A&E care team is a multidisciplinary one, comprising nurses, doctors, surgeons, administrators and so on. Obviously, all the clinical staff are involved in assessing newly admitted patients. There will be some assessment and treatment issues that are more or less the responsibility of certain members of the team. For example, the final decision to give a child a blood transfusion will be taken by the doctor, but that decision is inherently informed by the assessments and observations that the nurses and others have made on the patient and fed into the final decision-making process regarding whether or not the child should have a blood transfusion. Even the background laboratory scientists who test the patient's blood for its haemoglobin content and blood group to determine the blood group match for a safe blood transfusion are part of the care team. So, when reasoning what might be done in the case of the scenario issues described above, please operate on the level of principles, considering the most appropriate steps to take, not so much about which of the professionals (for example doctor or nurse) will undertake the tasks once the decision has been made. So here are my thoughts, which you are free to take issue with and challenge if you will, so long as you can offer a justification for disagreeing with my analysis of the issues in the scenario and the answers I advance with the supporting justification.

The first point I wish to make in respect to the scenario issues is legal. Section 2(1) of the Children Act 1989 as amended or modified by the 2004 Children Act tells us that where the child's mother and father were 'married to each other at the time of his birth, they shall have parental responsibility for the child'. The 2004 Act brings in a new section F2 (1A), where a child:

    a has a parent by virtue of s 42 of the Human Fertilisation & Embryology Act 2008; or

    b has a parent by virtue of s 43 of that Act and is a person to whom s 1(3) of the Family Law Reform Act 1987 applies, that child's mother and the other parent shall each have responsibility for the child.

Where a child's father and mother were

not married to each other at the time of his birth –

    a the mother shall have parental responsibility for the child [s 2(a)]

    b the father shall not have parental responsibility for the child, unless he acquires it in accordance with the provisions of this Act [s 2(b)].

The meaning of 'parental responsibility' under the 1989 Act 3(1) 'means all rights, duties, powers, responsibilities and authority which by law a parent has in relation to the child and his property'. 'Parental responsibility' also includes 'the rights, powers and duties which a guardian of a child's estate (appointed, before the commencement of s 5, to act generally) would have had in relation to the child and his property'.

Having or not having parental responsibility does not affect:

    a any obligation which he may have in relation to the child (e.g. statutory duty to maintain the child) b any rights which, in the event of the child's death, he (or any other person) may have in relation to the child's property.

Most crucially for the scenario in Box 14.10, Section 3(5) of the 1989 Act reads:

A person who –
  a Does not have parental responsibility for a particular child; but
  b Has care of the child,
May (subject to the provisions of this Act) do what is reasonable in all the circumstances of the case for the purpose of safeguarding or promoting the child's welfare. [Crucial to the obligations of the father in the Box 14.10 scenario.]

If we go to section 4 of the Act we will find some of the provisions under which a father not married to the mother of the child in question at the time of his birth can actually later acquire parental responsibility, as follows:

    4 Acquisition of parental responsibility by father:
  4(1) father shall acquire parental responsibility . . . if –
    a he becomes registered as the child's father under any of the enactments specified in subsection (1A);
- A court of law had subsequently granted the father parental responsibility;
- The father and mother may have a 'parental responsibility agreement' for the father to have parental responsibility for the child.

What does the above law mean in relation the father and child identified in Box 14.10? Let us start with the unmistakable principle, the necessity to treat the child in his/her best interest; to meet his immediate needs in this emergency context. The child may well be capable of consenting to his/her own treatment under 'Gillick/Fraser' competence. In any case healthcare professional responsibility and obligation, as well as common sense, indicate that, irrespective of the father's status regarding parental responsibility, the overriding concern is the child's care to the highest professional standard. Moreover, in respect to the father, section 3(1) of the 1989 Act tells us that a person who does not have parental responsibility but has care of the child may (subject to provisions of the Act) do 'what is reasonable in all the circumstances of the case for the purpose of safeguarding or promoting the child's welfare'. Clearly in the scenario it would be reasonable to expect even a father without parental responsibility to consent to his child having a life-saving blood transfusion.

    The man who describes himself as the child's father may well have parental responsibility and can consent to his child having the blood transfusion. Even if he has not got such a responsibility the fact that he is the current carer gives him a right to protect the interest

---

BOX 14.10 Student reflection scenario

A father who was unmarried to the mother at the time of the child's birth brings his 11-year-old child into the A&E unit, bleeding severely from a facial laceration. When the child's medical history is taken the father's matrimonial relationship to the child's mother at the time of birth comes to light. He says the child's mother is at work. Can he give consent for the child to have a blood transfusion or has he got to get the child's mother to come in and give consent? (See below for my commentary on this scenario.)

and welfare of his under-aged child. If health professionals in the context described in Box 14.10 have 'hang-ups' about parental responsibility in the heat of the moment to carry out a life-saving care intervention, then all one needs to do is to sensitively communicate with the father and son to establish parental responsibility.

Unlike the father in the appeal case of *David Moore* [1995] 16 Cr. App. R. (S)65, explained below, the dad in the above scenario had acted promptly and responsibly to get medical help for his son, which is the most crucial issue to address in the scenario. In the *Moore* case the father was found guilty of child cruelty for failing to secure immediate medical help for the burn suffered by the child through his own carelessness.

The concern of the healthcare professional in this exigency to act quickly, in the child's best interest, and moreover to save his/her life is a professional, legal, ethical and moral responsibility as well as obligation.

Reflect on your professional code of conduct, and on relevant ethical and moral principles of care in order to support the last point made.

Ethically, as healthcare professionals we owe it to the child to ensure our professional actions achieve the ethical principle of *beneficence* – in other words what we do for the child should *benefit* him/her. Our actions should not prejudice the child's chances of effective urgent treatment. Undue hesitation in giving the right care in any emergency situation is a move away from the ethical principle of *non-maleficence* – that we should do nothing to jeopardise, harm or hurt our patients. The child as a minor, who is also very ill, is unlikely to be able to exercise the ethics of *autonomy* and *self-determination*, even if (s)he is 'Gillick/ Fraser' competent. In the present context, under the Children Act 1989 (as amended) the NHS Trust to which the child has been taken for treatment has a duty to ensure (s)he gets the best treatment without undue delay.

Under Part II of the Children Act 1989 (as amended), section 27 provides for *cooperation between authorities*, where each authority means the persons in these authorities, section 27, sub-section (3), citing 'the persons' to include 'any health authority'. As nurses, doctors and other clinicians looking after the child concerned are servants of the Health Authority or NHS Trust they work for they are legally bound to protect the child, seeing to his/her health needs and welfare by giving him/her the best treatment. This includes acting urgently to save his/her life.

The second point I wish to make is that a father who takes his child into hospital on realising he needs medical care should be judged in the first place to be a responsible and caring person, unless there is evidence to the contrary. You may be thinking that he may have consciously damaged or injured the child himself, and you could be right about that. However, even if he did he has still demonstrated enough of a caring attitude to take his son for emergency care. In any case a good and discerning history and careful observation and analysis of the information being presented to the health professional by the father and his son will help that professional in determining whether there are sinister elements to this case.

Indeed standard 1 of the *National Service Framework for Children, Young People, and Maternity Services* (NSFfC,YP&MS) (DoH, 2007) lays down provisions for the acute and chronic care of children to be met, including children who suffer injuries. Health authorities working collaboratively with other services are obliged to do their part. The framework also stresses the importance of parents getting all the help and support they need in their attempt to provide the best care for their children. The father in the above scenario is trying to do just this for his 11-year-old. It is not for health authority staff to waste precious time doubting his parental status whilst the child he has brought into the accident and emergency department suffers or dies for lack of emergency treatment. The ethic of *justice* demands that we treat the child, foremost, and his father fairly and with due respect.

Professionally, the NMC (2010a) requires all nurses to play their part in 'safeguarding the public' and in doing so 'consistently deliver high quality healthcare'. Indeed the NMC (2010a) states that core principles within the (2008a) Code are about nurses *making patients' care their first concern*; *working with others to promote the health and wellbeing of service users, their families and carers*; and *providing a high standard of care at all times*. Nurses are told not to discriminate against those in their care. This includes the 11-year-old child and his father, whether or not he was married to the child's mother at the time of the child's birth. It could be argued that as a healthcare professional you are not there to judge the father; neither is the doctor there to do so. The main concern in this emergency is that the child gets the life-saving blood transfusion unless there are clinical contra-indicators. Nurses are told by the NMC to listen to service users, respond to their concerns, and 'work in partnership with people, their families and carers' (NMC, 2010a, guidance no. 15, p. 13).

Under *Competences for Children's nursing, Domain 1, Professional values,* the NMC (2010a) states that: 'All nurses must practise in a holistic, non-judgmental, caring and sensitive manner that avoids assumptions, supports social inclusion; recognises and respects individual choice; and acknowledge diversity, . . . challenge inequality, discrimination, and exclusion from access to care' (p. 40). This means that even if the child's father was single and not married to the child's mother, it would make no difference to the respectful, high standard of treatment he and his child should receive. 'Children's nurses must work in partnership with children, young people and their families to negotiate, plan and deliver child and family-centred care' (NMC, 2010a).

In the introductory chapter to this book I pointed out the fact that all health professionals have their own code of conduct. However, we noted that there are many overlapping code principles, whether we are dealing with nurses, doctors, or other therapists. Therefore, the doctors involved with the care of the 11-year-old in the above scenario should, under their code of conduct, be as concerned as you the nurse to make sure this child is given the best emergency treatment and that the father's caring role is respected. An NHS Trust cannot turn away those who turn up for emergency care. In *Cassidy v Ministry of Health* [1951] 2 KB 343, Lord Denning established the precedent that where and when a hospital holds out itself as offering hospital care the patient expects to receive the appropriate treatment.

The third point I wish to make is that an 11-year-old child who is conscious may be 'Gillick/Fraser' competent (*Gillick v West Norfolk and Wisbech AHA*) to give a good history and a good account of him-/herself, and to understand the purpose and possible effects of a proposed medical intervention. As a health professional in the present context, you should be able to ascertain from the child, if (s)he is conscious and can communicate, how (s)he acquired the injury, his/her relationship to the man who brought him/her to hospital, and whom (s)he lives with.

The fourth point I wish to make is that, since the child's mother is at work, she should be easily contactable by telephone so she could be informed of her child's admission to hospital and whether she needs to get to the hospital *urgently*. You may not wish to frighten the mother unduly by telling her on the phone that her child is critical and at death's door, and requires a blood transfusion that depends on her. However, you may want to urge her to get to the hospital as soon as possible, reassuring her at the same time that the child is being seen to by the medical staff. A mention that the child's father is with him/her may bring out some reaction from the mother that indicates whether or not everything is fine between her, her husband and the child. Be alert and observant and weigh up the information you are collecting. As a health professional you are expected to acquire the knowledge, skills, competence and correct caring attitudes to analyse simple as well as complex patient care issues quickly, efficiently and effectively.

The fifth point I wish to make is that the overriding consideration in this scenario is for you the health professional to ensure that your professional actions are in the child's *best interest*. Your clinical assessment of the child is crucial in determining the most appropriate course of treatment, so that if this child is perceived to need an emergency blood transfusion (s)he should have it without undue delay unless there are clinical contra-indicators. If the father is judged to be unable to give the necessary consent, then the mother should be urged to come to the hospital at once. If the child's condition is so critical that if the transfusion if not given at once it could lead to the child's death, then a couple of common-sense decisions could be taken. For example, two members of the medical staff could listen to a telephone consent from the mother to proceed with the transfusion. At the earliest opportunity after her arrival in the hospital the mother could be asked to formalise the consent by signing the necessary forms. This could be seen as risky as one cannot be sure one is speaking to the mother and no one else. However, the father would recognise the mother's voice. The *phone consent* may be seen as a little retrospective, but the courts will be likely to be sympathetic with the next best action taken to save the child's life. It would be important to get the mother to sign the consent form immediately she arrived in the hospital. It is a case of life or death and the child's *best interest* must be paramount.

If the child is conscious, (s)he must be informed of what the staff are about to do for him/her. A sensible 11-year-old child, though (s)he may be a little scared of a needle, can be persuaded to have the transfusion without much fuss and objection, following clear, sympathetic explanation of the life-saving nature of the blood transfusion. If the child is unconscious, the court will always take the view that the health professional, in this case, a doctor, must take action in the *unconscious patient's best interest*. Such a doctrine of 'best interest' clearly exists in this scenario.

My seventh point is this: if the father has not got parental responsibility for this child, he may well have on him a written authority from the child's mother or from a proper legal authority to make decisions of the nature of the consent needed for the blood transfusion. It has been my experience that sometimes teachers, foster parents or other child minders have parents' written permission to take their child for medical care and to make decisions such as giving consent to treatment.

My final point on the blood transfusion issue is that law court judges are very smart, clever and really practical people. They will always view a situation with care and within the context of the law, considering whether at the time of the professional healthcare decision making the decision was taken in the *child's best interest*.

The Children Act 1989 as amended by the 2004 Act also sets out rights, powers and duties of appointed *guardians* to a child and his/her estate; including powers to receive and recover in his/her own name, for the child's benefit, property to which the child is entitled. See further information below on appointment of guardians. As indicated above, the Children Act 1989 (as amended) charges local authorities and the courts to protect the welfare of children. Under section 47, Local Authorities have a duty to 'investigate' if they have reasonable suspicion a child in their area is suffering or at risk of suffering 'significant harm'. The authority must also provide 'services for children in need, their families and others' (section 17). Section 31 gives powers to the NSPCC to apply direct to the courts for an Order if it suspects a child is suffering or likely to suffer significant harm. As we have seen above the Act defines 'harm' in terms of ill-treatment and abuse [e.g. sexual, non-physical, or impairment of health (physical or mental) or development (physical, intellectual, social or behavioural)] (section 31).

What is significant harm?

'Significant' harm has not been defined by the 1989 Act. However the Act indicates to the Court that it must compare the health and development of the child with that which could be reasonably expected of a similar child. This is an example of an exercise in 'individual' assessment. This is a good assessment criterion that nurses and other health professionals can and hopefully do safely adopt. Although as a nurse you treat children from different cultural, religious, social class and ethnic groups, perhaps using measurement indicators that are culturally sensitive, at the end of the day the emphasis must be on *individual* assessment of each child.

Important guidance documents that could be helpful to the nurse

As a nurse you should know that three important *guidance documents* exist to help you and other professionals in England identify children at risk. These documents are as follows:

*   The National Institute for Health and Clinical Excellence (NICE, 2011) published *Using New NICE Guidelines on Child Maltreatment in Safeguarding Children Training*. These were first published July 2009 and may be found online at http://www.nice.org.uk.
*   *Working Together to Safeguard Children: A Guide to Interagency Working to Safeguard and Promote the Welfare of Children* (DCSF, 2010). This guide defines child abuse and neglect and guides agencies on steps to follow to make children safe. As the NSPCC (2010) points out, the guidance points to *roles* and *responsibilities* of *local safeguarding boards* and *Serious Case Reviews* (occurring after the death or serious injury of a child, as in the case of Victoria Climbie).
*   *The Framework for the Assessment of Children in Need and Their Families* (DoH, 2000). This non-statutory guidance provides professionals with a systematic direction to follow when assessing children in need and the helping approaches that should be instituted.

As a nurse you may want to look at another useful non-statutory guidance document, *What to Do if You're Worried a Child Is Being Abused* (DfES, 2006). This very important document outlines the children protection processes and systems contained within the two guidance documents (DoH, 2000; DCSF, 2010) mentioned above.

Which countries does the Children Act 1989 cover?

The Act legislates only in England and Wales. However, current guidance for Wales is set out under *Safeguarding Children: Working Together under the Children Act 2004* (Welsh Assembly Government, 2006). This may be found online at http://wales.gov.uk/topics/childrenyoungpeople/publications/safeguardingunder2004act/?lang=en.

Northern Ireland has a guidance framework under the *Children (Northern Ireland) Order 1995* (http://www.opsi.gov.uk/si1995/Uksi_19950755_en_1.htm). The Children (Scotland) Act 1995 can be found at http://www.hmso.gov/uk/acts/acts1995/Ukpga_19950036_en_1.htm.

It is to be noted that the above pieces of legislation in Scotland and Northern Ireland share the same child-safeguarding and protection principles, having their own guidance, under *Cooperating to Safeguard Children* (DHSSPS, 2003) and *Protecting Children: A Shared Responsibility: Guidance on Interagency Co-operation* (Scottish Office, 1998).

Wallace and Bunting (2007) and the NSPCC (2010) point out that, whereas Local Authorities are legally bound to investigate reports of children at risk, there is no specific mandatory or legal child abuse reporting laws in the UK that compel professionals to report their suspicion to the authorities. As a nurse, however, you have a professional, ethical and moral duty of care to give the highest standard of care to all patients in your care, and this includes children, who are amongst the most vulnerable of the service users' groups. So if in nursing a child you have reasonable ground to believe (s)he is being abused you should draw this to the attention of an appropriate authority. As a student, report the matter to your placement mentor or another senior member of staff. If you live in Northern Ireland it is an offence not to report an 'arrestable' crime to the police, and of course this group of wrongdoing includes crimes against children. There is no similar measure in England and Wales (Wallace and Bunting, 2007).

Other child protection measures set out in the Children Act 1989 as amended by the 2004 Children Act

- *Appointment of guardians*, such as court appointment of guardians, for example where the child has no parent with parental responsibilities; parental formal appointment of guardian to look after a child after death of the parent; or a guardian formally appoints another individual to look after a child in the event of his/her death.
- *Revocation and disclaimer* in respect to the appointment of guardians, meaning the appointment of guardians can be terminated.
- *Welfare reports*: under the 1989 Act (as amended by the 2004 Act) courts may seek welfare report on behalf of children under the Act, for example from a probation officer or other Local Authority professionals.
- *Residence, contact and other orders in respect to children. Residence orders* determine with whom a child will live [Part II, section 8(1) of the 1989 Act]. A *contact order* requires the person with whom the child will reside to allow the child to visit or be visited by persons named in the order, or that person and the child can otherwise have contact with each other. *Prohibited steps order* also comes under section 8(1) of the 1989 Act and means 'an order that no step which could be taken by a parent in meeting his parental responsibility for a child, and which is of a kind specified in the order, shall be taken by another person without the consent of the court'.
- *Restriction on making section 8 orders*: for instance, no court can make any section 8 order, other than residence order, with respect to a child who is in the care of a Local Authority. No application may be made by a Local Authority for a residence order or contact order and no court shall make such an order in favour of a Local Authority.
- *Power of the court to make section 8 orders*: it sets out the provisions under which the court can make section 8 orders, who may apply for the order to be made, and the timescale relating to application for orders.
- *Residence order and parental responsibility*: it sets out who will have parental responsibility in matters of residence orders.
- *Change of a child's name or removal from jurisdiction*: Part II of the Act, section 13 sets out the conditions under which a child under a residence order may or may not have his/her surname changed, and conditions under which (s)he may be removed from the jurisdiction. This means that, if a child is subject to a residence order, the person with whom (s)he resides cannot change his/her surname or remove him/her from the jurisdiction (e.g. England) without either the written consent of every person who has parental responsibility for the child or the leave of the court.
- *Orders for financial relief with respect to children*: this makes provision for financial relief for children.
- *Local authority provision of services for children in need and their families and others*: such provisions include safeguard, promotion of child and family welfare, and promoting the upbringing of the child by its family.
- *Day care for pre-school and other children*: every Local Authority shall provide day care for children in need within its area who are aged five or under and not yet attending

schools. Local Authorities may also provide facilities such as training, advice, guidance and counselling to those caring for children in day care.

- *Provision of accommodation for children*: Local Authorities must provide accommodation for children within their area who are in need of accommodation as a result of:
  - there being no person with parental responsibility for the child, for example an abandoned child or homeless children;
  - his/her being lost or abandoned;
  - trafficked children;
  - the person with parental responsibility being prevented for whatever reason from providing accommodation, for example in cases of abuse by the parents.
- General duty of Local Authority (LA) in relation to children looked after by them (Part II, section 22 of the Act).
- Cooperation between the relevant authorities to ensure child safety and welfare, for example between LA, Local Education Authority, Housing Authority, Health Authority and any person authorised by the Secretary of State for the purposes of this section of the Act. As noted earlier in this chapter, these last points are key features and requirements of the 2004 Children Act.

What is interesting, I think, is the fact that, although the above provision was made under the 1989 Children Act, we still had the situation where a child such as Victoria Climbie was ruthlessly murdered by her great-aunt and her boyfriend owing to failure in collaboration and proper working partnerships between the different services that could have saved her. The Victoria Climbie case is summarised in Box 14.2. Before (re)reading it, *please reflect on each of the protective measures of the 1998/2004 Children Acts outlined by bullet points immediately above and decide what implications if any each has for you as a nurse or other healthcare professional.*

Victoria's murder led to a public inquiry chaired by Lord Laming, hence the report of this review is referred to as the *Laming Report* (2003). What was so disturbing about the Victoria case was the catalogue of institutional failures that preceded Victoria's untimely death at the hands of her abusers, one of whom as you will have noted was Victoria's great-aunt, who to all intents and purposes was, at the time of the abuse and Victoria's death, the child's guardian. The inquiry revealed that up to Victoria's death local churches, the NHS, the police, the social services departments of four local authorities and the NSPCC all had contact with Victoria and noticed signs of abuse. Yet, as the judge in the trial case following Victoria's murder remarked, 'blinding incompetence' led to failure of all the services involved to properly investigate her situation and take appropriate protective or preventative action. Both Manning and Kouao were tried in the criminal court and found guilty of murdering Victoria. Both were sentenced to life imprisonment.

Positives that came out of the Victoria Climbie public inquiry

The report of the public inquiry seriously criticised the services involved with the care of Victoria. It noted that many opportunities to save Victoria had been missed because of poor organisation and running of many of the services and organisations involved in the child's care. Laming discussed the racial aspects surrounding the case, noting that many of the participants were black. Lord Laming made several recommendations aimed at improving child protection in England. Some of the good things that resulted from the Laming report were:

- the Every Child Matters initiative;
- the introduction of the Children Act 2004;

- the setting up of the 'Contact Point', which is a government database to accommodate information on all children in England;
- the creation of the Office of the Children's Commissioner, chaired by the Children's Commissioner for England.

Recognising child abuse and neglect

If you are astute in recognising signs of child abuse you may be the one to save the life of a child. As a nurse you should be able to identify signs of abuse and take appropriate action. The RCN (2007) writes: 'Nurses are well placed to identify children and young people who may be at risk and act to safeguard their welfare'. In addressing signs of abuse and neglect in Box 14.3, I have taken the view that as a nurse you may be working with children in settings such as schools, hospitals, social clubs, nurseries and other care settings. I would also ask you to be aware of the fact that a single sign may not be enough to confirm child abuse; a number of factors may be necessary to consider before a suspected case of child abuse can be confirmed.

Let us therefore focus on some possible family and child indicators in terms of child neglect, physical, emotional, sexually, domestic violence and bullying. Again one would point out that an individual item in any of the lists below may not be sufficient to confirm child abuse. However a combination of factors will help.

The child:

- shows sudden changes in behaviour, mood, school performance;
- has language, communication and learning difficulties, physical disabilities and learning difficulty that cannot be explained with reference to specific psychological or physical causes;
- is always quiet, jumpy, watchful as if anticipating something to happen; cowers in the presence of adults;
- is unable or reluctant to communicate his/her distress;
- is noticeably compliant, passive, withdrawn, sad or aggressive and lashes out at other children;
- shows reluctance to go home from hospital, school, church, clubs and the like;
- shows fear of adults, perhaps adopting defensive postures as though (s)he perceives (s)he is about to be hit;
- touches the parent/guardian rarely or reluctantly during visiting times;
- says (s)he does not like his/her parent/guardian; relates domestic violence in the home.

The family:

- shows a lack of interest in their child, perhaps rarely visiting their sick child;
- rarely if ever enquires about their child's recovery progress, or may even want to take the child out of the caring situation prematurely, for example before the child gets better from his/her illness;
- asks nurses and teachers to apply sharp and harsh discipline to their child;
- may have been abused as children themselves;
- sees the child as entirely useless, bad, worthless, hopeless, and a burden;
- demands exceptionally high standard of conduct, discipline and behaviour;
- demands unrealistic levels of academic and physical performance that the child cannot measure up to;

- looks to the child for attention, their emotional and physical needs, rather than giving such to the child;
- give little attention to the child, maybe in comparison with the level of attention given to other siblings in the family;
- states openly they do not like their child, or wish (s)he were as able, clever and as upstanding as other children they admire;
- rarely touch their child, both family and child rarely making eye contact with one another.

The case of physical abuse of a baby by its young mother is illustrated in Box 14.5 above. The offender in the *Barraclough* case was only 16 when she had the baby. The child was only two and a half months old when it was taken to hospital and found to have a number of serious fractures to the left femur and skull, which the court noted had been inflicted over a period of time. The baby, it seems, was some six weeks premature. As a nurse you should be aware that prematurity at birth, coupled with the factor of a young single unsupported mother, tends to increase the risk of abuse.

The two sex abuse cases in Box 14.6 are interesting because both had been brought a very long time after the alleged offences had taken place. One appellant failed at appeal whereas the other had his conviction quashed. But what is real is that child abusers can take no comfort that long years will prevent them being brought to trial if their abusers recall the abuse and have good evidence to support their claim of abuse. Once it is reported the police are obliged to investigate it.

Neglect and its manifestations

Neglect is a common form of child abuse which is often characterised by guardians/parents deliberately or unwittingly failing to provide for the child's basic needs: shelter, food, clothing, hygiene, emotional support warmth, security and supervision. It may also involve parents/guardians failing to get the child medical attention when needed, or denying the child social and psychological relationships and stimulation that are so profoundly essential for normal physical, emotional, social and psychological growth and development.

'Neglect is persistent failure to meet the child's basic physical and/or psychological needs, likely to result in the serious impairment of the child's health or development' (RCN, 2007). Severe neglect of young children can have adverse effects on their ability to form attachments, grow normally and develop intellectual skills. It can result in serious impairment of health, long-term difficulties with social functioning, relationships, educational progress, formation of positive self-esteem, and can lead to the child feeling unloved and isolated. In extreme case neglect can result in death (Daniel *et al.*, 2009; Stein *et al.*, 2009; HM Government, 2010, p. 258). For a fuller picture of the research evidence of effects of maltreatment on children's health and development see DCSF (2010).

How can we identify neglect?

Although not easy to spot, there are a few key indicators of child neglect. These include:

- child often by himself, for example on the road, no parental accompaniment;
- poor attendance or missing from school;
- consistently poor personal hygiene (e.g. offensive body odour, unwashed and matted hair, unbathed);

- unkempt, poor and dirty state of clothing, ill-fitting clothes inappropriate for the weather;
- long, filthy hair and nails;
- emaciation and other signs of poor state of health, medical problems/diseases, physical injuries for which medical help has not been sought; no immunisations received, poor dental state;
- isolation and lack of social relationships;
- scavenging behaviour, for example for food, cigarettes or toys;
- homelessness and aimless wandering, begging, stealing;
- destructive behaviour;
- sometimes a normal outward appearance as the child covers up the neglect;
- sometimes evidence of parental physical and mental disability – depression, anxiety states, mental illness, learning disability;
- alcohol and drug abuse by the child's parents impairing their ability to take proper care of the child;
- the child may expressly say (s)he is not being cared for, or that (s)he looks after him-/ herself and/or his/her parents (depending on age of child);
- child loitering at other people's houses and in public places, such as parks, playing fields, shops – anywhere where the child can scavenge food, get some attention – or playing in unsafe places;
- a vicious circle of circumstances where according to HM Government (2010, p. 258) the neglect, combined with other forms of maltreatment, leads to immediate and long-term impact of 'anxiety, depression, substance misuse, eating disorders and self-destructive behaviours, offending and anti-social behaviour';
- domestic violence in the family.

The Amina Banu and Portab Ali case (Box 14.11) is particularly interesting for a number of reasons. The victim (Shezul) whom they were convicted of starving and neglecting was not their child, although they had children of their own. Shezul was cousin to Amina Banu, who, on the death of one of her own children (Parvaz, her youngest of only six months, during a family holiday to Bangladesh) had brought Shezul back to England with her from Bangladesh, from where the couple originated. On the death of their own child whilst on holiday, Portab Ali returned to England by himself, leaving his wife, Amina Banu, in Bangladesh. Members of her family had persuaded her to bring her cousin's child, Shezul, back to England with her, possibly as substitute for the child she had just lost. Shezul, who apparently was being breast fed by his natural mother, did not bond with Amina. In March

---

BOX 14.11 A child neglect case

Case of *R v Banu* [1995] 16 Cr App R (S) 656

In this case the convicts (Amina Banu and Portab Ali) pleaded guilty (at Snaresbrook Crown Court, 1 June 1994) to wilfully neglecting a child (Shezul) for a period of about four months, but denied physically attacking the child. Their offence came under section 1(1)(a) of the Children & Young Persons Act 1933. They were both sentenced to three years' imprisonment, appealed and lost the appeal. The court held that the child had been starved and neglected.

1993 a social worker visited the family's accommodation. Thinking Shezul was Parvaz, she found him in a very neglected state, with a black eye, a badly bruised right ear, swollen mouth and skin lesions. He was listless and unresponsive. Amina kept up the pretence that Shezul was Parvaz and claimed the older children had pushed him into a sewing machine. The family's other two children were not neglected.

Shezul was taken to hospital on a number of occasions by a social worker. He was found to have 'numerous fractures' and to have been neglected over a long period of time. It is interesting to note that on the first occasion of Shezul's visit to hospital the doctors who examined him had unfortunately concluded that his injuries were consistent with the 'parental' explanation. Child abuse can sometimes be difficult to diagnose. In the present case the medical staff had missed an opportunity to diagnose abuse and so he was sent home to his tormentors. A missed opportunity that condemned the poor child to further abuse and neglect. The appeal judgement records that no radiography or close examination of the state of Shezul's limbs or skeleton had been performed. Noticeably, though, Shezul was found to be dirty and lethargic. With increasing cause for concern the social worker took him back to hospital some time later. On this occasion a more thorough examination and radiography revealed fractures to his skull, ribs, hands, legs and right foot, no fewer than 14 fractures in total. 'He had clearly suffered severe neglect and physical abuse for a long time', with the consultant who examined him saying it was the worst case he had seen in 10 years. It was hardly surprising therefore that at their appeal hearing the couple's conviction and sentence of three years' imprisonment stood.

As a nurse, you must be alert to unexplained bruises, black eyes and other signs of overt swelling on children's bodies. Even well-explained signs of injuries may not be what they seem. Some parents can be very plausible and convincing in their explanations of their children's injuries. If you have reason to think a particular injury is not accidental, you must bring your observation to the attention of a senior member of staff. You should also write your observation in the patient's records. Your astute and acute observation may get a child removed from the source of abuse and may even save his/her life.

It may help to reinforce your learning about the nature of this particular type of child abuse and to alert you to what could happen to a child if I draw your attention to some critical, carefully considered and weighed remarks of the trial judge in this case. At p. 4A the judge said:

> It seems clear to me that whilst that child was under their care, neither had any affection for this young helpless child. . . . He lost weight because he was not being fed adequately. That was one aspect of gross neglect . . . it lasted over a period of months.

At p. 9A the judge said:

> There are three different aspects of the wilful neglect in this particular case; one, the omission to feed the child adequately, resulting in its deteriorating health and . . . loss of weight, its visible lethargy and weakness; secondly, the deliberate omission to consult the social workers and the doctors with its aggravating feature of the social worker on occasion being fobbed off by the wife; and thirdly, the neglect which resulted in, whatever their cause, these appalling fractures to the body of this young child. That means that this child suffered appallingly, sustained appalling injuries as a result of appalling neglect.

There are other notable examples of parents being convicted of cruelty to children. In the appeal case of *Paul John Cameron and Jacqueline Rosemary Senior* [2000] 2 Cr. App.

R.(S) both appellants had earlier (on 12 July 1999) been convicted in Leeds Crown Court on three counts of cruelty to children. They had left the children at home unsupervised from 3.30 p.m. to 9.30 p.m., during which time the oldest, a 13-year-old, had consumed the drug, methadone, belonging to the first appellant, who was a drug addict. The child died from taking the methadone. Both appealed against the length of their 12-month prison sentence, but lost the appeal. They court said that the length of sentence was not excessive.

From the point of view of a healthcare professional you may find the appeal case of *David William Moore* [1995] 16 Cr. App.R.(S) of great interest since it involves an appeal against the length of sentence for cruelty to a child through failure to secure medical treatment for a child following an accident. At the Crown Court in Bury St Edmunds on 24 January 1994 the appellant, David Moore, had pleaded guilty to cruelty to his own three-year-old son, having failed to secure medical help for the child after he had sustained a painful burn from an iron the appellant had used to iron a shirt. He was sentenced to six months' imprisonment. Would the Court of Appeal (Criminal Division) reduce the length of his sentence?

> Held: (considering [the appeal case of] Gerald (1987) 9 Cr. App. R. (S) 425) the appellant had waited for a long period of time facing far more serious charges than that to which he had pleaded guilty. If the sentence had been passed reasonably soon after the offence, it would have been incontrovertible, but in the circumstances the Court would substitute a sentence of four months.

In the above case the appellant was very lucky to have his sentence reduced from six to four months because, although the charge he pleaded guilty to was indeed serious (failure to secure medical treatment for a child), his delay in seeking medical treatment could have resulted in very serious consequences of the initial injury, for example the death of the child, resulting in even more serious charges, such as manslaughter, having a far more severe sentence.

It may interest you to read the appeal decision to see some of the mitigating factors on the side of the appellant that the court took into account in reducing the length of sentence: for example, it was an accidental superficial burn but nevertheless a very painful one; the father pleaded guilty to the offence at the trial court rather than denying the truth and telling lies and consequently wasting police and court time; the father was remorseful over his action not to seek medical help for a small child earlier; the father had not served a previous custodial sentence even though he had some previous antecedent convictions but 'mainly for motoring offences'; he had two young sons and, although he had since parted with the child's mother, he still had regular supervised access to the victim and there was no malice between them; he was employed and had been trying to put his life together with some success; he had given up drink and had a new supportive girlfriend; the report from the prison he had been held in indicated his general attitude had been good, as was his behaviour. It goes to show how far the court will go to take into account things such as pre-sentencing reports on behalf of a person found guilty of a crime, dependent on the nature of the crime, of course. At the heart of this case, however, was the issue of a father failing to get his child prompt medical attention.

Implications of the above case for nurses

Reflect on what you see in the above case as the implications for nursing/nurses of a father failing to act quickly to protect a child and get him/her speedy treatment following the father's own blunder. Write down your reflective thoughts in the law and ethics section of your professional development portfolio.

My own reflective thoughts are that the case reminds me of the many occasions when I have been teaching student nurses law and ethics and have said to them: if you are caring for a patient and find that you have made a mistake that has injured the patient, or has the potential to cause him injury, please own up at once so that the patient can be seen to and the matter put right. If you delay in getting help for a negligent act on your part, not only could your patient suffer acutely unnecessarily, but failure to address the mistake with due haste could cost a patient his/her life. Also, without speedy action on your part, what might have otherwise only amounted to a negligent act may well progress from a case in the tort of negligence to a more serious case of 'gross negligence' and therefore to a serious crime punishable by the criminal court. Try to reflect on the case of *R v (Dr) Adomaka* and see if there are any parallels.

What do I do if a child tells me (s)he is being abused?

This is not the easiest of problems to handle. It is even more difficult to handle if the health-care professional listening to the complaint has him-/herself been abused in childhood. Child abuse stories can cause some health professionals to become very emotional, even tearful. As a lecturer with pastoral responsibilities for undergraduate nursing students, I have on a number on occasions had to refer personal tutees to the counselling services when they have reported experiencing distress as patients relate childhood experience of abuse to them, coming as it were on top of their own experience of abuse in their childhood.

If a child tells you (s)he is/has been abused, try the suggestions below. You can use these whether you are a nurse or other health professional working with children in a hospital or in the community, or you have been approached on the road, in the shopping centre, a school, wherever the child chooses to talk to you. If you are a student nurse as opposed to being a qualified registered nurse you will need to adapt my suggested approach to fit your status, because as a student working under the direction of a mentor within a placement you will be expected to seek guidance from your mentor/supervisor. As a registered nurse practising in your own right you have more leeway in how much you can do on your own before referring to others, such as the doctor or consultant in charge of the patient, the senior nursing hierarchy, or other managers in charge of your organisation. Adapt the suggested approach below to the context:

- Be pleasant and calm and look interested in what the child has to say to you;.
- Tell him/her you would be pleased to hear the rest of what (s)he has to say and will endeavour to help him/her as best you can.
- If appropriate find a place where you can both talk uninterrupted, always demonstrating sympathy with the child and offering reassurance.
- Use positive body language, smile and nod your head in the right places so the child can be reassured you are really an interested listener who wants to help.
- Avoid looking distressed and worried about what the child tells you.
- Whilst demonstrating a relaxed body posture, get down to the child's height/level so you can engage him/her further with eye-to-eye contact.
- Demonstrate belief in what (s)he tells you.
- Maintaining eye contact and never looking at your watch to indicate you are in a hurry will be reassuring.
- Reassure the child your are pleased (s)he considered you a friend to tell you of his/her problems.
- Reassure him/her (s)he has done nothing to deserve the bad treatment and that it is the abuser who is at fault and has a problem, which (s)he is probably taking out on him/her.

- Tell the child you would like to help him/her but avoid making firm promises that you will be unable to keep later. In any case try to get him/her to trust you; that way (s)he is likely to reveal more than if (s)he did not have any trust in you. Avoid giving the impression or promising to keep what is told to you as a secret, because in the child's best interest and perhaps even that of other children/siblings, you may have to report to a proper authority the abuse reported.

- Be aware, though, that the child may first ask you to agree not to relate what (s)he tells you to anyone else. Be sure not to commit to this, but at the same time demonstrate sympathy and understanding.

- Be aware that sometimes children do not wish to repeat to a third party, for example other officials such as child care protection personnel, what they have told you. For this reason, you may have to indicate to the child that to be able to help him/her (s)he may need to tell his/her story to whoever you have managed to identify as the next professional to deal with the case and get him/her the help (s)he needs.

- You should also be aware that should a court case arise out of the abuse story the child tells you and some parent is put in the dock to answer for the abuse, the defence barrister could be quick to claim on behalf of the accused (the abuser) (s)he is defending that the child's complaint has been a rehearsed story based on fiction and that you may have played a part in making up or exaggerating the story. You could even be accused in court of encouraging the child to make a false allegation. You should therefore be able to stand your ground and testify to what the child told you. Following the meeting with the child, good note making and accurate record keeping of what the child told you is important.

- Reassure the child that you will do your best to get him/her help and support, reinforcing the need for him/her to trust you.

- Contact an appropriate care agency, depending on your assessment of the situation: it could be medical help, the police, local authority social services, the NSPCC or some other. Many child protection agencies may be located online.

- If this child is of school age and attending school you could contact the school, his/her teacher or the head teacher and have a discussion with them, explaining the child's situation as you heard and assessed it.

- If you are a hospital nurse, then you need perhaps to make contact with the school nurse, depending on the child's age and whether (s)he is at school. Clearly as a student you would first seek advice from your mentor, your tutor or some other senior person, perhaps even your trade union representative, on how to proceed.

- Most important of all, convey to the child the fact that the way (s)he is being treated or neglected is not his/her fault, so (s)he should not feel guilty; reassure him/her help will be sought.

- The child may tell you (s)he does not want his/her parents to know (s)he told you his/her problem. A very difficult one to handle, because at some point the parents will have to be told and will need to be part of any solution to the problem.

- Depending on the circumstances, you may, however, feel you should tell the child that it is possible that, in getting him/her the help (s)he needs, his parents or whoever the abuser is may eventually become part of the solution to the problem as they too may need help.

- You yourself may need some counselling and support to help you deal with the problem. As said above, if you have been abused yourself in childhood the challenge of helping a child get over his abuse can be that much more challenging, so you too may need psychological support.

If you are unsure what to do, Kidscape (http://www.kidscape.org.uk/professionals/childabuse.shtml) points out that there are many child welfare agencies and organisations you can contact for help and support, for example the police, the NSPCC, Children First, Irish Society for the Prevention of Cruelty to Children, Social Services children's welfare departments, Childline, the Samaritans and Parentline. The telephone numbers of most of these organisations can be found on the Kidscape website at http://www.kidscape.org.uk/professionals/chilabuse.shtml.

Legislation since the Children Act 1989

This final section of the chapter is to give you a speedy tour through post-1989 Children Act legislation designed to strengthen child protection.

- The *United Nations Convention on the Rights of the Child 1989* (United Nations, 1989) was ratified by the UK in December 1991. It gives children the rights to express their views and be listened to; it accords protection from abuse and the right of disabled children and children living away from home to services and care.
- The *Human Rights Act 1998* incorporated the *European Convention on Human Rights* into British law effectively since 2 October 2000. This Act does not *mention* children specifically, but in the sense that children are people then they are firmly covered by the Articles of the Human Rights Act 1998. We have drawn extensively on the Human Rights Act in other chapters of this book. However, so that children are put into the correct focus as to their rights under this very important Act I have summarised below the rights the Act bestow on everyone, children included, although you will find that there are some Articles of this Act that have a greater or lesser application to younger children:
  - right to life (Article 2);
  - prohibition of torture (Article 3);
  - prohibition of slavery (Article 4);
  - right to liberty and security (Article 5);
  - right to fair trial (Article 6);
  - no punishment without trial (Article 7);
  - right to respect for private and family life (Article 8);
  - freedom of thought, conscience and religion (Article 9);
  - freedom of expression (Article 10);
  - freedom of assembly and association, depending on age (Article 11);
  - right to marry, if of the right legal age, bearing in mind that 16- and 17-year-olds can legally marry under English law (Article 12);
  - prohibition of discrimination (Article 14);
  - derogation in times of war or public emergency (Article 15);
  - restrictions on political activity of aliens (Article 16).

Student reflection

Obviously some of the rights above have greater or lesser applicability to children, depending on factors such as age of the child, issues around marriage and so on. A portfolio reflective exercise for you is to consider the fundamental rights above and decide for yourself which of them may not be applicable particularly to younger children. Write up your reflection in your portfolio, giving your own justification why you have arrived as your particular conclusion. For more information on the Human Rights Act 1998 please visit http://www.opsi.gov.uk/acts/acts1998/19980042.htm.

- The *Children's Commissioner for Wales Act 2001* created the first children's commissioner post in the UK. The Commissioner's duty is to promote and safeguard children's rights and welfare.
- *Commissioner for Children and Young People (NI) Order 2003* created a children's commissioner for Northern Ireland.
- The *Commissioner for Children and Young People (Scotland) Act 2003* created a children's commissioner for Scotland.
- The *Children Act 2004*, a very important Act whose enactment was stimulated by the Victoria Climbie Inquiry report (Laming, 2003), has altered some parts of the Children Act 1989 and has since 2004 become a key piece of legislation on which many childcare administrative policy decisions have been made. (You will recall that Victoria Climbie was murdered by her great-aunt and her boyfriend in 2000.) The NSPCC (2010) notes that the government responded to the Climbie inquiry report by Lord Laming by producing two important reports: *Keeping Children Safe* (DfES, 2003a) and the *Every Child Matters* green paper (DfES, 2003b). Both these reports led to the enactment of the *Children Act 2004*.

  The main purposes of the Children Act 2004 are as follows:
  - It sets out the framework that integrates children's services so that all children can achieve the *Every Child Matters* outcomes: health, safety enjoyment, achievement and being able to make a contribution to society (NSPCC (2010).
  - It creates a *Children's Commissioner for England* to achieve parity with Wales, Scotland and Northern Ireland.
  - It puts an obligation on local authorities to appoint a director of children's services and an elected lead member for children's services with accountability to deliver children's services.
  - It puts an obligation on local authorities and the agents they work with for the protection and welfare of children (e.g. schools, police, health services, youth and justice organisations) to work in partnership and collaboration for the welfare of children.
  - It replaced the non-statutory *Area Child Protection Boards* with the new statutory *Area Child Protection committee*.
  - It revised the issue of physical punishment and makes it illegal to hit a child in such a way that it could leave a permanent mark or cause mental trauma.
- *Children and Adoption Act 2006*: makes it easier for Courts to facilitate child contact and enforce child contact orders in cases of parental separation and dispute.
- The *Children and Young Persons Act 2008* made the recommendations in the *Care Matters* white paper (DfES, 2007) achievable, for example recommendation to provide high-quality care and services to children in care.
- The *Borders, Citizenship and Immigration Act 2009* puts an obligation on the UK Border Agency to protect children's welfare, for example preventing children from being taken into and out of the country illegally.

Sex offenders, domestic violence and genital mutilation

There are a number of other high-profile Acts enacted to protect children especially from sexual abuse. I will only summarise these in Table 14.1 whilst giving you the respective websites where you can look them up.

Table 14.1 Other legislation to protect children

Legislation	Aim/purpose
Sex Offenders Act 1997 http://www.hmso.gov.uk/acts/acts1997/1997051.htm	Established Sex Offenders Register. Cautioned or convicted offenders notify police of names, addresses, change of address
Sexual Offences Act 2003 http://www.hmso.gov.uk/acts/acts2003/20030042.htm	Updates legislation relating to offences against children, e.g. it strengthened the Sex Offenders Act 1997, making it easier to monitor sex offenders. Covers offences such as grooming children for sex, abuse of trust, trafficking, sexual offences committed by British subjects whilst abroad
Sexual Offences (Scotland) Act 2009; Sexual Offences (N. Ireland) Order 2008 http://www.opsi.gov.uk/legislation/scotland/acts2009/asp_20090009_en_1 http://www.legislation.gov.uk/nisi/2008/1769/contents	Has similar judicial functions, aims and purposes to Sexual Offences Act 2003 above
Female Genital Mutilation Act 2003 http://www.legislation.gov.uk/ukpga/2003/31/conrents	Makes female genital mutilation by UK nationals or permanent UK residents a crime in the UK or abroad, even in a country where this is legal
Domestic Violence, Crime and Victims Act 2004 http://www.legislation.hmso.gov.uk/acts/acts2004/20040028.htm	Stops defendants in murder and manslaughter cases escaping conviction by each claiming the other had killed the child. The Act introduced a new offence of causing or allowing the death of a child or vulnerable adult
Home Office Circular (16/2005) Guidance on Offences against Children	Provides a list of offences that child care agencies can use in determining and identifying persons presenting risks to children
Serious Organised Crime and Police Act 2005	Improves vetting procedures for adults wanting to work with children; sets up framework for UK-wide Child Exploitation & Online Protection (CEOP) Centre
Safeguarding Vulnerable Groups Act 2006 (SVGA, 2006); Safeguarding V. Groups (NI) Act 2007; Protection of Vulnerable Groups (Scotland) Act 2007	Following the Bichard Inquiry into deaths of 10-year-old Jessica Chapman and Holly Wells, the SVGA 2006 was set up to centralise the vetting of people working with children
Forced Marriage Act (Civil Protection) 2007	Empowers courts to protect victims and potential victims of forced marriages and remove them from the situation. Does not make forcing someone into a marriage a crime, but makes contravening of a *Forced Marriage Protection Order* a crime
Criminal Justice and Immigration Act 2008	Allows people who commit sex offences against children abroad to face justice in the UK, even if the offence is legal in the foreign state

Conclusion

Hopefully you will have noted the plethora of UK legislation designed to protect children and ensure their health and social welfare. These pieces of legislation are by themselves not effective without the action of child care professionals and childcare agencies to reinforce them. Children, adult, mental health and learning disability nurses who work with children and young people, as well as other child care professionals, all have an obligation to protect children from abuse and neglect and to ensure that make a contribution to make sure children grow up healthily, stay safe and are able to enjoy life, achieve and make a positive contribution to their society, whilst also achieving economic well-being for themselves. You will have noted also in this chapter that children's rights not only are bestowed by Acts of Parliament, including the Human Rights Act 1998, Court Orders, Statutory Instruments, and case law, but also exist by virtue of children being people, vulnerable human beings for whom we all have a human, professional, ethical and moral obligation to care. Children are the adults of tomorrow. They have vulnerabilities that we all need to help in protecting.

15 Mental health law

(Written by Herman H. Wheeler and Christopher Waggstaff)

Objectives of this chapter

After reading this chapter you should be able to:

*   explain the rationale underlying the Mental Health Act (MHA) 1983 as amended by the 2007 MHA;
*   explain the aims, objectives and key changes of the 2007 amendments of the 1983 MHA by the 2007 MHA;
*   discuss formal and informal arrangements whereby patients with mental disorder may be admitted to a mental health hospital;
*   discuss legal safeguards of people with mental health problems and nurses' and other mental health professionals' responsibilities in ensuring these safeguards work in practice;
*   define 'mental disorder' within the terms of the MHA 1983 as amended by the 2007 Act;
*   use your portfolio to critically reflect on your learning from this chapter, address the student exercises built into the chapter, and reflect on the nurse's role and responsibilities when caring for people with mental health problems under the MHA.

Introduction

Healthcare professionals who care for people with mental health problems need to have an understanding of the legislation that is specific to people with mental health problems. It may be useful to revisit the work on *consent* in Chapter 5 looking at the rules governing people giving, or not giving, consent. The general rule of treating *mentally competent* patients is that they have exercised their autonomy to consent to treatment and this is encapsulated in the Mental Capacity Act (MCA) 2005 section 2(1) (hereafter referred to as the MCA 2005). Equally, the MCA 2005 allows competent people to refuse to consent if they so desire. Moreover, the common law makes it possible as well as clear that the right to consent in the matter of a person's medical treatment is essential (*R v Sullivan* [1984] AC 156). Even a competent patient with a mental disorder may be able to refuse to consent to treatment (*Re C (Adult: Refusal of Treatment)* [1994] 1 WLR 290). The general consent rule indicates that where a patient who has capacity temporarily becomes incapacitated, for example by a state of unconsciousness, that person may be given emergency treatment under common law under the principle of treating the patient in his/her *best interest*. With respect to the principle that a mentally competent adult must normally first consent to treatment before he is treated, there is a statutory exception to this rule, made possible by the Mental Health Act 1983 (hereafter referred to as the MHA 1983) as amended by the Mental Health Act 2007 (hereafter referred to as the 2007 Act).

The MHA 1983 (as amended by the 2007 Act), provides a comprehensive legal framework for the compulsory detention in hospital and for medical treatment of persons suffering from 'mental disorder'. The MHA protects the rights of people in England and Wales who have a mental disorder.

The focus of this chapter is an overview of the 1983 MHA and the key amendments made to it by the 2007 Act. Also the chapter examines the underlying political reasons for the amendments in the 2007 Act, and the issues that the key amendments were trying to resolve. The MCA 2005 was also amended by the 2007 Act to give added protection and safeguard to the human rights of some of the most vulnerable people in society. For this reason we will make references to some key issues in the MCA 2005, making links as appropriate with MHA 1983 as amended by the 2007 Act. This chapter does not offer a comprehensive account of the MHA 1983, which has over 100 parts (or sections), neither does it cover all the details of the 2007 amendments. However, the key sections and amendments are explained.

The 2007 amendments to the MHA 1983 came into force in October 2008. An important point to note is that the 2007 Act has not replaced the MHA 1983; it has amended it, meaning changing some parts of it. The Human Rights Act 1998 (hereafter referred to as the 1998 Act) (implemented in England on 2 October 2000) is also referred to in this chapter, because, whereas the 1998 Act gives greater protection to people's human rights, a series of English court decisions found that under section 4 of the 1998 Act certain provisions of the 1983 MHA have proved to be incompatible with Article 5 of the 1998 Human Rights Act (see *R(H) v Mental Health Review Tribunal* [2002] QB 1). The 2007 Act aimed to prevent incompatibility between the 1983 MHA and the Human Rights Act 1998.

Principles underlying the MHA and the 2007 amendments

One of the key principles underlying the MHA is *parens patriae*, under which the state has both a right and an obligation to treat sick people when it is necessary to do so. The formal admissions to mental health hospitals and the treatment provisions of the 1983 Act, prior to the 2007 Amendments, owe their origins to the *parens patriae* principle, which holds that the state acts as the parents of its citizens and as such must act to protect those citizens who are mentally ill and need treatment. The state also has responsibility, obligation and right to protect citizens who are themselves not mentally ill, but are at risk from those who are. The mentally unwell citizen may object to being detained in a mental hospital on the grounds that the state is interfering with his/her fundamental right to *liberty* and *freedom* within a democracy.

The *parens patriae* principle therefore takes the view that the state can justifiably override the citizen's right to freedom in order to protect that citizen from him-/herself and to protect other citizens from the mentally ill person. The philosopher John Stuart Mill argued in his essay *On Liberty* that restricting people's liberty and fundamental freedoms can only be justified where such restrictions 'prevent harm to others'. It is not sufficient to restrict people's freedoms on the grounds of the person's 'best interest'. Yet McHale and Fox (2007) note that the *parens patriae* justification is at the root of, and indeed formed critical bases to, the reform of both the MHA of 1959 and that of 1983.

In addition to the *parens patria* issue, Bowen (2007) points out that two important events in England expedited the 2007 amendments. One of them was the murder of Jonathan Zito, on 17 December 1992, by Christopher Clunis, a patient suffering from paranoid schizophrenia, who had stopped taking his medication whilst in the community under the care of the community mental health services, under section 117 of the MHA 1983. The second event was the murder of Lynn and Megan Russell, on 9 July 1996, by Michael Stone, a convicted man suffering from a severe 'personality disorder'. Stone had been refused admission to hospital just days before he committed the murders. The reason he was refused admission was because he was an 'untreatable psychopath' (Bowen, 2007, p. 6).

The Bournwood case outlined in Box 15.1 was another key driver behind the 2007 amendments of the 1983 MHA.

Bournwood safeguards

Prior to the 2007 amendment of the MHA 1983 a small number of patients who lacked capacity and who did not dissent from being admitted to psychiatric hospitals were admitted 'informally' under provisions of section 131(1) of the MHA 1983. The legal correctness of this practice was challenged in the *Bournwood* case (*R v Bournwood Community Mental Health NHS Trust ex p L* [1998] AC 458 (see Box 15.1).

Prior to the 2007 amendments, the problem for a small group of 'passive' informal patients (like Mr L) was that they had been admitted informally to hospital, because they lacked capacity and did not object to their informal admission status. However, on account of their informal status they had no protection under the provisions of the Mental Health Review Tribunal (MHRT), a statutory body set up to consider requests from formally detained patients to have their detention reviewed. Therefore, when this small group of 'passive' informal patients wished to leave hospital, or their carers decided to ask for their release, and their psychiatrists refused, they could not appeal to the MHRT. Thus they were in a 'no man's land' situation. The government was mindful of the lack of safeguard for such patients. Thus Parliament made sure that the 2007 Act amended the 2005 MCA, setting out new procedures for detention of so-called 'Bournwood' patients. (It should be noted that this type of amendment of the 2005 MCA comes under 'personal welfare' decisions covered by that Act. Indeed, the MCA 2005 also covers property and affairs, but these elements of the Act were not amended by the 2007 Act.)

BOX 15.1 The *Bournwood* case

Mr L, an adult with a learning disability, was admitted informally to a mental health unit. He was not formally detained under the MHA 1983, so had no protection under the Mental Health Review Tribunal (MHRT). His carers (Mr and Mrs E) asked for his discharge but the responsible psychiatrist refused, saying that the patient needed to remain in hospital in his 'best interest' (a common law measure). L's carers challenged the decision but lost in the High Court. However, the Court of Appeal said that section 131 of the MHA 1983 required a person to have mental capacity to agree to admission under the Act. Mr L could have been lawfully admitted and detained only under the formal provisions of the MHA 1983; he was not. In a subsequent appeal to the Lords, the Law Lords held that an adult lacking mental capacity could be detained and cared for in a psychiatric hospital under common law powers.

The ECHR ruled that L's right to freedom had been infringed under Article 5 of the 1998 Act. Materially, the detainment of incapacitated patients such as Mr L under the common law doctrine of necessity was incompatible with Article 5 of the Human Rights Act 1998.

Main objectives of the 2007 amendments to the MHA 1983 were:

- to provide adequate powers of control and treatment to ensure that patients continue to comply with their treatment whilst in the community;
- to make it easier to admit and re-admit and detain psychopaths even if they are considered untreatable; this is a measure to protect the public;
- to provide adequate safeguards for the detention and treatment of patients like Mr L., as an alternative to compulsory admission under the MHA 1983;
- to continue the policy of treating the vast majority of people with mental health problems within the community as opposed to in hospitals;
- to bring mental health services in line with major current thinking and philosophy about how patients with mental health problems should be treated, being free of unfair discrimination, prejudices and stigma, whilst creating a balance between protecting vulnerable mental health patients and at the same time ensuring public safety;
- to bring provisions of the MHA 1983 in line with its obligations under the ECHR and the Human Rights Act 1998, especially in relation to new provisions about 'nearest relatives';
- to introduce supervised community treatment and remove the old 'treatability' test, introducing instead a new 'therapeutic purpose' test;
- to introduce new safeguards for the admission and detention of children to mental health hospital;
- to cater for the need to place a child under 18 years old admitted to hospital in a 'suitable environment' [new section 131A(2)];
- to confer responsibility for people with mental health conditions on a broader range of mental health professionals, not just psychiatric social workers and RMOs.

Formal admission

Under the MHA 1983 (as amended by the 2007 Act) a mentally competent person may be *compulsorily detained* for treatment if (s)he has a *mental disorder*, even if (s)he objects to such a detention (cf. Box 15.2). *Formally* detained patients are referred to as being 'sectioned' under the MHA 1983 (as amended by the 2007 Act). Whether or not detained patients have capacity, they have been admitted to hospital because they have a mental disorder and have been unwilling to be admitted informally. There are many reasons why people may be reluctant to be admitted to a mental health hospital *informally*. Some patients with a mental disorder refuse to admit that they are ill or acknowledge the severity of the disorder. Some people may have a very real fear of stigma of being admitted to a psychiatric hospital, or have a fear for their own safety if admitted to one.

Compulsory admissions under the MHA 1983 (as amended by the 2007 Act) of patients suffering from 'mental disorder' (except patients coming through the courts from prison) take place under the following sections (in the list all durations are maximums):

section 2 – admission for assessment; duration 28 days;
section 3 – admission for treatment; duration six months; renewable for a further six months, and every 12 months thereafter;
section 4 – emergency admission for assessment; duration 72 hours;
section 5(2) – detention of patient already in hospital; duration 72 hours;
section 5(4) – emergency Nurse Holding Power of an 'informal' in-patient being treated for a mental disorder; duration six hours.

BOX 15.2 A brief scenario

Conditions under which a patient came to be 'sectioned' under the MHA

Juliette, 37, is under the care of a Community Mental Health team. She has a long-standing diagnosis of schizophrenia and is well known to mental health services. The team receives a phone call from the group home where Juliette lives saying that she has been pacing her room all night and can be heard shouting to herself. She is visited by two community psychiatric nurses (CPNs) and needs a lot of persuasion to open the door to her flat as she is very suspicious of the CPNs' intentions for being there. She becomes increasingly hostile towards the nurses, implying a conspiracy between mental health services, her mother and the Pope. Judging by the amount of medication that is in the flat it is clear that Juliette has not taken any of her prescribed oral anti-psychotic medication for a period of time. Given that their presence is making Juliette more agitated and more hostile, the CPNs soon leave, saying that they will return. The staff discuss the situation with Juliette's consultant psychiatrist and after considering her medical history and her previous risk history they decide that a Mental Health Act assessment needs to be done. In the meantime, Juliette has left her flat and gone to the local train station in a state of undress. There she is hostile and verbally aggressive towards station staff and commuters. She is picked up by police and taken to the police station as a place of safety. The consultant psychiatrist, her GP and an approved mental health professional complete a Mental Health Act assessment in the police station and, after consulting with her mother, decide that Juliette needs to be detained under section 3 of the Mental Health Act.

Student reflection

As well as being aware of the scenario above, outlining the conditions under which a patient came to be 'sectioned' under the MHA, please use your portfolio to reflect on possible implications and consequences that may arise from the above case, discussing the part you feel the nurses in the receiving hospital may have to play in relation to the care of the patient and her significant others.

Applicability of above sections

Section 2:   applied to patient suffering from mental disorder warranting detention for assessment. Detainment is in the interest of the patient's health and safety, or protection of others. Detention is based upon two medical recommendations and approval by an Advanced Mental Health Professional (AMHP).

Section 3:   patient's behaviour warrants detention for treatment, for the benefit of the patient's health and safety or the protection of others. Detention is based upon two medical recommendations and approval by an AMHP.

Section 4:   as for section 2 above, but accepting *only one medical recommendation from a doctor who knows the patient,* where waiting for two medical recommendations would introduce undue delay, and approval by an AMHP.

Section 5(2): applies where in-patient receiving treatment for a mental disorder needs to be detained in the interest of the patient's health and safety or the protection of others. This section contains powers for a doctor to prevent someone who is otherwise a voluntary patient from leaving hospital. Detention is based upon a report by a registered medical practitioner.

Section 5(4): a person who is a voluntary patient in a hospital can be legally detained there if it appears to a suitably qualified nurse that the conditions are met; that the patient is suffering from a mental disorder to such a degree that is necessary for his/her health or safety or for the protection of others for him/her to be immediately restrained from leaving hospital; and that it is not practicable to secure the immediate attendance of a medical practitioner for the purpose of furnishing a report under section 5(2).

It must be noted that *Special Mental Health Act Forms* for admission and record keeping are required in all the above instances. The receipt and the careful management of the paperwork is one of the most important roles and responsibilities that a nurse has in the process of a person being detained in hospital. An important factor to bear in mind is that the Mental Health Act is perhaps a unique piece of legislation in the UK, in that a person can be deprived of his/her liberty when (s)he has neither committed a crime nor appeared before a court. Once detained, a person can be subjected to treatment that would otherwise be regarded as assault. Therefore nurses must take great care and precision to make sure the paperwork relating to the person's detention is correctly filled out.

Another issue for ward-based nurses to be mindful of in relation to admitting someone who is detained under the Mental Health Act to a ward is the person must be informed that (s)he is detained under the Act and be informed of his/her right of appeal. In the first instance it is the nurse in charge of the ward's responsibility; however, it is not enough to tell the person once. The nursing staff on the ward must continue to tell the person that (s)he is detained and that (s)he has the right of appeal. The staff continues to inform the patient until they are satisfied that (s)he understands.

Powers to formally detain criminals

As Bowen (2007) has pointed out the criminal court is empowered to remand accused persons to hospital for reports (section 35) or for treatment (section 36) and to impose a hospital order [sections 37, 38 and 51(5)], with or without a restriction order (section 41) or a hospital limitation direction (section 45A) upon that person being convicted of a crime. Under section 47 the Secretary of State has administrative powers to transfer serving prisoners to psychiatric hospital. The Secretary of State can also transfer other detainees such as remand prisoners and immigration detainees to psychiatric hospital (section 48). These powers under the MHA 1983 were not amended by the 2007 Act.

Informal admissions

Not all patients being treated in hospitals for mental health problems are compulsorily detained (Dimond and Barker, 1996; Fennell *et al.*, 2009; Bowen, 2007). Most informal patients have capacity and consent to their 'informal' admission status and treatment. As Bowen (2007, p. 26) explains, 'compulsory detention under the MHA 1983 [as amended by the 2007 Act] is a measure of last resort'. It continues to be the case that some patients admitted and treated in mental health facilities are 'informal patients'. Although technically these people are being admitted *under provisions* of Part 2, section 131 of the MHA 1983 (as amended by the 2007 Act) they are not 'sectioned' or detained under the MHA.

Informal patients leaving hospital

'Informal' patients have the right to leave hospital when they wish, day or night. However, if, in the professional judgement of the nurse taking care of such 'informal' patients, the patient who is about to discharge him-/herself is at risk to him-/herself or others then the nurse must exercise his/her professional judgement to persuade the patient to stay until the patient is less distressed. This is seen as good practice under both the MHA Code of Practice and NMC (2008a) Code of conduct that requires nurses to put patients *at the centre of care*, always making the patient's needs your primary concern. Furthermore, the *ethic of beneficence* requires nurses to act in a way that protects and benefits the patient.

Nurse holding powers

Sometimes the situation requires the nurse to have more legal protection, both for him-/herself and for the patient. In these instances then, it is appropriate that *specific prescribed* nurses use the *emergency holding power* (the *Nurse's Holding Power*) to detain 'informal' patients being treated for mental disorder, if the situation warrants it [section 5(4)]. This detention must be for a maximum of six hours and aimed at ensuring the health and safety of the patient or the protection of others.

The following are suggestions about how the nurse in the scenario in Box 15.3 could proceed. The first thing that needs to be done is to try and persuade Gill to stay. The nurse may want to speak with her in a quiet part of the ward, where they will not be disturbed, perhaps offering to make a drink. The nurse needs to convey to Gill his/her concern for her welfare, perhaps trying to persuade her to sleep on her decision. If, in spite of the nurse's best efforts, Gill still seems to want to go home then the nurse, acting in Gill's best interests, may try to persuade her to wait to be seen by the Responsible Clinician (RC). However, Gill may tell the nurse that she does not want to wait to see the RC. The next step for the nurse may be to persuade Gill to wait until the nurse has had the opportunity to ring a duty doctor to come to see her. Gill may reluctantly agrees to. However, the nurse has problems contacting the doctor and Gill remains determined to leave the hospital. In this instance the nurse may feel that the only option that (s)he has left is to invoke the emergency nurse holding power under section 5(4). The detention can only be for a maximum of six hours. No medical recommendation is necessary for this to happen. Under section 5(5) the prescribed nurse who has exercised the holding power must report the detention to the hospital managers. The necessary Statutory Mental Health Act Forms 13 and 16 must be used to effect the nurse holding power (Box 15.4). It is imperative that the RC see the patient within this six-hour window. If the nurse has exercised section 5(4) and the RC has decided to apply section 5(2)

BOX 15.3 Nurse holding power scenario

Gill, aged 28, who is suffering from depression, is an 'informal' patient in a mental health hospital. She is suicidal and known to harbour a hate of her husband, whom she has reported to have cheated on her with another woman, known to Gill. It is 12 midnight and Gill tells the nurse in charge of her ward that she is going home immediately and has in fact already called a taxi. What would your reaction be and why?

Imagine that you are the nurse in charge of the ward. Use your law and ethics portfolio to come up with an answer as to what you would do under the circumstances and why. In other words justify any action you take.

BOX 15.4 Student reflective exercise

Whilst on clinical placement, locate examples of the Statutory Mental Health Act Forms 13 and 16 and insert them in your portfolio. Write out a reflective piece about what difficulties you foresee about (a) trying to persuade an informal patient to stay in hospital and (b) the differences between keeping a patient on the ward using common law and keeping a patient on the ward using the Mental Health Act.

---

then a 72-hour detainment begins under this section at the time the nurse made out his/her report under section 5(4). Remember, it is not necessary for a nurse to use section 5(2) or 5(4) if the patient is already detained under the 1983 MHA.

Main changes to the 1983 MHA by the 2007 Act

Although the objectives of the 2007 amendments are enshrined in law it is perhaps too early to say whether all the objectives are being met in practice. Below is a brief overview of the main changes to the Mental Health Act 1983, as amended by the 2007 Act.

1. *Definition of mental disorder*: The 2007 Act widens the definition of 'mental disorder'; a single definition now applies and categories of disorder are abolished.
2. *Detention criteria*: It introduces a new appropriate medical treatment test in all longer-term detention. Consequently it is not possible for patients to be compulsorily detained, or their detention continued, unless appropriate medical treatment and all other circumstances of the case are known to the patient. The treatability test has been abolished.
3. *Nearest relative*: Patients can now displace their nearest relative if they consider them unsuitable. They can do so by application to the court. County courts can also displace a nearest relative they consider unsuitable. Civil partners can now be nearest relative.
4. *Supervised community treatment (SCT)*: The 2007 amendments introduced SCT for patients following hospital detention. SCT will allow certain patients with a mental disorder to be discharged from detention subject to the possibility of recall to hospital if necessary. SCT orders are also designed to reduce mental health patients' non-compliance with medication following their discharge from hospital. These orders also aim to reduce the tendency towards deterioration in patient's health, requiring further detention and leading to the 'revolving door' situation.
5. *Care professionals*: It widens the group of practitioners able to assume functions previously performed by approved social workers (ASWs) and responsible medical officer (RMO).
6. *Electro-convulsive therapy [ECT]*: It introduces new safeguards for patients; for example, a competent person with a mental disorder cannot be forced to have ECT.
7. *Tribunal*: It reduces periods after which hospital managers must refer certain patients' cases to the MHRT if they do not apply themselves. It introduces an order-making power to make further reductions in due course.
8. *Independent mental health advocacy*: It places a duty on the appropriate national authority to arrange help by independent mental health advocates.
9. *Age-appropriate services*: It requires hospital managers to ensure that children (under 18 years old) who are admitted to hospital for mental disorder are accommodated in age-appropriate environments, subject to the patient's needs.

10. *Additional safeguard for admission and detention of children*: The 2007 Act amends the MHA 1983 to provide additional safeguard for the admission and detention of children. Capable children 16 or 17 years of age with capacity cannot be admitted *informally* without their consent. As was the case before the 2007 Act, 16- and 17-year-old children with capacity can consent to their informal admission notwithstanding parental objection. Under a new s 131(2–5), introduced by the 2007 Act, a competent child (i.e. one having capacity) cannot be admitted informally on the basis of the consent of the person with parental responsibility. This replaces the common law rule in the case of *Re C (Detention: Medical Treatment)* [1997] 2 FLR 180. However, parents can still consent to their *incapable* child of any age being admitted informally to hospital.

The Mental Health Act Code of Practice: implications for mental health professionals

All health professionals who work with and care for people with mental illness under the 1983 MHA as amended by the 2007 Act need to be aware of the principles of the MHA Code of Practice. Under section 118 of the MHA 1983 a *Code of Practice* must be prepared and, from time to time, revised by the Secretary of State and, in Wales, by the National Assembly for Wales, to provide key principle guidance to be followed by health professionals in respect to caring for people detained under the MHA 1983. The Code of Practice was reviewed and amended in 2008 and came into force on 3 November of that year. Under the 2007 Act a new section 118(2D) requires people performing functions under the Mental Health Act to 'have regard' to the code. What does this mean? The House of Lords in *R (Munjaz) v Mercy Care NHS Trust* [2005] UKHL 58 stated that: 'Statutory guidance of this kind is less than a direction. But it is more than something to which those to whom it is addressed must "have regard to"'. Lord Hope went on to say that those who choose to depart from the code 'must give cogent reasons':

> these reasons must be spelled out clearly, logically and convincingly. I would emphatically reject any suggestion that they have discretion to depart from the Code as they see fit. Parliament by enacting s 118(1) has made it clear that it expects that the persons to whom the Code is addressed will follow it, unless they can demonstrate that they have a cogent reason for not doing so.

The House of Lords' message to health professionals in the above quotation is that they must follow the MHA Code of Practice. The Code therefore has a *statutory* status and must be followed by all healthcare professionals caring for people with mental health problems under the 1983 Act (as amended) unless there are compelling good reasons for not following the Code. Dimond and Barker (1996) have stated that any objection or reasons the mental health professional has for not following the Code must be clearly stated, preferably in writing. As a mental health professional you should also be aware that a court of law could cite the Code as evidence in legal proceedings against you or your employer. Such proceedings could, for example, be against a nurse who was cited for failure to provide appropriate suitable care for his/her patient. It could be against the hospital management for failure to provide suitable age-appropriate mental healthcare facilities for minors. It is therefore important for mental health professionals such as nurses and doctors to understand the Code's aims and underlying principles and follow them, since a departure from the Code could give rise to legal challenges. Courts reviewing departure from the Code are most likely to scrutinise the reasons for the departure, in order to ensure that there is sufficiently convincing justification in the circumstances. This source also points out that the Code is also useful to the police, ambulance services, health and social service staff, including voluntary sector workers who provide services to patients who are treated under the MHA 1983 as amended by the 2007 Act. The Code will also be helpful to patients, their representatives, carers, families and friends and others who support them.

Guiding principles of the Mental Health Act Code of Practice

When professionals are making decisions about patients detained under the MHA they must operate according to the following principles of the MHA Code of Practice:

Purpose principle

- Invoke the powers of the MHA only where and when necessary. In other words, only if a person's mental health is considered serious enough to warrant his/her detention should (s)he be compulsorily detained. This makes good sense, given that such detention actually amounts to a loss of fundamental liberty and freedom.
- Seek to minimise the undesirable effects of mental disorder by maximising patients/ clients' mental and physical safety and well-being, and by promoting recovery and protection from harm.
- Keep a focus on the need for review of the patient's detention, always being mindful of the need to enhance the detained patient's social and civil status.
- Detained patients have a right of appeal to the MHRT. Even mental health patients admitted for assessment (as opposed to treatment) have a right of appeal to the MHRT under the MHA 1983, as amended by the 2007 Act.

Least restriction principle

- Professionals making decisions about patients with mental health problems must aim to minimise the restrictions placed on the patient's liberty.
- The restrictions imposed must be purposive and not imposed for the sake of imposition.

Respect principle

- Recognise and respect the diverse needs, values and individual circumstances of each client, taking into account their ethnicity, religion, culture, age, gender, sexual orientation and any disability.
- Take into account the patient/client's views, wishes and feelings when dealing with them, and as far as it is possible to do respecting mental health patients' right to their own views and their rights under the Human Rights Act 1998.
- Do not unlawfully discriminate against the patient and his/her relatives/significant others.

Participation principle

- As far as is practicable, involve patients in decision making relating to their care: its assessment, planning, implementation, review and evaluation.
- The above includes giving patients the opportunity to be involved in the multidisciplinary review of their condition and treatment, ensuring that the delivery of treatment is appropriate and effective.

- As far as possible involve family members and significant others who have an interest in the patients' welfare, unless there are factors pointing to the undesirability of doing so.

Effectiveness, efficiency and equity principle

- Use resources effectively, efficiently and equitably, to meet patients' need and achieve the purpose for which the care decision was taken.

Using the principles

- Ensure care decisions are lawful and informed by sound evidence based professional practice.
- Lawfulness must comply with the principles of the Human Rights Act 1998.
- The principles of the Code of Practice must inform decisions, not determine them.

See the exercise in Box 15.5 to consider these principles. It is also worth stating that although the 1983 MHA and the MCA 2005 each have their own *Code of Practice*, for want of space only the MHA Code of Practice is covered in this chapter by way of a mere overview. The Mental Capacity Act 2005 Code of Practice can be located online at http://www.justice.gov.uk/docs/mca-cp.pdf.

Definition of mental disorder

Prior to the 2007 amendments, mental disorder was defined in section 1(2) as follows: 'mental disorder means mental illness, arrested or incomplete development of mind, psychopathic disorder, and any other disorder or disability of mind and "mentally disordered" shall be construed accordingly'. Thus there were three categories of mental disorder in the MHA 1983: (1) mental illness, (2) psychopathic disorder and (3) arrested or incomplete development of mind. The third was subdivided into 'mental impairment' and 'severe mental impairment', thus effecting a fourth classification of mental disorder. 'Mental illness' is given no further definition, whereas the other three are. Learning disability was regarded as part of 'mental impairment' and 'severe mental impairment'.

The amendment of the 1983 Act gave a wider definition of 'mental disorder', whereby section 1(2) now defines 'mental disorder' as any disorder or disability of the mind; and 'mentally disordered' shall be construed accordingly. Thus the *four classifications* or categories of mental disorder have been *removed*, wherever they had appeared throughout the MHA 1983.

For patients suffering from learning disability (previously classified as 'mental impairment' or 'severe mental impairment' a new classification has been introduced in *a new section 1(2A)* to read:

> But a person with learning disability shall *not* be considered by reason of that disability to be
> (a) suffering from mental disorder for the provisions mentioned in subsection (2B) below; or
> (b) requiring treatment in hospital for mental disorder for purposes of sections 17E and 50–3 below,
> unless that disability is associated with abnormally aggressive or serious irresponsible conduct on his part'

**BOX 15.5 Scenarios encompassing some of the principles of the MHA
Code**

Using the case studies in Boxes 15.2 and 15.3, please think about how the principles
of the MHA Code should be applied in both these cases.

The 2007 Act defines learning disability thus: 'learning disability means a state of
arrested or incomplete development of the mind which includes significant impairment of
intelligence and social functioning' (section 2B). So the MHA 1983 does cover people with
learning disability. If a patient suffering from learning disability has a mental disorder that
renders him/her seriously aggressive and irresponsible, to the extent that (s)he is a danger to
him-/herself or to others (s)he can be formally detained in a mental health hospital. Issues
raised by the *Bournwood* case have resonance for people with learning disability.

Dependency on alcohol and drugs

A new section 1(3) states that dependency on alcohol or drugs is not regarded as a disorder
or disability of mind for the purposes of subsection (2) above. The old section 1(3) has been
repealed, so that exclusion for promiscuity or other immoral conduct or sexual deviancy has
been removed. Bowen (2007, p. 51) argues that the removal of these forms of conduct from
the 'exclusions' to the definition of 'mental disorder' is unlikely to have a weighted effect
because:

> it was always the case that any such behaviour which either causes, or is caused by,
> a mental disorder which otherwise meets the criteria will justify . . . detention and
> treatment . . . Such patients were detained in the past and will continue to be detained.

Nearest relative under the 2007 Amendments

The role of the 'nearest relative' (as defined by the 1983 MHA) is important. The nearest
relative has a significant role to play. There are changes to 'nearest relative' in the 2007 Act.
Section 26–30 of the MHA 1983 determines the appointment and removal of the nearest
relative, who have the following powers:

- to apply for a patient to be detained under section 2 or 3;
- to veto applications for admission under section 3 [section 11(4)];
- to exercise power to effect the patient's discharge from detention under sections 2 and
  3 (section 23);
- to apply to the MHRT on the patient's behalf (section 66).

The above provisions have been amended by the 2007 Act to bring about compatibility of
the MHA with the European Convention Rights. Under the MHA 1983 there were a number
of flaws relating to the nearest relative. For example, their appointment was automatic, giving
the patient no choice over appointment or removal of nearest relative even if the latter were
considered unsuitable, or the patient simply did not wish them to act on his/her behalf. Patient
choice was therefore excluded. These provisions brought about incompatibility with Article
8 of the Human Rights Act (*JT v United Kingdom* [2000] 1 FLR 909; *R (M) v Secretary of
State for Health* [2003] 1 MHLR 88). The 2007 Act has remedied these flaws as follows:

- It has defined 'relative' and 'nearest relative' to include civil partners.
- Under section 29(1)(2) a patient can now displace his/her nearest relative as being unsuitable by working through the courts. The courts can also initiate the removal of an unsuitable 'nearest relative'.

Treatment amendments under the 2007 Act

General principle of informed consent

A notable example of where deviating from the common law norm of obtaining patients' consent for treatment would not constitute a trespass to the patient ('battery') or an assault is where, for example, a patient is being detained under the Mental Health Act 1983. If a patient detained under the 1983 MHA (as amended by the 2007 Act) is unable to consent or refuses to consent to treatment it is possible under defined circumstances to treat that patient under Part IV of the Act.

Medical treatment under the MHA 1983 has been amended by the 2007 Act

Under the MHA 1983, as amended, Part IV confers power to treat patients under the Act. Equally, Part IV also places safeguards to protect patients against unnecessary treatment. In contrast to the situation at common law where mentally competent adults need to consent before they can be treated, Part IV of the 1983 MHA confers power to treat competent patients with mental disorder even when they object to such treatment. This is done under sections 58 and 63 and, in emergencies, under section 62. Bowen (2007, p. 28) asserts that:

> The fact the patient has capacity is a relevant factor that the RMO is to take into account, but it carries no more weight than any other factor. The fact that the treatment requires to be imposed by force, upon a capable or incapacitated patient, is likely to carry more weight.

Under the 2007 amendments, section 57 provides that under certain circumstances more intrusive treatments *cannot* be imposed without consent. Section 58A gives additional safeguards against electro-convulsive therapy (ECT). For example, ECT can no longer be given without the consent of the patient with capacity. In the case of an incapacitated patient who has a bona fide *advanced decision* in place (ruling out ECT), ECT cannot be given to him/her. In the case of an incapacitated patient, ECT may also be ruled out by a donee having a lasting power of attorney to make healthcare decisions in the best interest of the donor of the power who is now the incapacitated patient with mental disorder. ECT may also be ruled out for a patient lacking capacity by a deputy, or the Court of Protection under the 2005 Mental Competency Act. As noted earlier in this chapter, like competent adults, competent children admitted to psychiatric hospitals cannot be treated with ECT if they object to this therapy.

Under the 2007 amendments of the MHA 1983 a new Part IVA has been created in the MHA 1983, setting out the conditions under which treatment may be given to 'community patients' who are subject to Community Treatment Orders (CTOs) under section 17A. The 2007 amendment of Part IV has:

- A new definition of 'medical treatment', section 145(1), and new treatability conditions, section 145(4). Under section 145(1) 'medical treatment' includes nursing, psychological intervention and specialist mental health rehabilitation.

- Removed the 'treatability' test in sections 57 and 58 and introduced a new 'appropriate treatment' test for the Second Opinion Appointed Doctor. The new 'Appropriate Treatment Test', section 64(3), states that 'it is appropriate for treatment to be given to a patient if the treatment is appropriate to his case, taking into account the nature and degree of the mental disorder . . . and all other circumstances of his case'.

- Applied treatability to all forms of mental disorder. Removal of the 'treatability test' for psychopaths means that psychopathic disorder can now be treated under the Act. It is now sufficient that the purpose of the treatment is to alleviate or prevent a worsening, rather than it having to be 'likely' the treatment would have that effect. A responsible clinician making recommendation for treatment under sections 3, 37, 45A and 47 now just needs to satisfy him-/herself the treatment has the purpose of benefitting the patient, not that the treatment is 'likely' to have a beneficial effect.

  Reflection on Michael Stone's 1996 killing of the Russells: If the new treatability test in the 2007 Act had been around in 1996, perhaps Mr Michael Stone, the then 'untreatable' psychopath, would have been brought into hospital before he had time to kill Megan and Lynn Russell. Today he might have been admitted under the 2007 amendment as the new 'treatability' test is that the purpose of the treatment is to alleviate or prevent worsening, not that it is 'likely' to have that effect; a totally new emphasis. The new 'treatability test' now applies to all forms of mental disorder, including psychopaths and learning-disabled patients (Bowen, 2007, p. 51). To reiterate, a learning disability patient with mental disorder who is abnormally aggressive with serious irresponsible conduct on his/her part could be brought into hospital compulsorily under the MHA for treatment.

- Made it possible for treatment to be given by or under direction of a non-medically qualified 'responsible clinician'.

Supervised Community Treatment Order (SCT)

Under the MHA 1983, provisions existed to care for and control patients with mental disorder in the community under guardianship, aftercare supervision, release of patients on section 17 leave and conditional discharge of patients restricted under sections 42 and 73. The 2007 Act has repealed *aftercare supervision*, replacing it with the new SCT. Furthermore section 17 is amended to allow a patient to be released on section 17 leave for no longer than seven days. Under the 2007 amendments conditional discharge of restricted patients stands.

Conclusion

The chapter has, hopefully, enabled you to get to grips with the main changes to the Mental Health Act (MHA) 1983 as amended by the 2007 MHA. As can be seen the 2007 Act has amended not only the MHA 1983 but the MCA 2005 as well, to give added protection and safeguard to the human rights of people detained under the MHA, and to prevent clashes and incompatibility between the MHA and the MCA 2005.

The key principles underlying the MHA 1983 and its amendments in 2007 have been outlined and described, as are the objectives and main changes to the 1983 Act. Time will tell whether in practice these amendments are working. Some implications of the amendments have been pointed out.

Both formal and informal admissions to mental health hospitals have been covered, including explanation of the various sections relating to formal detention. The formal admission of criminals under the MHA was also covered.

It is hoped that all healthcare professionals treating patients under the MHA will read and understand the principles and aims of the MHA Code of Practice as it offers 'statutory' guidance principles on how best to maintain standards of care when treating patients with mental health problems under the MHA. No mental health nurse or other mental health professional can afford to ignore the principles of the MHA Code of Practice. If you do, you do so at your own peril. It can be seen that the 2007 amendments have given extra safeguards to people being treated under the MHA.

There is a definite healthy tension between the MHA 1983 as amended by the MHA 2007, the Mental Capacity Act 2005 and the Human Rights Act 1998. I leave you with the key thought below:

An important factor to bear in mind is that the MHA is perhaps a unique piece of UK legislation, in that it can deprive a person of his/her liberty even when that person has neither committed a crime nor appeared before a court. Once detained, a person can be subjected to treatment that would otherwise be regarded as assault. Therefore, nurses and other mental healthcare professionals must take great care and precision to make sure the paperwork relating to the person's detention is correctly filled out.

References

Agard A, Hermeren G and Herlitz J (2000) Should cardiopulmonary resuscitation be performed on patients with heart failure? The role of the patient in the decision-making process. *Journal of Internal Medicine*, 248: 279–286.

Age Concern (2007) What is ageism? Online at: http://www.ageconcern.org.uk, accessed 18 October 2011.

Age UK (2010a) Factsheet 78. April 2010: Safeguarding older people from abuse. Online at: http://www.ageuk.org.uk/Documents/EN-GB/Factsheets/FS78_Safeguarding_older_people_from_abuse_April_2010_fcs.pdf?dtrk=true, accessed 10 January 2011.

Age UK (2010b) Legal issues, living wills. Online at: http://www.ageuk.org.uk/money-matters/legal-issues/living-wills/, accessed 10 January 2011.

Aristotle (1976) *The ethics of Aristotle: the Nicomachean ethics.* Translated by Thompson J A K, revised by Tredennick H. Harmondsworth: Penguin.

Aveyard H (2005) Informed consent prior to nursing care procedures. *Nursing Ethics*, 12(1): 19–29.

Bandura A, Ross D and Ross S A (1961) Transmission of aggression through imitation of aggressive models. *Journal of Social Psychology*, 63: 575–582.

Banerjee R (2005) Family and child development: Moral behaviour. Online at: http://www.open2.net/healtheducation/family_childdevelopment/morality2.html, accessed 16 January 2011.

Banja J D (1996) Ethics, values and world culture: impact on rehabilitation. *Disability and Rehabilitation*, 1: 279–284.

Baskett P J F (1990) The ethics of resuscitation. In Evans T R (ed.) *ABC of resuscitation* (2nd edn). London: British Medical Journal Publications.

Batty D (2004) Timeline: the history of child protection. *Guardian Society*. Online at: http://www.guardian.co.uk/society/2004/apr/23/childrenservices.childprotection, accessed 24 March 2011.

BBC News (13 January 2004) Harold Shipman: The killer doctor. Online at: http://news.bbc.co.uk/1/hi/uk/3391897.stm, accessed 3 January 2011.

BBC News (8 March 2006) Nurse killed patient with drug. Online at: http://news.bbc.co.uk/1/hi/england/humber/4787492.stm, accessed 3 January 2011.

BBC News (20 November 2010) Have your say: Will the Pope's condom comments change the Catholic Church? Online at: http://www.bbc.co.uk/blogs/haveyoursay/2010/11/will_the_popes_condom_comments.html?page=6, accessed 2 November 2011.

BBC News Channel (18 April 2006) Nurse guilty of killing patients. Online at: http://news.bbc.co.uk/hi/england/491846.stm, accessed 8 December 2010.

Beauchamp T L and Childress J F (2001) *Principles of biomedical ethics* (5th edn). Oxford: Oxford University Press.

Beauchamp T L and Childress J F (2008) *Principles of biomedical ethics* (6th edn). Oxford: Oxford University Press.

BIS (Department for Business Innovation and Skills) (2011) Default retirement age. Online at: http://www.bis.gov.uk/policies/employment-matters/strategies/default-retirement, accessed 1 November 2011.

BMA (2002) *Medical ethics today: Its practice and philosophy*. London: BMA Publishing Group.

BMA (2005) Confidentiality as part of the bigger picture: Executive summary. Online at: http://www.bma.org.uk/ethics/confidentiality.ConfidentialityBiggerPicture.jsp, accessed 22 March 2011.

BMA (2010) Confidentiality and disclosure of health information toolkit. Online at: http://www.bma. org.uk/ethics/confidentiality/confidentialitytoolkit.jsp, accessed 23 March 2011.

Bowen P (2007) *Blackstone's guide to the Mental Health Act 2007*. Oxford: Oxford University Press.

Bytheway B and Johnson J (1990) On defining ageism. *Critical Social Policy*, 27: 27–30.

Cherniack E P (2002) Increasing use of DNR orders in the elderly worldwide: Whose choice is it? *Journal of Medical Ethics*, 28: 303–307.

Chiu W C K, Chan A W, Snape E and Redman T (2001) Age stereotypes and discriminatory attitudes towards older workers: An East–West comparison. *Human Relations*, 54(5): 629–661.

Cobbe S M, Dalziel K, Ford I and Marsden A K (1996) Survival of 1476 patients initially resuscitated from out of hospital cardiac arrest. *British Medical Journal*, 312: 1633–1637.

Costello J (2002) Do not resuscitate orders and older patients: Findings from an ethnographic study of hospital wards for older people. *Journal of Advanced Nursing*, 39(5): 491–499.

Courtney M, Tong S and Walsh A (2000) Acute care nurses' attitudes toward older patients: A litera-ture review. *International Journal of Nursing Practice*, 6(2): 62–69. Also available online at: http://eprints.qut.edu.au/, accessed 25 February 2011.

Crain W C (1985) *Theories of development*. Englewood Cliffs: Prentice Hall, pp. 118–136. Also avail-able online at: http://faculty.plts.edu/gpence/html/kohlberg.htm, accessed 18 October 2011.

Curzon L B (1998) *Dictionary of law* (5th edn). London: Financial Times Pitman Publishing.

Daily Record (25 October 2009) Killer nurse Colin Norris trapped by arrogance. Online at: http://www.dailyrecord.co.uk/news/scottish-news/2008/03/04/killer-nurse-colin-norris-trapped-by-arrogance-86908-20339733/, accessed 17 March 2011.

Daily Telegraph (4 March 2008) Colin Norris, 'Angel of Death' nurse, jailed for life. Online at: http://www.telegraph.co.uk/news/1580651/Colin-Norris-Angel-of-death-nurse-jailed-for-life.html, accessed 8 December 2010.

Daily Telegraph (9 June 2000) Cost of NHS negligence doubles in 10 years. Online at: http://www.telegraph.co.uk/news/uknews/1341694/Cost-of-NHS-negligence-doubles-in-10-years.html, accessed 18 October 2011.

Daily Telegraph (3 August 2010) Negligence claims will cost £15bn. Online at: http://www.telegraph.co.uk/healthnews/7622845/nhs-legal-claims-will-cost-1, accessed December 2010.

Daniel B, Taylor J and Scott J (2009) *Noticing and helping the neglected child: Literature review*. London: Department for Children, Schools and Families.

Data Protection Act (1998) Online at: http://www.legislation.gov.uk/ukpga/1998/29/contents, accessed 18 November 2010.

Davis N (1991) Contemporary deontology. In Singer P (ed.) *A companion to ethics*. Oxford: Blackwell.

DCSF (Department for Children, Schools and Families) (2010) *Working together to safeguard chil-dren: A guide to inter-agency working to safeguard and promote the welfare of children*. London: Department for Children, Schools and Families. Also available online at: http://publications.dcsf. gov.uk/eOrderingDownload/000305–2010DOM-EN.PDF, accessed 24 March 2011.

De Vos R, Koster R W, De Haan R J, Oosting H, Van der Wouw P A and Schoenemaeckers A J (1999) In hospital cardiopulmonary resuscitation: Pre-arrest morbidity and outcome. *Archives of Internal Medicine*, 159: 845–850.

DfES (Department for Education and Skills) (2003a) Keeping Children Safe: The Government's response to the Victoria Climbie Inquiry. Online at: http://www.education.gov.uk/consultations/downloadableDocs/KeepingChildrenSafe.pdf, accessed 1 November 2011.

DfES (2003b) Every Child Matters. Online at: http://www.education.gov.uk/consultations/down-loadableDocs/EveryChildMatters.pdf, accessed 1 November 2011.

DfES (2006) What to do if you're worried a child is being abused. Online at: http://www.dcsf.gov.uk/everychildmatters/resources-and-practice/IG00182/, accessed 24 March 2011.

DfES (2007) Care Matters: Time for change. Online at: https://www.education.gov.uk/publications/eOrderingDownload/Cm%207137.pdf, accessed 1 November 2011.

DHSSPS (2003) *Cooperating to safeguard children*. Belfast: Department of Health, Social Services and Public Safety. Also available online at: http://www.dhsspsni.gov.uk/show_publications?txtid=14022, accessed 18 October 2011.

Dicey A V (1959) *Introduction to the study of the law of the constitution* (10th edn). London: Macmillan.

Dimond B (2005) *Legal aspects of nursing* (4th edn). Harlow: Pearson Longman.

Dimond B (2008) *Legal aspects of nursing* (5th edn). Harlow: Pearson Education.

Dimond B and Barker F H (1996) *Mental Health Law for Nurses*. Oxford: Blackwell Science Ltd.

Disability Discrimination Act (1995) Online at: http://www.hmso.gov.uk/acts/acts1995/1995050.htm, accessed 20 November 10.

Dogan H, Tschudin V, Hot I and Ozkan I (2009) Patients' transcultural needs and carers' ethical responses. *Nursing Ethics*, 16(6): 683–696.

DoH (Department of Health) (1996) Department of Health NHS indemnity: Arrangements for clinical negligence claims in the NHS (1996). Cat No. 06 HR 0024.

DoH (1998) *HSC 1998/217: Preservation, retention and destruction of GP general medical services records relating to patients (replacement for FHSL(94)30)*. London: Department of Health.

DoH (2000) *Framework for the assessment of children in need and their families*. London: The Stationery Office. Also available online at: http://www.dh.gov.uk/assetRoot/04/01/44/30/04014430. pdf, accessed 18 October 2011.

DoH (2003a) *Confidentiality: NHS code of practice*. London: Department of Health.

DoH (2003b) *Making amends: Clinical negligence reform*. Online at: http://webarchive.national-archives.gov.uk/+/www.dh.gov.uk/en/Consultations/Closedconsultations/DH_4072363, accessed 20 January 2011.

DoH (2004) *Better health in old age*. London: Department of Health.

DoH (2005a) NHS Research and Development Forum. Online at: http://www.rdforum.nhs.uk, accessed 18 October 2011.

DoH (2005b) Elimination of mix-sex accommodation in hospital. Online at: http://www.dh.gov.uk/ prod_consum_dh/groups/dh_digitalassets/@dh/@en/documents/digitalasset/dh_4112141.pdf, accessed 8 February 2011.

DoH (2005c) Research governance framework for health and social care. Online at: http://www.dh.gov. uk/prod_consum_dh/groups/dh_digitalassets/@dh/@en/documents/digitalasset/dh_4122427.pdf, accessed 8 February 2011.

DoH (2006) Records management: NHS Code of Practice: Part 1. Online at: http://www.dh.gov.uk/ publications, accessed 15 January 2011.

DoH (2007) National Service Framework for Children, Young People, and Maternity Services: Core standards DH, 23 March 2007. Online at: http://www.dh.gov.uk/en/Publicationsandstatistics/ Publications/PublicationsPolicyAn, accessed 24 March 2011.

DoH (2008) Annex. Online at: http://www.dh.gov.uk/prod_consum_dh/groups/dh_digitalassets/@ dh/@en/documents/digitalasset/dh_088288.pdf, accessed 14 November 2011.

DPP (Department of Public Prosecutions) (2010) *Assisted suicide*. Online at: http://www.,cps.gov.uk/, accessed 15 January 2011.

Ebrahim S (2000) Do not resuscitate decisions: Flogging dead horses or a dignified death? *British Medical Journal*, 320: 1155–1156.

Fagerlin A and Schneider CE (2004) Enough: The failure of the living will. *Hastings Center Report*, 34: 30–42.

Fennell P, Williamson T and Yeates V (2009) Law and ethics of mental health nursing. In Norman I and Ryrie I (eds) *The art and science of mental health nursing* (2nd edn). Maidenhead: Open University Press.

Ferner R E (2000) Medication errors that led to manslaughter charges. *British Medical Journal*, 321: 1212.

Gerteis M, Edgman-Levitan S, Daley J and Delbanco T L (1993) *Through the patient's eyes: Understanding and promoting patient centered care*. San Francisco: Jossey-Bass Publishers.

Gibbs G (1988) *Learning by doing: A guide to teaching and learning methods*. Oxford: Further Education Unit, Oxford Brookes University.

Gilligan C (1982) *In a different voice: Psychological theory and women's development*. Cambridge, MA: Harvard University Press.

Gillon R (2003) *Philosophical medical ethics*. Chichester: John Wiley & Sons.

GMC (General Medical Council) (1985) Professional conduct and disciplines: Fitness to practise. London: GMC, 1985: 19–21. Cited in Gillon R (2003) *Philosophical Medical Ethics*. Chichester: John Wiley & Sons.

Griffin J (1986) *Well-being: Its meaning, measurement and moral importance*. Oxford: Clarendon Press.

Haidt J (2001) The emotional dog and its rational tail: A social intuitionist approach to moral judgment. *Psychological Review*, 108(4): 814–834.

Havard J (1985) Medical confidence. *Journal of Medical Ethics*, 11: 8–11.

Hawley G (1997) *Ethics workbook for nurses: Issues, problems and resolutions*. Sydney: Social Science Press.

Hawley G (2007) *Ethics in clinical practice: An interprofessional approach*. Harlow, Essex: Pearson Educational.

Help the Aged (2002) *Age discrimination in public policy: A review of the evidence*. London: Help the Aged.

Henderson V (1960) *Basic principles of nursing care*. London: International Council of Nurses.

Henderson V (1966) *The nature of nursing*. New York: Macmillan.

Hendrick J (1997) *Law and ethics in nursing and health studies*. Cheltenham: Stanley Thornes.

Hendrick J (2000) *Law and ethics in nursing and health studies*. Cheltenham: Nelson Thornes.

Herring J (2008) *Medical law and ethics*. Oxford University Press: Oxford.

Higgins I, Riet P Van Der, Slater L and Peek C (2007) The negative attitudes of nurses towards older patients in the acute hospital setting: A qualitative, descriptive study. *Contemporary Nurse*, 26(2): 225–237.

HM Government (2006) *Working together to safeguard children: Guide to inter-agency working to safeguard and promote the welfare of children*. London: The Stationery Office.

HM Government (2010) Chapter 9: Lessons from research. In *Working together to safeguard children: Guide to inter-agency working to safeguard and promote the welfare of children*. Online at: http://publications.dcsf.gov.uk/default.aspx?PageFunction=productdetails&PageMode=publications&ProductId=DCSF-00305-2010.

Homer A C and Gilleard C (1990) Abuse of elderly people by their carers. *BMJ*, 301(6765): 1359–1362. Also available online at: http://www.ncbi.nlm.nih.gov/pmc/articles/PMC1664522/, accessed 18 October 2011.

Hope T, Savulescu J and Hendrick J (2003) *Medical ethics and law: The core curriculum*. Edinburgh: Churchill Livingstone.

Human Rights Act (1998) Online at: http://www.legislation.gov.uk/ukpga/1998/42/schedule/1, accessed 17 November 2010.

The Independent (11 April 2000) Male nurse 'drugged and raped patients'. Online at: http://www.independent.co.uk/life-style/health-and-families/health-news/male-nurse-drugged-and-raped-patients-720087.html, accessed 18 October 2011.

The Independent (8 July 2000) Rapist who drugged victims is given seven life sentences for manslaughter and rape. Online at: http://www.independent.co.uk/news/uk/this-britain/rapist-who-drugged-victims-is-given-seven-life-sentences-for-manslaughter-and-rape-707025.html, accessed 18 October 2011.

International Council of Nurses (2006) *Code of ethics for nurses*. Geneva: ICN.

JCAHO (Joint Commission on Accreditation of Healthcare Organisations) (2005) *Health care in the cross-roads: Strategies for improving the medical liability system and preventing patient injury*. Oakbrook Terrace, IL: Author.

Johnson M-J (2008) *Bioethics: A nursing perspective*. London: Elsevier Health Sciences.

Jones J (1981) *Bad Blood*. New York: Free Press.

Kant I (1998) *Groundwork of the metaphysics of morals*. Translated and edited by Gregor M. Cambridge: Cambridge University Press.

Kearney N, Miller M, Paul J and Smith K (2000) Oncology healthcare professionals attitudes toward elderly people. *Annals of Oncology*, 11: 599–601.

Khan M and Robson M (1997) *Medical negligence*. London: Cavendish Publishing.

Kohlberg L (1980) *The philosophy of moral development*. San Francisco: Harper and Row.

Kolb D A (1984) *Experiential learning: Experience as the source of learning and development.* Englewood Cliffs: Prentice Hall.

Laakkonen M, Pitkala K H, Strandberg T E, Berglind S and Tilvis R S (2005) Old peoples reasoning for resuscitation preferences and their role in the decision-making process. *Resuscitation*, 65(2): 165–171.

Laming L (2003) *The Victoria Climbie inquiry: Report of an inquiry by Lord Laming.* Cm 5730. Norwich: The Stationery Office.

Landon L (2000) CPR: When is it acceptable to withhold it? Hospital survey of 'Not for CPR' orders. *Age & Ageing*, 29(S1): 9–16.

Lidz C W, Meise A, Zerubavel E, Carter M, Sestak R M and Roth L H (1986) *Informed consent: A study of decision making in psychiatry.* New York: Guilford Press.

Marik P E and Zaloga G P (2001) CPR in terminally ill patients. *Resuscitation*, 49(1): 99–103.

Marquis B L and Huston C (2008) *Leadership and management functions in nursing.* Philadelphia: Lippincott Williams & Wilkins.

Mason J K, McCall Smith R A and Laurie G T (1999) *Law and medical ethics* (5th edn). London: Butterworths.

Mason J K, Laurie G T and Aziz M (2006) *Mason and McCall Smith's law and medical ethics* (7th edn). Oxford: Oxford University Press.

McDonald A and Taylor M (2006) *Older people and the law.* Bristol: Policy Press.

McHale J V (2010) Nurse prescribing: Does more responsibility mean more litigation? *British Journal of Nursing*, 19(5): 315–317.

McHale J and Fox M (2007) *Health care law: Text and materials* (2nd edn). London: Sweet and Maxwell.

McHale J and Tingle J (2001) *Law and nursing.* Oxford: Butterworth.

Mello M and Jenkinson C (1998) Comparison of medical and nursing attitudes to resuscitation and patient autonomy between a British and an American teaching hospital. *Social Science & Medicine*, 46(3): 415–424.

Meyers R, Lurie N, Breitbutcher R and Waring C (1990) Do-not-resuscitate order in an extended-care study group. *Journal of the American Geriatrics Society*, 38: 1011–1015.

Miller J M and Bersoff D M (1992) Cultural and moral judgement: How are conflicts between justice and interpersonal responsibilities resolved? *Journal of Personality and Social Psychology*, 62: 541–554.

Muldowney M (1999) Case Comment: Medical negligence – Liability on hospital records – passage of time. *Medico-Legal Journal of Ireland*, 5(2): 86.

Murphy M (2008) The natural law tradition in ethics. In Zalta E N (ed.) *The Stanford Encyclopedia of Philosophy*. Online at: http://plato.stanford.edu/archives/fall2008/entries/natural-law-ethics/, accessed 18 October 2011.

National Audit Office (2001) *Handling Clinical Negligence Claims in England.* Online at: http://www.nao.org.uk/publications/0001/handling_clinical_negligence.aspx, accessed 2 March 2011.

National Health Service (2007) National Service Framework for Children Young People and Maternity Services. Online at: http://www.dh.gov.uk/en/Publicationsandstatistics/Publications/PublicationsPolicyAndGuidance/Browsable/DH_4866860, accessed 14 November 2011.

Newham R and Hawley G (2007) The relationship of ethics to philosophy. In Hawley G (ed.) *Ethics in clinical practice: An interprofessional approach.* Harlow: Pearson Educational.

NHSLA (NHS Litigation Authority) (2010) *Report and Accounts 2010.* HC52. London: The Stationery Office.

NHSLA (2011) *Care and compassion? Report of the Health Service Ombudsman on ten investigations into NHS care of older people.* HC778. London: The Stationery Office. Also available online at: http://www.ombudsman.org.uk/_data/assets/pdf_file/0016/7216/Care-and-Compassion-PHSO-0114web.pdf, accessed 2 November 2011.

NICE (National Institute for Health and Clinical Excellence) (2011) *Using new NICE guidelines on child maltreatment in safeguarding children training.* Online at: http://www.nice.org.uk.

Nightingale F (1859) *Notes on nursing: What it is and what it is not.* London: Harrison.

NMC (Nursing and Midwifery Council) (2004) *Code of professional conduct: Standards of performance, conduct and ethics*. London: NMC.

NMC (2006) A–Z advice sheet: Medicines management. Online at: http://www.positive-options.com/news/downloads/NMC_-_Medicines_management_A-Z_advice_sheet_-_2006.pdf, accessed 11 November 2011.

NMC (2007) Covert administration of medicines: Disguising medicine in food and drink. Online at http://www.nmc-uk.org/Nurses-and-midwives/Advice-by-topic/A/Advice/Covert-administration-of-medicines/, accessed 11 November 2011.

NMC (2008a) The code: Standards of conduct, performance and ethics for nurses and midwives. Online at http://www.nmc-uk.org/aHeader.aspx, accessed 21 October 2008.

NMC (2008b) The code in full. Online at: http://www.nmc-uk.org/Nurses-and-midwives/The-code/The-code-in-full/, accessed 2 November 2011.

NMC (2009a) Record keeping guidance for nurses & midwives. Online at http://www.nmc-uk.org/Documents/Guidance/nmcGuidanceRecordKeepingGuidanceforNursesandMidwives.pdf, accessed 10 March 2011.

NMC (2009b) Guidance for the care of older people. Online at: http://www.nmc-uk.org/General-public/Older-people-and-their-carers/Care-and-respect-every-time-new-guidance-for-the-care-of-older-people/, accessed 10 March 2011.

NMC (2010a) Standards for pre-registration nursing education. Online at: http://standards.nmc-uk.org/PublishedDocuments/Standards%20for%20pre-registration%20nursing%20education%2016082010.pdf, accessed 23 March 2011.

NMC (2010b) *Guidance on professional conduct for nursing and midwifery students* (2nd edn). London: NMC. Also available online at: http://www.nmc-uk.org/, accessed 10 March 2011.

NMC News 29 (2009) Record keeping interview with Martine Tune. Online at: http://www.nmc-uk.org/Nurses-and-midwives/Record-keeping-interview-with-Martine-Tune/, accessed 2 November 2011.

Norman A (1985) *Triple jeopardy: Growing old in a second homeland*. London: Centre for Policy in Ageing.

Norman K (2011) Primary and community care. In: Hindle A and Coates A (eds) *Nursing care of older people*. Oxford: Oxford University Press.

NSPCC (2010) An introduction to child protection legislation. Online at: http://www.nspcc.org.uk/inform, accessed 11 November 2010.

NSPCC (2011a) Types of child abuse. Online at: http://www.nspcc.org.uk/, accessed 25 March 2011.

NSPCC (2011b) Prevalence and incidence of child abuse and neglect. Online at: http://www.nspc.org.uk/Inform/research/statistics/prevalence_and_incidence_of_chil, accessed 25 March 2011.

O'Neil O (2003) Some limits of informed consent. *Journal of Medical Ethics*, 29: 4–7.

Oxford Paperback Dictionary (1979) Hawkins J M (ed.). Oxford: Oxford University Press.

Palmer G R and Short S D (1994) *Health care and public policy: An Australian analysis* (2nd edn). Melbourne: Macmillan Education Australia.

Payne S, Hardey M and Coleman P (2000) Interactions between nurses during handovers in elderly care. *Journal of Advanced Nursing*, 32: 277–285.

Pence G (2004) *Classic cases in medical ethics*. New York: McGraw-Hill.

Pfeifer J E, Sidorov J E, Smith A C, Boero J F, Evans A T and Settle M B (1994) The discussion of end-of-life medical care by primary care patients and physicians: A multicenter study using structured qualitative interviews. The EOL Study group. *Journal General Internal Medicine*, 9: 82-88.

Pozgar D P (2007) *Legal aspects of health care administration* (10th edn). Boston: Jones and Bartlett.

Rawls J (1972) *A theory of justice*. Oxford: Oxford University Press.

RCN (Royal College of Nursing) (2003) *Defining nursing*. London: Royal College of Nursing.

RCN (2007) Safeguarding children and young people: Every nurse's responsibility. Online at: http://www.rcn.org.uk, accessed 18 October 2011.

RCN, Resuscitation Council (UK) and BMA (2007) Decisions relating to cardiopulmonary resuscitation: A joint statement from the British Medical Association, the Resuscitation Council (UK) and the Royal College of Nursing, October 2007. Online at: http://www.resus.org.uk/pages/dnar.pdf, accessed 13 October 2011.

Report of the Royal Liverpool Children's Inquiry (2001) Online at: http://www.dh.gov.uk/en/ Publicationsandstatistics/Publications/PublicationsPolicyAndGuidance/DH_4009030 (summary and recommendations) and http://www.rlcinquiry.org.uk/download/chap1.pdf (full report to the House of Commons) , accessed 31 October 2011.

Rest J R and Narvaez D (2009) *Moral development in the professions: Psychology and applied ethics*. Englewood Cliffs: Lawrence Erlbaum Associates.

Roberts E (2000) *Age discrimination in health and social care*. London: Kings Fund.

Rolf G, Jasper M and Freshwater D (2011) *Critical reflection in practice* (2nd edn). Houndmills, Basingstoke, Hampshire: Palgrave Macmillan.

Rosenfeld K E, Wenger N S and Kagawa-Singer M (2000) End-of-life decision making: A qualitative study of elderly individuals. *Journal of General Internal Medicine*, 15: 620–625.

Ross W D (1930) *The right and the good*. Oxford: Oxford University Press.

Royal College of Psychiatrists (2005) *Who cares wins: Improving the outcomes for older people admitted to the general hospital: Guidance for the development of liaison mental health services for older people*. London: Royal College of Psychiatrists.

Ryan A (ed.) *Utilitarianism and other essays*. Harmondsworth: Penguin.

Saha S, Beach M C and Cooper L A (2008) Patient centeredness, cultural competence and healthcare quality. *Journal of the National Medical Association*, 100(11): 1275–1285.

Schon D A (1983) *The reflective practitioner*. London: Temple Smith.

Scott P D (1975) The tragedy of Maria Colwell. *British Journal of Criminology*, 15: 88–90.

Scottish Office (1998) *Protecting children: A shared responsibility: Guidance on interagency co-operation*. Edinburgh: The Stationery Office.

Selvin M (1984) Changing medical and societal attitudes toward sexually transmitted diseases: A historical overview. In King K, Holmes P-A, Mardh P, Sparling F and Wiesner P J (eds) *Sexually transmitted diseases*. New York: McGraw-Hill.

Siegler M (1982) Confidentiality in medicine: A decrepit concept. *New England Journal of Medicine*, 307: 1518–1521.

Shipman Inquiry (2002) Online at: http://www.the-shipman-inquiry.org.uk/6r_page.asp?ID=3401, accessed 20 January 2011.

Silveira M J, Kim S Y H and Langa K M (2010) Advance directives and outcomes of surrogate decision making death. *New England Journal of Medicine*, 362: 1211–1218.

Simpson E L (1974) Moral development research: A case study of scientific cultural bias. *Human Development*, 17: 81–106.

Slevin O D (1991) Ageist attitudes among young adults: Implications for a caring profession. *Journal of Advanced Nursing*, 16: 1197–1205.

Smart J J C and Williams B (1998) *Utilitarianism, for and against*. Cambridge: Cambridge University Press.

Smith A P (2005) As we lie in the bed: The malpractice and regulatory consequences of failing leadership. *Nursing Economics*, 23(2): 97–99.

Smith J (2000) *Smith and Hogan criminal law* (9th edn). London: Butterworths.

Snape J (1986) Nurses attitudes to care of the elderly. *Journal of Advanced Nursing*, 11: 569–572.

Stein M, Rees G, Hicks L and Gorin S (2009) *Neglected adolescents: A review of the research and the preparation of guidance for multi-disciplinary teams and a guide for young people*. London: Department for Children, Schools and Families.

Stevens J and Crouch M (1995) Who cares about care in nurse education? *International Journal of Nursing Studies*, 32: 233–242.

Superson A (2009) *The moral skeptic*. Oxford: Oxford University Press.

Surrey County Council (2011) Every Child Matters guidance for professionals. Online at: http://www. surreycc.gov.uk/sccwebsite/sccwspages.nsf/LookupWebPagesByTITLE_RTF/Every+Child+Matt ers+guidance+for+professionals?opendocument, accessed 2 November 2011.

Teno J M, Gruneir A, Schwartz Z, Nanda A and Wetle T (2007) Association between advance directives and quality of end-of-life care: A national study. *Journal of American Geriatric Society*, 55: 189–194.

The Times (31 May 1973) Stepfather's preferential treatment. Issue 58796, p. 2, col. F.

312   *References*

The Times (11 October 1973) Girl was like a living skeleton, neighbour tells inquiry. Issue 58910, p. 3, col. A.

The Times (23 October 1973) Foster-parents not told of decision to move girl. Issue 58920, p. 3, col. A.

The Times (15 February 2006) Nurse killed patients for kicks: 18 victims injected with lethal drugs so that hospital worker could enjoy the thrill of reviving them. Online at: http://www.timesonline. co.uk/to1/news/uk/article7308898.ece, accessed 8 December 2010.

Treharne G (1990) Attitudes towards the care of elderly people: are they getting better. *Journal of Advanced Nursing*, 15: 777–781.

UKCC (United Kingdom Central Council for Nursing, Midwifery & Health Visiting) (1999) *Fitness for practice: The UKCC Commission for Nursing & Midwifery Education*. London: UKCC.

UKCC (2001) UKCC position statement on the covert administration of medicines: Disguising medicine in food and drink. UKCC Registrar's letter 26/2001. London: UKCC.

United Nations (1989) Convention on the Rights of the Child adopted under General Assembly Resolution 44/25, United Nations 20 November 1989. Geneva: UN. Online at: http://www2.ohchr. org/english/law/crc.htm, accessed 18 October 2011.

Vandrevala T, Hampson S, Daly T, Arber S and Thomas H (2006) Dilemmas in decision-making about resuscitation: A focus group study of older people. *Social Science & Medicine*, 62(7): 1579–1593.

Wallace I and Bunting L (2007) *An examination of local, national and international arrangements for the mandatory reporting of child abuse: The implications for Northern Ireland*. Belfast: NSPCC. Also available online at: http://nspcc.org.uk/Inform/research/Findings/mandatoryreportingN1_wda51129.html, accessed 10 March 2011.

Welsh Assembly Government (2006) Safeguarding children: Working together under the Children Act 2004. Online at: http://wales.gov.uk/topics/childrenyoungpeople/publications/safeguardingunder2004act/?lang=en, accessed 18 October 2011.

Wheeler H (2011) The law and the older person. In Hindle A and Coates A (eds) *Nursing care of older people*. Oxford: Oxford University Press.

Whitehead J and Wheeler H (2008) Patients' experience of privacy and dignity. Part 2: An empirical study. *British Journal of Nursing*, 17(7): 458–464.

Wierenga E (1983) A defensible divine command theory. *Nous*, 17(3): 387–407.

Willard C (2000) Cardiopulmonary resuscitation for palliative care patients: A discussion of ethical issues. *Palliative Medicine*, 14: 308–312.

Williams G and Smith A T H (2006) *Learning the law* (13th edn). London: Sweet and Maxwell.

Wood C (2003) The importance of good record-keeping for nurses. *Nursing Times*. Online at: http://www.nursingtimes.net/nursing-practice-clinical-research/the-importance-of-goo, accessed 7 December 2011.

World Health Organization (1994). *Declaration of promotion of patients' rights in Europe*. A WHO European Consultation on the Rights of Patients; 1994 Mar 28–30; Amsterdam. Copenhagen: WHO Regional Office for Europe.

World Health Organization (2011) World Health Organization definition of child abuse. Online at: http://www.yesican.org/definitions/WHO.html, accessed 25 March 2011.

Index